T0315321

Functional Atlas of the Human Fascial System

Senior Content Strategists: *Alison Taylor, Rita Demetriou-Swanwick*
Content Development Specialists: *Sheila Black, Nicola Lally*
Project Manager: *Joanna Souch*
Designer: *Christian Bilbow*
Illustration Manager: *Brett MacNaughton*
Illustrator: *Electronic Publishing Services*

Functional Atlas of the Human Fascial System

CARLA STECCO MD

Orthopaedic Surgeon;
Professor of Human Anatomy and Movement Science,
University of Padua, Italy

English Language Editor
Warren Hammer DC MS

Postgraduate Faculty,
New York Chiropractic College, NY,
and Northwestern Health Sciences University,
Bloomington, MN, USA

Forewords by
Andry Vleeming PhD

Professor, Department of Anatomy,

Center of Excellence in Neuroscience,

University of New England, Maine, USA;

Professor, Department of Rehabilitation and Kinesiotherapy,

University of Ghent, Belgium; Program Chairman,

World Congress Lumbopelvic Pain

Raffaele De Caro MD

Full Professor of Human Anatomy,
Director, Institute of Human Anatomy,
Department of Molecular Medicine,
University of Padua, Italy;
President, Italian College of Anatomists

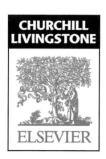

Edinburgh   London   New York   Oxford   Philadelphia   St Louis   Sydney   Toronto 2015

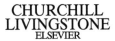

ISBN 978-0-7020-4430-4

Notices
Knowledge and best practice in this field are constantly changing. As new research and experience broaden our understanding, changes in research methods, professional practices, or medical treatment may become necessary.

Practitioners and researchers must always rely on their own experience and knowledge in evaluating and using any information, methods, compounds, or experiments described herein. In using such information or methods they should be mindful of their own safety and the safety of others, including parties for whom they have a professional responsibility.

With respect to any drug or pharmaceutical products identified, readers are advised to check the most current information provided (i) on procedures featured or (ii) by the manufacturer of each product to be administered, to verify the recommended dose or formula, the method and duration of administration, and contraindications. It is the responsibility of practitioners, relying on their own experience and knowledge of their patients, to make diagnoses, to determine dosages and the best treatment for each individual patient, and to take all appropriate safety precautions.

To the fullest extent of the law, neither the Publisher nor the authors, contributors, or editors, assume any liability for any injury and/or damage to persons or property as a matter of products liability, negligence or otherwise, or from any use or operation of any methods, products, instructions, or ideas contained in the material herein.

your source for books, journals and multimedia in the health sciences

www.elsevierhealth.com

Working together to grow libraries in developing countries

www.elsevier.com • www.bookaid.org

The publisher's policy is to use paper manufactured from sustainable forests

Printed in Great Britain

Last digit is the print number: 10

Contents

Companion website: www.atlasfascial.com (videos)

Foreword by Andry Vleeming

Before me is a new anatomical atlas of the human fascial system. Its focus is on the integration of the fascial and muscular tissues and their relevance in mutual interactions for effectively transferring loads through the body. I believe it will help us to better appreciate how we function as humans.

Classical topographical atlases divide our bodies into regions and sections. This serves a crucial didactic purpose, to understand the constituents of our body. However, in complex constructs like our bodies, focusing on single tissues impedes a proper analysis of daily life functioning, because the interplay between these various tissues is also crucial. In addition, the mechanical load encountered in the body is distributed through this continuous network of fascia, ligaments and muscles, which support the entire skeleton.

Unlike standard topographic anatomy, functional anatomy should present the necessary information to incorporate the interrelationships between muscle, its internal fascial skeleton and the surrounding external fascial network into which it is integrated. Such an approach can be easily missed in traditional anatomical dissection. Moments and reaction forces, generated by muscles and their associated passive structures, provide an equilibrium in the multiple degrees of freedom of our joints. The passive structures also interact with the muscular system through their role as sensory organs, thereby adding a component of feedback control to the system.

The various myofascial structures with differing elastic moduli, contribute to the formation of composites in our body: from the superficial skin, to the bones, we find connective tissues with very different abilities to be pulled and strained. Describing the physical properties and functions of these composite arrangements is a necessary prerequisite for understanding the many complex roles of our body.

This new atlas helps us to appreciate the unique architecture of our bodies and how we are able to express ourselves through so many different forms of movement. By necessity, we will gain a deeper respect of its miraculous architecture.

The first chapter gives an effective overview on what we can expect from this new atlas. The wish to create a complete overview of the fascial structure of the body, took the author more than 10 years to finalize.

As readers of this book, we see a new anatomical universe enfolding before our eyes in the form of superb dissections and drawings, combined with an accurate text, describing the consequences of this new anatomical integrated approach.

This book is conceived by an author with a great scientific and medical family tradition. Prof. Dr. Carla Stecco, created many respectable articles on integrating fascia into a realistic functional concept of our locomotorsystem.

I have had the great honor to know Dr. Stecco for many years and realize that her benchmark for quality has been raised to a very high level. The excellence of this book can be recognized from the first to last chapter. From the people who donated their body to science, to the precision of which the dissections were performed, not to mention the ability to photograph this all in a way that helps us appreciate the complexity of the human body.

Dissection with precision needs very specific skills, both academically as well as outstanding dexterity. Characteristics which have not often been combined in fascial research studies. In fact, the author must have explored and refined her approach many times, finding the best form of dissection to present the amazing pictures and drawings.

The author has composed a lucid and fascinating atlas of fascia and connective tissue in relation to muscles, bones, joints and organs.

Reading this book will not only enhance your anatomical knowledge and skills, but will also reveal how the body is able to allow sliding of superficial and deep tissues when we are in motion.

Perhaps we needed an Italian orthopedic surgeon and anatomist like Carla Stecco, who by nature understands the double connotation of the Latin word 'E motione' meaning literally 'in motion'. And that is what we can see in the beautiful pictures: functional anatomy showing specific anatomical layers of tissue enabling 'in movement'.

I can assure you that the pictures in this book are one of the finest I have ever seen. Although by necessity 2 dimensional pictures, they are dissected so precisely and carefully on fresh specimen, it almost seems that we get a 3D look of the bodies as if the energy of this fine tuned system of a moving and sliding fascia is still palpable in these pictures!

This book can be regarded as a new standard atlas for understanding integrated anatomy of the locomotorsystem and connective organization of our body. It is the epitome of superclass dissection labor, primarily focusing on the role of the fascial system.

Colleagues reading this book can enroll in an easy to follow academic script of how the different connective tissue layers are interrelated with muscles and bone.

This is an engaging and fascinating book. Dr. Stecco is presenting the true architecture of our body in a marvelous way. I would highly recommend this book to all of you!

Prof. Dr. Andry Vleeming,
Department of Rehabilitation Sciences and
Physiotherapy.
Faculty of Medicine and Health Sciences
Ghent University, Belgium

Department of Anatomy
Medical College of the University of New England,
Biddeford, Maine, USA.

Foreword by Raffaele De Caro

To write the preface of a book is always a source of satisfaction and pride, but this one, written by my colleague Carla Stecco, is a particular honour. I have known Carla Stecco for years, and have always admired her dedicated study of the fasciae and her devotion to research. Over the years, she has acquired a deep knowledge of the fasciae and has become a world-class dissection expert. Dr Stecco began as a promising anatomy student. As a child, she and her father would dissect small animals to have an in-depth knowledge of the fasciae. Later, as a medical student, she started to research the human fasciae. Beginning at age 26, she spent extended periods of time at the University of Paris, where she was permitted to perform dissections of unembalmed cadavers. With a dedicated focus on her dissections, she was able to explain for the first time the various fasciae of the human body and their connections with muscles, joints, vessels and nerves. Upon first acquaintance I was struck by her curiosity about anatomy and her remarkable talent in dissection. I have come to realize her potential as a teacher and as a true academician. Her experience in teaching, her interest in research and her passion to publish in scientific journals have made her an accomplished and admired author. Over the years, I have appreciated first hand her devotion to research and her way of thinking outside the bounds of convention. She was always strongly convinced of the truth of her findings, even when they did not conform to current orthodoxy. The publication of this book and the success of her ideas in recent years have demonstrated the truth of her conclusions.

This Atlas is the first accurate description of the human fasciae. It has revived the use of the scientific method for the study of human anatomy. Indeed, in recent years the fascial system has been recognized as significant by physiotherapists, osteopaths, chiropractors, manual therapists and athletic trainers. The photos in this book show for the first time in a systematic way what human fascia is. We now understand its borders and its macroscopic and microscopic features. An in-depth understanding of the fascial layers' structure and its relationship to the transmission of force and proprioception has helped to develop this original vision of myofascial-skeletal anatomy. The data in this book will be a standard for all future researchers. The understanding of fasciae from an anatomical point of view will suggest better ways to treat fascial syndromes.

The material is logically organized, beginning with the first three chapters that provide an overview of the connective tissues and of the superficial and deep fasciae. The next five chapters describe the fasciae from a topographic point of view. Throughout, care was given to explain the myofascial connections and the fascial continuities.

We must be grateful that Carla Stecco had the vision to conceive of and the industry to prepare such a useful text as *Functional Atlas of the Human Fascial System*.

Prof. Raffaele De Caro
Full Professor of Human Anatomy,
Director, Institute of Human Anatomy,
Department of Molecular Medicine,
University of Padua, Italy
President, Italian College of Anatomists

Preface

Major anatomical atlases describe in detail the organs and muscles of the body. However, the coverings of these structures, the fasciae, are generally left to the imagination of the readers. Typically, local areas of fasciae are described and they are characterized by only one of their minor functions: as an opaque covering. Similarly, anatomists understand connective tissue as something to be removed so that joints, muscles, organs and tendons may be studied carefully. Many dissect with preconceived notions based on their studies of previous anatomical texts. Unfortunately, these studies are destined to describe only part of the locomotor system. The fasciae, as an integral part of this system, are ignored or dismissed.

In recent years, research has revealed that bodily movement consists of far more than the actions of individual muscles in response to nerve stimulation. Muscles are now understood as part of a system that must be coordinated to function properly. It is the fasciae that are responsible for much of the coordination of the motor system. They act as a bridge passing over joints and septa to connect muscles, and muscles act in concert because of these attachments. Muscles move in relation to one another as a function of the fascial structures that give them form and permit the proper amount of glide. Pathologists who study the musculoskeletal system and disregard the fascial system often have difficulty discovering the aetiology of pain and classify it as 'nonspecific'. The traditional approach that studies the muscles as independent units, has been a barrier to understanding the bigger picture of fascial function. We now know that understanding the fascial system, its composition, form and function, permits a more precise understanding of anatomy.

Just as descriptive anatomists have omitted important fascial structures in their research, so has medical treatment when it focuses only on muscles, joints and ligaments. This has meant less effective treatment of pathologies arising from contraction and tightness in the fascia. Only an in-depth understanding of the fascial layers and their connections can guide the practitioner in the selection of the proper technique for a specific fascial problem and the correct hand pressure during treatment. Such knowledge can only enhance manual methods. In addition, surgeons need a rigorous understanding of the fascia they must cut, not only to create effective fascial flaps but also to pinpoint the best, bloodless surgical access. This understanding enables the surgeon to respect the whole tissue they are dealing with and also improves patient recovery.

This book is based on the dissection of hundreds of fresh, human cadavers over the past 10 years. I performed these dissections myself in order to attain the closest possible observation of natural, living fasciae, their connecting paths, the gliding they permit and their fascial planes. The latter of which are impossible to learn from embalmed cadavers. My dissections have given me a unique vision of the human fasciae. Formerly, the fascial system was studied as a distinct and isolated aspect associated with specific, separate regions of the body. This suggests that fasciae begin and end in a single segment, which is not the case.

In this book, I stress the continuity of the fascial planes and an understanding of the function of the fasciae as connections between muscles, nerves and blood vessels. My own understanding of the fascia is as a proper organ system with its unique macroscopic and histological aspects, and its own functions and pathologies. Remaining consistent with this view, I have employed a restrictive definition of fascia. I exclude joint capsules, ligaments, tendons and the loose connective tissue from this definition. True, the fasciae are continuous with all of these but they have distinct microscopic features and functions.

I have tried to include the various definitions and descriptions of the fasciae presented in the literature, for the reference of scholars in this area. Ideally, an agreed upon definition for fascial tissue, and its various layers and their characteristics, will benefit future research in this field and will ultimately enhance clinical practice and allow easier, more precise approaches to fascial studies.

My work owes a great deal to the support of Professor De Caro (Padua University, Italy) and to the collaboration of Professor Delmas (Paris, Descartes University, France). I must also thank my colleagues: Professor Veronica Macchi and Professor Andrea Porzionato. Their work and help enabled my study of the fasciae both microscopically and in vivo. Comparing cadaver findings with in vivo studies revealed much about the fasciae. I ascertained that researchers could successfully evaluate the fasciae with common imaging techniques (ultrasound, CT and MRI). It is my hope that information in this book will inspire practitioners to include the fasciae in their imaging examinations.

The first chapter classifies connective tissue and explains its composition in terms of percentages of fibres, cells and extracellular matrix. This composition defines the histological and mechanical features of the different types of connective tissue, in particular the fasciae. The second chapter describes the general characteristics of the superficial fascia from both a macroscopic and microscopic point of view. In the third chapter the deep fascia is analysed in the same manner. The subsequent five chapters describe the fasciae from a topographical perspective. In this part of the atlas, common anatomical terminology is used to refer to the various fasciae. However, I am careful to highlight the continuations between the fasciae of the different body segments. Care is also taken to specify the connections between fasciae and muscles. This is important in understanding the key role of fascia in coordinating muscular activity and acting as a body-wide proprioceptive organ. Fascial connections can provide an alternative explanation for referred pain distribution and emphasize the connections between the lower limbs, the trunk and the upper limbs. Here again, a whole-body conception of the fascial system is essential. For years, manual medical practitioners have understood intramuscular connections using illustrative descriptions, functional screening and physical testing. I hope that this book will also provide a photographic understanding of these connections.

Carla Stecco

Acknowledgements

To my dear husband, Giuseppe, and children, Elettra and Jago, for the time that I have stolen from them to write this book.

To my father for inspiring me to look beyond classical anatomy, and for an enduring fascination with the fascial system.

To Warren Hammer and his assistant, Martha Cook Hammer, for their suggestions for improving this book and for helping to make it clear.

Don't be trapped by dogma – which is living with the results of other people's thinking. Don't let the noise of others' opinions drown out your own inner voice. And most important, have the courage to follow your heart and intuition.

Steve Jobs, Stanford Report, 2005

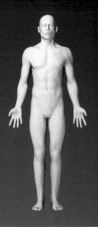

1

Connective Tissues

Composition of the Connective Tissues

Connective tissue (CT) is one of the four major classes of tissue (the others being epithelial, muscle and nerve tissue). It maintains the form of the body and its organs, and provides cohesion and structural support for the tissues and organs. CT derives its name from its function in connecting or binding cells and tissues. It is ubiquitous in the body and can be considered the 'glue' that holds the body parts together.

CT has three main components: cells, fibres and extracellular matrix (ECM) (Fig. 1.1). The cells provide the metabolic properties of the tissue, the fibres the mechanical properties, and the ECM the plasticity and malleability of the tissue. The most common cell types are fibroblasts, which produce collagen fibres and other intercellular materials. Cells such as adipocytes and undifferentiated mesenchymal cells are also present. The proportions of these three components vary from one part of the body to another depending on the local structural requirements. In some areas, the CT is loosely organized and highly cellular; in others, its fibrous components predominate; and in still others, the ground substance may be its most conspicuous feature. The consistency of the ECM is highly variable

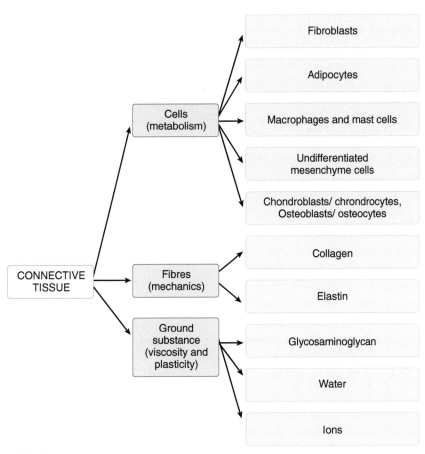

FIGURE 1.1 Composition of the CTs.

and ranges from gelatin like to a more rigid material. Consequently, the CT ranges in consistency from the gel-like softness of loose CT to the hardness of bone. The anatomical classification of the various types of CT is based largely upon the relative abundance and arrangement of these components. For example, strong CTs, such as tendons and ligaments, require a greater proportion of collagen fibres and fewer cells. Whereas, a CT composed mostly of cells like adipose tissue (fat) would not be very strong.

The CT has many functions:

- Structural support: it provides a structural framework for the body and maintains the anatomical form of the organs and systems. It forms the skeleton and the capsules surrounding the organs.
- Connection of body tissues: such as ligaments, tendons and fasciae.
- Protection of organs: it cushions and envelops the organs and separates them from surrounding structures. It permits necessary motilities between organs and fills the spaces between organs, preventing friction, pressure and damaging collisions among the mobile structures.
- Metabolical functions: provides a nutritive role. All the metabolites from the blood pass from capillary beds and diffuse through the adjacent CT to cells and tissues. Similarly waste metabolites from the cells and tissues diffuse through the loose CT before returning to the blood capillaries. The CT mediates and controls the various exchanges.
- Storage of energy: in the adipose tissue (a specialized CT).
- Regulation of diffusion of substances.
- Formation of scar tissue: it has a fundamental role in the recovery of the tissues following traumatic damage.

All CT cells are derived from mesenchymal cells. Mesenchymal cells are found in embryos and are, for the most part, derived from the middle germ layer of the embryo (mesoderm), but some of the CTs of the head region are derived from the neural crest (ectodermal in origin). Mesenchymal cells are only found in embryos, although some mesenchyme-like cells persist in adult CT and retain their capacity to differentiate in response to injury.

Extracellular Matrix

The ECM refers to the extracellular components of CT and supporting tissues. This matrix distributes the mechanical stresses on tissues and provides the structural environment for the cells embedded in it. It forms a framework to which cells adhere and on which they can move (Standring 2008), and is composed of a ground substance and fibres. The ground substance is composed of water, extracellular proteins, glycosaminoglycans (GAGs) and proteoglycans, in varying proportions. It is clear, colourless and viscous. The fibres are of different types, but the principal ones are collagen and elastin and these define the mechanical properties of the tissue.

GROUND SUBSTANCE

Ground substance is an amorphous gel-like substance surrounding the cells. It does not include fibres (e.g. collagen and elastic fibres), but does include all the other components of the ECM and is also known as the extrafibrillar matrix. The ground substance is responsible for the support and nutrition of cells. It determines the compliance, mobility and integrity of the CT and is a lubricant and binder for the diverse elements of the ECM (Hukinsa & Aspden 1985). The presence of macromolecules in the ground substance allows the collagen fibres to slide with little friction, when force is applied, providing relative mobility until the interfibrillar cross-links are tensioned. Both collagens and water molecules have electric conductive and polarization properties, as do the matrix molecules. Polarization waves are possible and protons can 'jump' along the collagen fibres much faster than electrical signals conducted by nerves (Jaroszyk & Marzec 1993).

Proteoglycans

The ground substance contains proteoglycans that are very large macromolecules consisting of a core protein to which many GAG molecules are covalently attached, somewhat like the bristles around the stem of a bottle brush. GAGs are long-chained polysaccharides made up of repeating disaccharide units and one of the sugars in each disaccharide unit is a glycosamine, hence the name GAG. Many of the sugars in GAGs have sulfate and carboxyl groups, which makes them highly negatively charged. A family of seven distinct GAGs is recognized, based on differences in the specific sugar residues, nature of the linkages and degree of sulfation. These GAGs are hyaluronan, chondroitin-4-sulfate, chondroitin-6-sulfate, dermatan sulfate, keratin sulfate, heparin sulfate and heparin.

GAGs are not flexible enough to assume a globular form and stay extended occupying an ample surface in relationship to their volume. The high density of negative charges attracts water forming a hydrated gel; this gel is responsible for the turgidity and viscoelasticity of the CT and controls the diffusion of various metabolites. In particular, it permits the rapid diffusion of water-soluble molecules but inhibits the movement of large molecules and bacteria. Its viscoelasticity allows the tissue to return to its original form after stress, and enables the collagen fibres to move without friction against each other, to absorb forces that affect the tissue and to protect the collagen network from excessive stress. The various levels of water determine if the ground matrix is a sol or gel and subsequently the mobility of the collagen fibres that are embedded inside. Smaller proteoglycans such as decorin, which has a single GAG chain, could play a role in the organization and disposition of collagen fibres. Proteoglycans are also found in cellular membranes and inside cells, and mediate the interactions of the cells and ground substance.

Hyaluronan

Hyaluronan (HA) is the GAG most represented in loose CT and is the only one that has no sulfate groups. It differs from the typical GAG because it is extremely long and rigid: consisting of a chain of several thousand sugars, as compared to several hundred or less found in other GAGs. It also does not bind to a core protein to become part of a proteoglycan; instead, proteoglycans indirectly bind to HA via special linker proteins to form giant macromolecules. These hydrophilic macromolecules are particularly abundant in cartilage ground substance and are responsible for the turgor pressure that gives cartilage its shape. HA provides the structure as well as turgor to the aqueous of the eye and protects fetal vessels from compression in the Wharton's jelly of the umbilical cord (Fig. 1.2).

HA provides moisture for the skin by means of its large volume of solvent water (as much as 10,000 times the volume of the original material). It also provides a lubricant for muscles and tendons as they glide over skeletal or under aponeurotic fasciae. It is likely that these gliding interactions are influenced by the composition and efficacy of the HA-rich ECM. This HA-rich layer also protects muscles and supports recovery from injury, and stimulates satellite cell proliferation following loss of muscle fibres. Changes in this HA-rich matrix contribute to pain, inflammation and loss of function. HA is abundant during the earliest stages of wound healing and functions to open up tissue spaces through which cells can travel. By binding to

cell receptors and interacting with the cytoskeleton it confers motility to the cells.

HA is particularly plentiful during embryogenesis and in tissues undergoing rapid growth, and is present wherever repair and regeneration occur. Depending on its chain length, especially when it becomes fragmented, HA has recently been shown to have a wide range of opposing biological functions: such as becoming angiogenic, inflammatory and immunostimulatory.

The turnover of HA is about 2–4 days compared to 7–10 days for the other sulfated GAGs. This means that the HA cells must remain active, otherwise there is the risk of reduction in the quantity of ground substance. The residual products of the GAGs have a feedback effect on the cells and this controls synthesis. It has been established that mechanical distortion of CT cells represents a stimulus for ECM synthesis (Adhikari et al 2011).

Link proteins

Link proteins stabilize the aggregates of proteoglycans in the ground substance and form large bottle-brush-like configurations. Of the link proteins, the most well known are vinculin, spectrin and actomyosin. They represent the constituents that mediate the interactions among cells, fibres and other components of the matrix and their primary tasks are the binding of collagen fibres to the cell membrane and the organization of the elastic fibres in the ECM. Other specific functions for individual link proteins are to guide mobile cells through the CT, to control the activity of the cell nucleus, mitochondria, and Golgi apparatus, and to connect the cytoskeleton with the ECM. During the

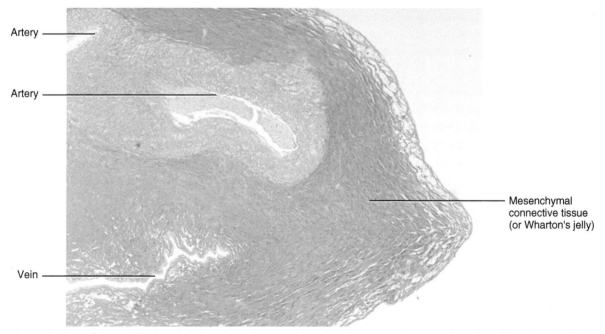

FIGURE 1.2 Histology of the umbilical cord, Alcian blue, enlargement 50×. Note how much the mesenchymal CT stains blue, highlighting the abundance of hyaluronan in the ECM of the umbilical cord.

aging process the quantity of link proteins increases and this reduces the mobility of the CT.

FIBRES

There are two types of fibres secreted by CT cells: collagen fibres and elastic fibres. The abundance and preponderance of different types of fibres varies according to the type of CT. Both types of fibre are formed from proteins consisting of long peptide chains.

Collagen fibres

The collagen fibres are flexible with a high tensile strength. Generally, each collagen fibre is made up of thread-like subunits called collagen fibrils. Each fibril in turn is made up of collagen molecules that are aligned head to tail in overlapping rows. The fibril's strength is due to covalent bonds between collagen molecules of adjacent rows. The collagen molecule (called tropocollagen) is composed of three intertwined polypeptide chains (each of which is called an alpha chain) that form a right-handed triple helix. Except for the ends of the chain, every third aminoacid is a glycine. Sugar groups are associated with the triple helix, so collagen is properly called a glycoprotein. The alpha chains that form the helix are not all alike and, based on differences within the chains, many types of collagen have been identified. They are classified by Roman numerals on the basis of chronology of discovery and the most important types are:

- Type I is the most prevalent type of collagen and constitutes about 90% of body collagen. It is the collagen found in the dermis of the skin, bone, tendon, fasciae, organ capsules and many other areas. These fibrils aggregate to form thick bundles of 2–10 μ in diameter and give the CT high tensile strength (500–1000 kg/cm^2).
- Type II is the main constituent of cartilage and these fibres are finer.
- Type III or reticular fibres have a narrow diameter and typically do not form bundles to become thick fibres. They are arranged in a mesh-like pattern and provide a supporting framework for the cellular constituents of various tissues and organs, e.g. the liver. These fibres are also found at the boundary of the epithelium, in loose CT, and around adipocytes, small blood vessels, nerves, tendons and intramuscular CTs (Fig. 1.3). They are the first to be secreted during the development of all the CTs and in the formation of new CT, as in a scar.
- Type IV forms a web rather than fibrils and is a fundamental component of the basal lamina of epithelia.

The synthesis of collagen fibrils is performed by the fibroblasts. Type III fibres which support the stroma of the haemopoietic and lymphatic tissues are made by reticular cells, and the endoneurium of peripheral nerves is produced by Schwann cells. The smooth muscle cells (present in the tunica media of blood vessels and the muscularis externa of the alimentary canal) are able to secrete all of the CT fibre types.

Single collagen fibres usually align along the main lines of a mechanical load. Under pathological circumstances, due to changes in the density of ground substance, the collagen fibres get closer to each other and may form pathological cross-links. This may prevent the ability of a normal collagen network to develop.

Collagen fibre turnover is normally about 300–500 days. Carano and Siciliani (1996) demonstrated that stretching fibroblasts could increase turnover by increasing the secretion of collagenase, an enzyme that plays an important role in the degradation of collagen fibres. These authors demonstrated that cyclical stretching is more effective than a continuous stretch. Stretching or compressing delivers an immediate and proportional deformation of the fibroblasts, but after 10–15 min the cell morphology readapts to the new mechanical environment, causing a loss of the biological activation. This suggests that a new mechanical stimulus is necessary to induce a new biological reaction.

Elastic fibres

Elastic fibres are thinner than collagen fibres and are arranged in a branching pattern to form a three-dimensional network. They give tissues the ability to cope with stretch and distension, and the elastic fibres are interwoven with collagen fibres in order to limit distensibility and to prevent tearing. The elastic fibres are composed of two structural components: elastin and fibrillin:

- Elastin is a protein related to collagen but with an unusual polypeptide backbone that causes it to coil in a random way. The configuration of a molecule's coiling is not permanent since it can oscillate from one shape to another. The coiled elastin molecule can be stretched, and when the force causing the stretch is withdrawn the molecule recoils back to its former state. Two large aminoacids unite to elastin, called desmosine and isodesmosine, cause elastin molecules to covalently bond to one another

---

CLINICAL PEARL 1.1 EHLERS–DANLOS SYNDROME

Etiology: a defect in the synthesis of type I or III collagen fibres that causes progressive deterioration of collagens. Different sites of the body could be affected, such as joints, heart valves, organ walls and arterial walls, and give different Ehlers–Danlos syndrome types. Symptoms such as joint hypermobility, pain and reduced muscle strength are common. Clayton et al (2013), by demonstrating that these patients have proprioceptive impairment, supports our hypothesis that CT impairment is a key element in proprioception (see Chapter 3).

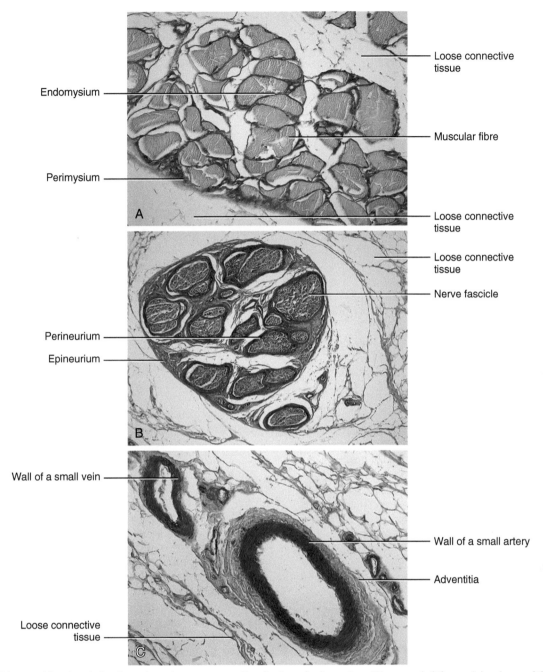

Endomysium

Perimysium

A

Loose connective tissue

Muscular fibre

Loose connective tissue

Perineurium

Epineurium

B

Loose connective tissue

Nerve fascicle

Wall of a small vein

Loose connective tissue

C

Wall of a small artery

Adventitia

FIGURE 1.3 Immunohistochemical stain to show the presence and localization of collagen type III in a muscle **(A)**, a peripheral nerve **(B)** and small vessels **(C)**. Note the abundance of collagen type III fibres in the endomysium and perimysium, in the perineurium and in the wall of the small arteries and veins.

and form an elastin matrix. The entire matrix is engaged during the stretch and recoil of elastic tissue.

- Fibrillin is a fibrillar glycoprotein. In developing elastic tissue, it appears before the elastin, and is believed to serve as an organizing structure.

In most cases, elastic fibres are produced by fibroblasts; however, elastic artery fibres are produced by the smooth muscle cells of the tunica media. The elastic material produced by the smooth muscle cells does not contain fibrillin, only elastin, and as a result does

not form elastic fibres. Instead, the elastin is laid down in fenestrated sheets or lamellae arranged in concentric layers between layers of smooth muscle.

Connective Tissue Cells

Many different kinds of cells can be found in CT. The more important cells are the fibroblasts, but also adipocytes and undifferentiated mesenchymal cells can be found. If the adipocytes are numerous and organized into lobules, the CT is referred to as adipose tissue. The fibroblasts can differentiate into cells responsible

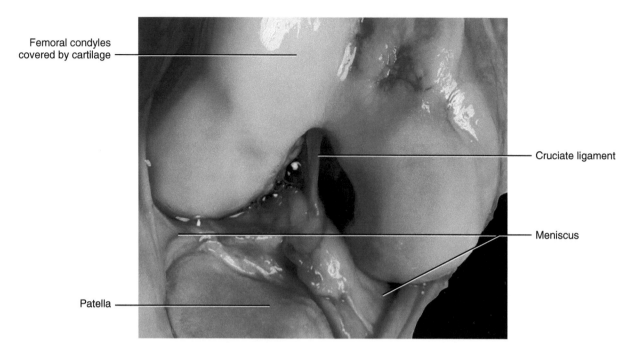

Femoral condyles covered by cartilage

Cruciate ligament

Meniscus

Patella

FIGURE 1.4 Macroscopic aspect of the knee cartilage: femur condyles and patellar surface. The cartilage forms a smooth surface. Note the cartilage degeneration at the patellar articular surface.

CLINICAL PEARL 1.2 MARFAN'S SYNDROME

Marfan's syndrome is a hereditary disorder of CT and is due to mutations in the fibrillin-1 gene (FBN1). Marfan's syndrome has a range of expressions from mild to severe. Patients with Marfan's tend to be tall with long limbs and long, thin fingers. In addition to skeletal features, patients with Marfan's syndrome have involvement of the eyes, heart valves and aorta, skin, lungs, and muscle tissues. Over the past 30 years, evolution of aggressive medical and surgical management of cardiovascular problems, especially mitral valve prolapse, aortic dilatation, and aortic dissection, has resulted in considerable improvement in life expectancy.

for producing several different kinds of CT: including chondroblasts, which are responsible for making cartilage (Fig. 1.4), and osteoblasts, which produce bone. Finally, always present in the CT are macrophages, mast cells, and transient migrant cells, such as lymphocytes, plasma cells and the white blood cells.

FIBROBLASTS

Fibroblasts are the principal cells of CT. The main function of fibroblasts is to maintain the structural integrity of CTs by continuously secreting precursors of the ECM, such as the collagen and elastic fibres and all the complex carbohydrates of the ground substance. They contribute to the organization of the matrix and, indeed, the organization of their cytoskeleton influences the disposition of the matrix that they produce.

Fibroblasts also have a role in the remodelling of the matrix through the processes of degradation and synthesis of new fibres and proteins. Unlike epithelial cells lining the body structures, fibroblasts do not form flat monolayers and are not restricted by a polarizing attachment to a basal lamina on one side.

Like other cells of the CT, fibroblasts are derived from primitive mesenchyme and their lifespan, as measured in chick embryos, is 57 ± 3 days. Tissue damage stimulates fibrocytes and induces fibroblastic mitosis. Fibroblastic proliferation and degradation is a normal occurrence in everyday mechanical loading such as walking, running and most forms of movement. Even mechanical loading during rest and sleep stimulates CT function. Collagen synthesis in the patellar tendon increases by nearly 100% as a result of just a single bout of acute exercise, and the effect is still evident three days later. In the initial training period, collagen turnover in tendons (i.e. the balance between synthesis and degradation) is increased and there is a net loss of collagen. This enables a tendon to restructure and adapt to an increased loading pattern. It is not until training continues that there is a net gain in collagen synthesis.

Fibroblasts also play an essential role in wound healing. After an initial injury to CT and blood vessels, growth factors cause an increased amount of fibroblasts to enter the wound and to start synthesizing new collagen, creating new granulation tissue and assisting in remodelling. The ECM of granulation tissue is both created and modified by fibroblasts. Initially, the fibroblasts produce type III collagen, a weaker form of the structural protein; later, they produce the stronger, long-stranded type I collagen that appears in the scar

CLINICAL PEARL 1.3 BENEFICIAL RESULTS FROM MECHANICAL LOAD ON FIBROBLASTS AND CIRCULATION

Mechanical load strongly influences the activity of the fibroblasts and the deposition of collagen fibres. After a sprain or another trauma of the locomotor system, new collagen fibres will be produced; however, if the patient is immobilized the collagen fibres will have an irregular disposition. This will cause restricted movement and prolong recovery time. Only early movement permits the correct formation of collagen fibres along the functional lines of force.

Loghmani and Warden (2009) injured bilaterally the medial collateral ligaments (MCL) of 51 rodents and used instrument-assisted, cross-fibre massage on the contralateral ligaments of 31 rodents one week following injury. They cross-friction massaged the injured area three sessions per week for one minute per session. Treatment was introduced unilaterally with the contralateral, injured MCL serving as an internal control (nontreated). Results showed that the treated ligaments were 43.1% stronger (P < 0.05), 39.7% stiffer (P < 0.01), and could absorb 57.1% more energy before failure (P < 0.05) than the contralateral, injured, nontreated ligaments at four weeks postinjury. On histological and scanning electron microscopy assessment, the treated ligaments appeared to have improved collagen fibre bundle formation and orientation within the scar region when compared with nontreated ligaments.

In a similar study, Loghmani and Warden (2013) used cross-friction massage on injured MCLs and found that there was not only a temporary increase in vasodilation within the ligament, but an alteration of microvascular morphology in the vicinity of the healing knee ligaments, including a larger proportion of blood vessels in the diameter range of arterioles. These changes persisted for one week after final intervention.

tissue. A scar is collagen deposited by fibroblasts during repair.

Tendons that undergo high rates of stretching may be more susceptible to inflammation and eventual degeneration due to the stretching of fibroblasts. Cyclic stretching of fibroblasts, and especially increasing the frequency of the stretching, increases the production of proinflammatory cyclooxygenase enzyme (COX-1, COX-2) and prostaglandin-E2 (Yang et al 2005). Therefore, overstimulation of fibroblasts may be responsible for repetitive-motion problems. Recent studies (Kaux et al 2013) have shown how eccentric exercises may be more beneficial than concentric exercises regarding the rehabilitation of muscles and tendons. There is reason to believe that the effect of the load pattern of eccentric exercise creates greater stimulation of fibroblasts, which increases collagen synthesis and thereby stimulates the healing of the injured tissue. Stretching also causes an increase in tendon fibroblast alignment.

Abbott et al (2013) theorize that CTs, especially fibroblasts, are part of a whole body cell-to-cell communication-signalling network. They state that fibroblasts exhibit active cytoskeletal responses within minutes of tissue lengthening:

Analogous cell-to-cell signalling involving calcium and/or ATP may exist within CT and may be accompanied by active tissue contraction or relaxation. One can envisage a whole-body web of CT involved in a dynamic, body-wide pattern of cellular activity fluctuating over seconds to minutes reflecting all externally and internally generated mechanical forces acting upon the body.

A particular type of fibroblast called the myofibroblast is found in tendons, fasciae and scars (Hinz et al 2012). These cells have in their cytoplasm actin fibres allowing them to contract. During wound repair it is necessary for fibroblasts to convert into myofibroblasts that then create extracellular collagen fibre deposition. They express a smooth muscle type actin–myosin complex that closes wounds and speeds up their repair by contracting the edges of the wound. Upon resolution of the injury, these myofibroblasts undergo apoptosis (programmed cell death). In wounds that fail to resolve and become keloids or hypertrophic scars, myofibroblasts may persist, rather than disappearing by apoptosis. According to Schleip (Schleip et al 2006), these cells also have an important role in determining the basal tone of CT.

ADIPOCYTES/FAT CELLS

Adipocytes can be present in many types of CT as isolated cells or as small aggregates. They form a specialized CT, called adipose tissue, when they become the predominant cell and their main function is the storage of energy as fat. Although the lineage of adipocytes is still unclear, preadipocytes are undifferentiated fibroblasts originating from mesenchymal stem cells that when stimulated form adipocytes.

We can distinguish two types of adipose cells:

- Unilocular adipocytes: these are large cells (their diameter varies from 50 to 100 μ) characterized by the presence of a large lipid droplet surrounded by a layer of cytoplasm. The nucleus is flattened and located on the periphery. A typical fat cell is 0.1 mm in diameter although some are twice that size and others half that size. The fat stored is in a semi-liquid state, and is composed primarily of triglycerides and cholesteryl esters. These fat cells secrete many proteins such as resistin, adiponectin and leptin, and they can synthesize estrogens from androgens. Their number can increase in childhood and adolescence, while it remains constant in adulthood. When fat cells have increased in size, about fourfold, they begin to divide, increasing the absolute number of fat cells present. After marked weight loss the number of fat cells does not decrease, but rather they contain less fat.

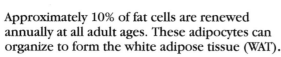

Approximately 10% of fat cells are renewed annually at all adult ages. These adipocytes can organize to form the white adipose tissue (WAT).

- Multilocular cells: these are little cells characterized by the presence of numerous smaller lipid droplets in the cytoplasm and also contain a large quantity of mitochondria. These fat cells can organize to form the brown adipose tissue (BAT).

MULTIPOTENT STROMAL CELLS

These cells retain the potential of embryonic mesenchymal cells with the capability of differentiating into a variety cell types, including osteoblasts, chondrocytes, adipocytes, myocytes and neurons. They have a great capacity for self-renewal while maintaining their multipotency.

Classification of Connective Tissue

There are three subtypes of CTs: specialized, proper and embryonic. The specialized CT includes adipose tissue, bone and cartilage. Regarding the specialized CT, we will be discussing only the adipose tissue due to its strong relationship to the superficial fascia. Please refer to other textbooks for information on bone and cartilage.

Proper CT is a very large group of tissues comprising both loose and dense CT (Fig. 1.5). It encompasses all organs and body cavities and connects one part with another. Equally important, it separates one group of cells from another. All fasciae have been classified as proper CT, but some authors exclude either the loose or the dense from this definition. The embryonic CT includes the mesenchyme (Fig. 1.6) and mucous CT (Fig. 1.2). In the following discussion we will describe the pertinent features of the proper CT so that we can correctly classify fasciae.

Loose Connective Tissue

Loose CT (or areolar tissue) is the most widespread CT of the body. It is characterized by an abundance of ground substance, plus thin and relatively few fibres and cells (Fig. 1.7). The main cellular elements are fibroblasts and a smaller amount of adipocytes. Fat cells are a normal constituent of loose CT, but when they are abundant and organized into large lobules for storage purposes the tissue is better classified as adipose tissue. The adipocytes present in loose CT are generally isolated cells or small aggregations that do not function as storage depots, and their principle function is to facilitate gliding and to act as interstitial filler. The adipocytes of the loose CT usually do not increase in volume when individuals gain weight. Collagen is the principal fibre of loose CT and is arrayed in all directions to form a loose network in the intercellular material. Many elastic fibres are also present.

The loose CT has a viscous, gel-like consistency and its consistency may fluctuate in different parts of the body due to variations in temperature or pH. This CT allows gliding between the various muscles and organs (Figs 1.8 and 1.9) and permits the diffusion of oxygen/nutrients from small vessels to the cells and the diffusion of metabolites back to the vessels. It is the initial site where antigens, bacteria and other agents that have breached an epithelial surface can be destroyed. It also forms a mesh-like tissue with a fluid matrix that supports the epithelia, such as the skin and other membranes. This CT fills the spaces between various organs and thus holds them in place while cushioning and protecting them; it also surrounds and supports the blood vessels.

A particular type of loose CT is the reticular tissue that contains only reticular fibres made of type III collagen. The reticular cells have a stellate shape and long processes that make contact with neighbouring cells, and the subsequent tissue supports a number of bodily

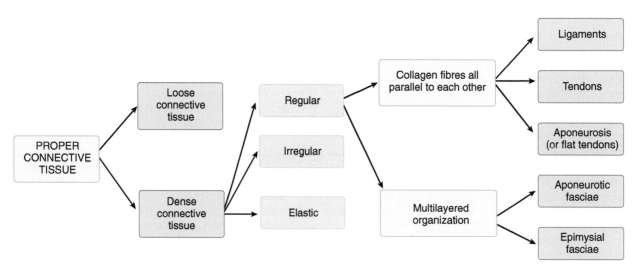

FIGURE 1.5 The proper CT classifications.

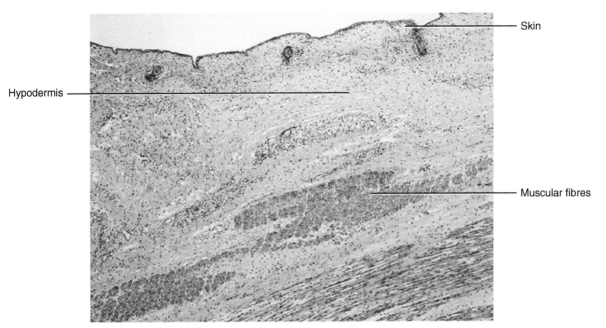

Skin

Hypodermis

Muscular fibres

FIGURE 1.6 Histological section of the abdominal wall of an embryo of 19 weeks, hematoxylin and eosin stain, enlargement 50×. Note the high cellularity and absence of well-defined fascial planes.

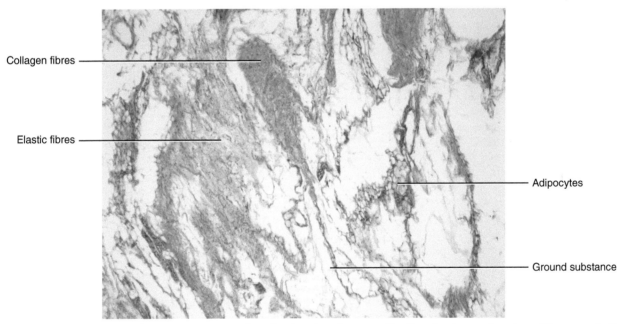

Collagen fibres

Elastic fibres

Adipocytes

Ground substance

FIGURE 1.7 Histological section of the loose CT, hematoxylin and eosin stain, enlargement 50×. Note the absence of any type of tissue organization. The collagen and elastic fibres are disposed in many directions and some adipocytes are present.

structures, such as the liver, spleen, bone marrow and lymphatic organs.

Adipose Tissue

Adipose tissue is not merely a tissue designed to passively store excess carbon in the form of triacylglycerols. Mature adipocytes synthesize and secrete numerous enzymes, growth factors, cytokines and hormones that are involved in overall energy homeostasis. There are different types of adipose tissue, for example: adipose tissue is commonly distinguished in WAT and BAT (Smorlesi et al 2012). The WAT is divided into two major types according to localization: subcutaneous white adipose tissue (SWAT) and visceral white adipose tissue (VWAT). Sbarbati et al (2010) used the structural and ultrastructural features of the adipose cells to classify the WAT into three different

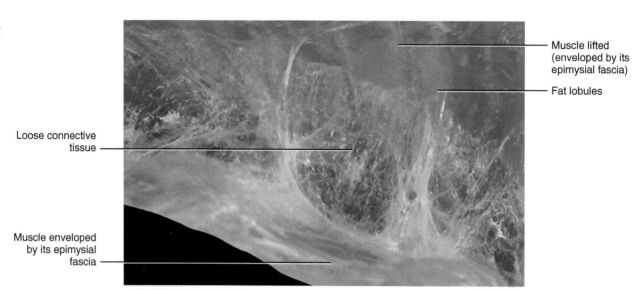

FIGURE 1.8 Macroscopic aspect of the loose CT between pectoralis major and minor muscles. The loose CT creates a gliding surface between the two muscles and permits their independent contraction. The white lines are the collagen fibres. The empty space between them is occupied in the living by water linked to the GAGs.

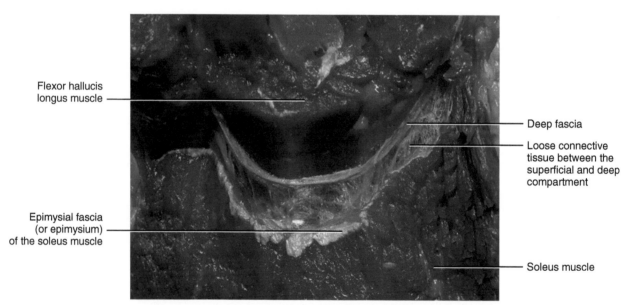

FIGURE 1.9 Transverse section of the middle third of the leg. The fascia of the flexor hallucis longus is detached from the underlying muscle while the soleus is strongly adhered to its own fascia. Tractioning the soleus muscle distally simulates a contraction and its fascia follows the muscle. Note the loose CT between the fascia of the soleus and the flexor hallucis longus. This creates a gliding surface between the two fasciae allowing an independent contraction and/or passive stretch of the two muscles.

types: deposit WAT (dWAT), structural WAT (sWAT) and fibrous WAT (fWAT).

WHITE ADIPOSE TISSUE (WAT)

WAT is the major form of adipose tissue in mammals (commonly referred to as 'fat'). It is composed of adipocytes held together by a loose CT that is highly vascularized and innervated. White adipocytes are rounded cells that contain a single large fat droplet that occupies over 90% of the cell volume and the mitochondria and nucleus are squeezed into the remaining cell volume. There are differing microscopic features of subcutaneous adipose tissue in different parts of the body. In the subcutis of the abdomen, the fat cells are tightly packed and linked by a weak network of isolated collagen fibres. These collagen fibres are very meager with large cells and few blood vessels (Fig. 1.10). In the SWAT of the limbs, the stroma is fairly well represented with adequate vascularity and its cells are wrapped by a basket of collagen fibres (Figs 1.11 and 1.12). In the foot and in areas where a severe mechanical stress can occur, the SWAT has a significant fibrous

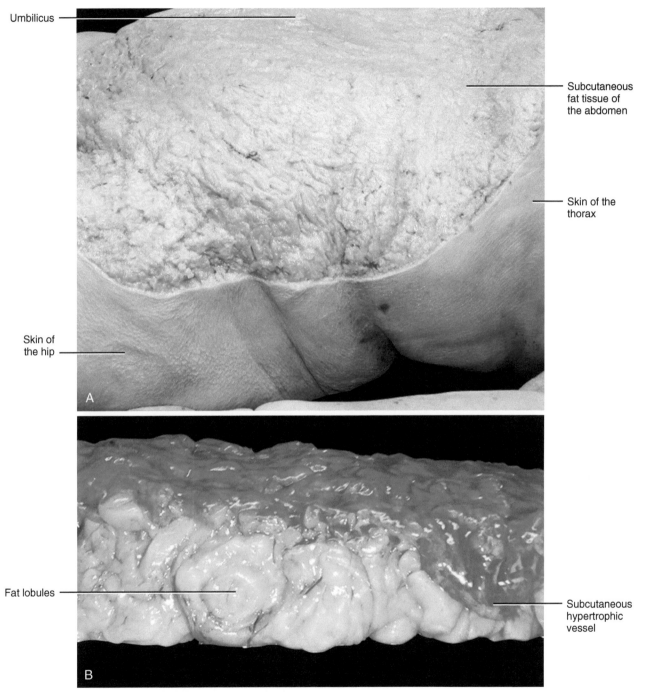

Umbilicus

Subcutaneous fat tissue of the abdomen

Skin of the thorax

Skin of the hip

A

Fat lobules

Subcutaneous hypertrophic vessel

B

FIGURE 1.10 (A) Macroscopic aspect of the adipose tissue from the abdomen of a fatty cadaver. **(B)** Adipose tissue of the abdomen removed from an obese person. Note the large lobules of fat and the paucity of fibrous tissue support. The vessels cross the tissue perpendicularly and are hypertrophic.

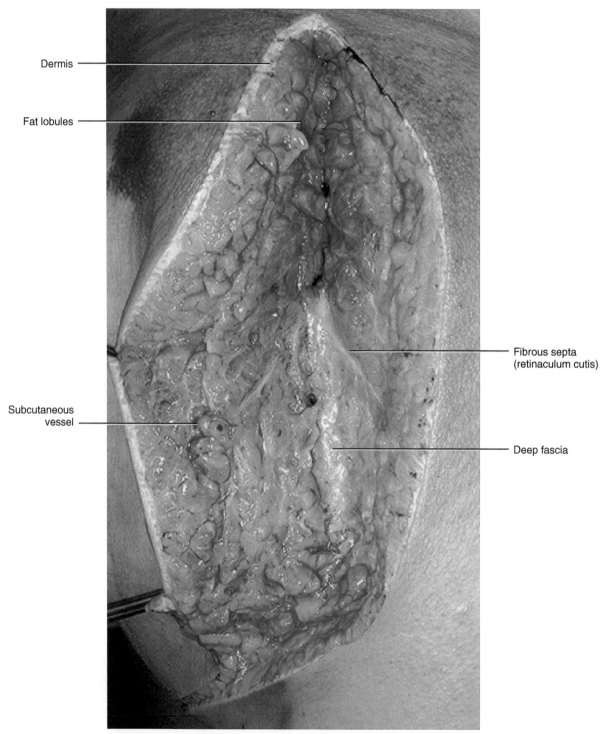

Dermis

Fat lobules

Fibrous septa
(retinaculum cutis)

Subcutaneous
vessel

Deep fascia

FIGURE 1.11 Macroscopic aspect of the thigh adipose tissue of a standard cadaver. The fat lobules are small and the supporting fibrous tissue is well represented. The vessels are small and numerous and are sufficient to vascularize the adipose tissue in a homogeneous manner.

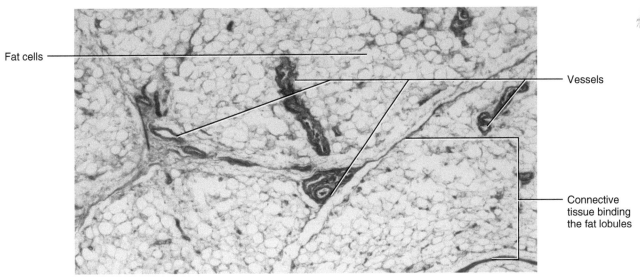

Fat cells

Vessels

Connective tissue binding the fat lobules

FIGURE 1.12 Histology of the adipose tissue of the thigh. The adipocytes are small and form regular lobules. Each lobule is supported by CT. The vessels are numerous. Hematoxylin and eosin stain, enlargement 25×.

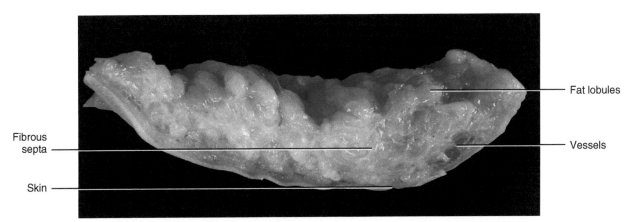

Fat lobules

Fibrous septa

Vessels

Skin

FIGURE 1.13 Macroscopic aspect of the fat pad of the heel. In the weight bearing areas the fibrous component (with a white appearance) of the adipose tissue (with a yellow appearance) increases with each adipocyte having its own thick fibrous shell. This type of fat functions as a cushion and does not increase in thickness when a person gains weight.

component containing adipocytes with thick distinct fibrous shells (Fig. 1.13). We can recognize a different composition of the SWAT based on its relationship with the superficial fascia. The WAT between the skin and the superficial fascia is true fatty tissue and usually increases when a person fattens, while the WAT between the superficial fascia and the deep fascia is usually looser and generally does not increase in thickness (see Chapter 2) (Fig. 1.14).

VWAT is composed of several adipose depots, including mesenteric, epididymal and perirenal depots (Fig. 1.15). VWAT tissue is associated with insulin resistance, diabetes mellitus, dyslipidaemia, hypertension, atherosclerosis, hepatic steatosis, and overall mortality.

The primary function of the WAT is to store energy and act as a cushion. However, it also plays important roles as an endocrine/immune organ by secreting

adipokines, such as inflammatory cytokines, complement-like factors, chemokines, and acute phase proteins. Its endocrine function includes participating in the regulation of appetite, glucose and lipid metabolism, the inflammatory process and reproductive functions. Subcutaneous and visceral adipocytes originate from different progenitor cells that exhibit different genetic expression patterns. SWAT, compared to VWAT, responds better to the antilipolytic effects of insulin and other hormones, secretes more adiponectin and less inflammatory cytokines, and is differentially affected by molecules involved in signal transduction as well as drugs. According to Sudi et al (2000), the quantity of subcutaneous adipose tissue from the upper body is significantly and positively correlated to the level of leptin, suggesting that leptin is under the control of certain subcutaneous adipose tissue depots from the upper body.

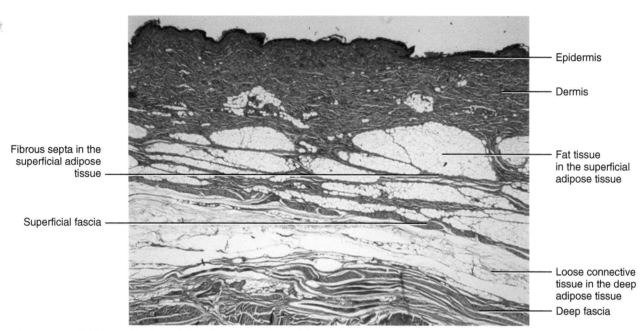

Epidermis

Dermis

Fibrous septa in the
superficial adipose
tissue

Fat tissue
in the superficial
adipose tissue

Superficial fascia

Loose connective
tissue in the deep
adipose tissue

Deep fascia

FIGURE 1.14 Full-thickness histology of the subcutaneous tissue of the thigh, Mallory–Azan stain, enlargement 16×. It is evident that the white adipose tissue between the skin and the superficial fascia is true fatty tissue, and is formed by adipose lobules surrounded by fibrous septa. Between the superficial and deep fascia the tissue is looser and the fibrous septa are scarce.

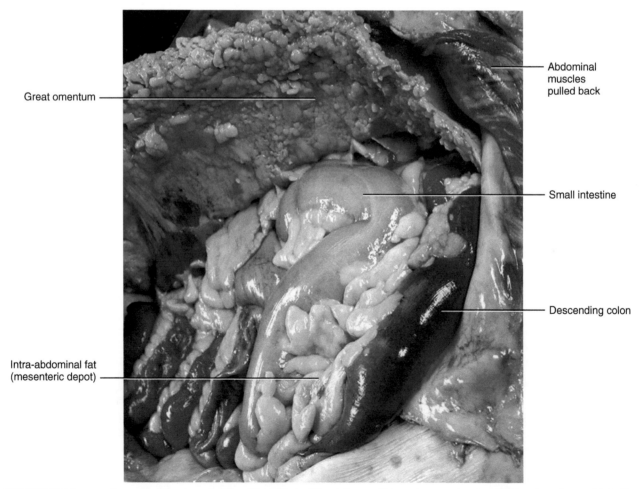

Great omentum

Abdominal
muscles
pulled back

Small intestine

Descending colon

Intra-abdominal fat
(mesenteric depot)

FIGURE 1.15 Macroscopic aspect of the visceral white adipose tissue of the abdomen. The greater omentum was lifted to show the small intestine with the fat all around the loops. The fat lobules are large and scantily vascularized. The fibrous CT, with its function of support, is almost absent.

BROWN ADIPOSE TISSUE (BAT)

The BAT is a specialized adipose tissue and its primary function is thermogenesis. BAT is so-called because it is darkly pigmented due to the high density of mitochondria rich in cytochromes. It specializes in the production of heat (adaptive thermogenesis) and lipid oxidation and is especially abundant in newborns and in hibernating mammals, but could be found also in human adults in the neck, around the aorta and in the supraclavicular, mediastinal and interscapular areas. BAT contains more capillaries than white fat since it has a greater need for oxygen than most tissues. Brown adipocytes are smaller in overall size compared to white adipocytes and are polygonal in shape and contain numerous large mitochondria. Whereas, white adipocytes contain a single large fat droplet, brown adipocytes contain several small lipid droplets. Brown adipocytes are molecularly Thermogenin + (UCP1$^+$) and leptin$^-$. BAT is highly vascularized and contains a very high density of noradrenergic nerve fibres. BAT is essential for classical nonshivering thermogenesis; this phenomenon does not exist when functional BAT is absent. In addition, it is essential for cold acclimation-recruited, norepinephrine-induced thermogenesis. Heat production from BAT is activated whenever the organism is in need of extra heat, e.g. postnatally, during entry into a febrile state, and during arousal from hibernation. Feeding also results in activation of BAT. A series of diets, apparently all characterized by being low in protein, would result in a leptin-dependent recruitment of the tissue. When the tissue is active, high amounts of lipids and glucose are combusted in the tissue. The development of BAT, with its characteristic protein, UCP1 was probably essential for the evolutionary success of mammals, as its thermogenesis enhances neonatal survival and allows for active life even in cold surroundings. Ito et al (1991) demonstrated that human brown fat cells begin to show a transformation into white fat cells at the infantile stage. This change occurs from the peripheral towards the central portion of the lobule, so that various functioning cell types remain only in the central area of the lobules. In contrast to humans, in hibernating animals the white fat cells never occur within the brown fat tissue. According with Bartness et al (2010), the BAT presents both a sympathetic innervation and a sensory innervation, which probably has the role of perceiving the temperature changes and monitoring the lipolysis. It has also been demonstrated that in some BAT depots, a parasympathetic innervation exists.

Dense Connective Tissue

Dense CT is characterized by large, robust collagen fibres that provide a considerable amount of strength to this tissue. Fibres are so numerous that the key identifying trait of this tissue is the absence of open spaces between cells or fibres. Since the protein fibres are the dominant component of these tissues, the types of fibres and their orientation within these tissues is the basis for the naming scheme. Dense CTs contain either collagen or elastic protein fibres; therefore, there are dense collagenous CTs and dense elastic types. The collagenous types are far more abundant and are called fibrous or 'white' CT. Elastic fibres, on the other hand, appear yellow in unstained tissues and are commonly referred to as 'yellow' CT (e.g. the yellow ligaments of the spine). Fibroblasts are the only cells visible and are arranged in rows between the fibres. Their function is to create the collagen fibres of the tissue.

The main roles of dense CT are to transmit forces over a distance and to connect different organs/muscles. Collagen fibres are disposed along the direction of mechanical loads present in that specific tissue. The capacity of dense CT to resist mechanical stress is directly related to the structural organization of the ECM and above all, the collagen fibres.

The dense CT is subclassified as follows:

- Dense, irregular CT has irregularly arranged collagen fibres and usually comprises the dermis and fasciae. In the last few years, it has been demonstrated that the irregular appearance of deep fasciae may be due to its multilayered structure, but in actuality each layer presents its own regularity (see Chapter 3). Consequently, the deep fasciae could be classified as dense regular CT.

- Dense, regular CT is a white, flexible tissue that contains tightly packed bundles of collagen fibres. All of these fibres run in one direction and are arranged parallel to the direction of forces exerted on the particular body part where the tissue is located. This arrangement is typical of tendons and ligaments, but according to recent studies (Benetazzo et al 2011) the deep fasciae could also be classified in this group. Purslow (2010) demonstrated that the epimysium and perimysium have a very specific organization that also may classify them as dense, regular CT, and Huijing and Baan (2003) demonstrated this tissue's role in force transmission (see Chapter 3). Finally, a specific discussion of the endomysium is necessary as it is not clear whether this has a structure similar to a microtendon (Purslow 2010) or if it is better classified as loose CT (Testut 1905). In the following chapters, the characteristics and functions of the deep fasciae, epimysium and perimysium will be described in greater detail.

We can further classify the regular CT according to its function:

- Dense CT connecting two bones: referred to as ligaments as they are composed of collagen fibres positioned parallel to each other and rich in elastic fibres (Fig. 1.16).

- Dense CT connecting muscles to bones: referred to as common tendons as they are also characterized by collagen fibres positioned parallel to each other (Figs 1.17 and 1.18), and

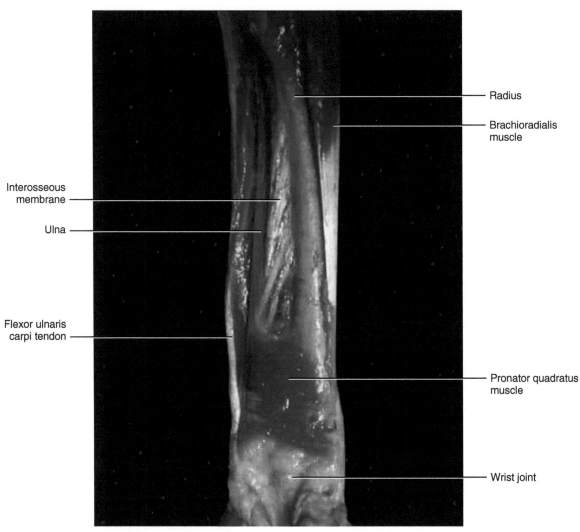

Radius

Brachioradialis
muscle

Interosseous
membrane

Ulna

Flexor ulnaris
carpi tendon

Pronator quadratus
muscle

Wrist joint

FIGURE 1.16 Dissection of the anterior region of the forearm (in a supine position). The interosseous membrane of forearm appears as a broad ligament joining radius and ulna bones with well evident collagen fibrous bundles. The interosseous membrane divides the forearm into anterior and posterior compartments, serves as a site of attachment for muscles of the forearm and transfers forces from the radius, to the ulna, and to the humerus.

there are very few elastic fibres. Tendons could be divided into two sub-categories: tubular tendons (e.g. biceps brachii tendon and patellar tendon) and flat tendons (or aponeuroses). In the past, the terms 'fascia' and 'aponeurosis' were used in an interchangeable way; however, based on their collagen fibre disposition, the aponeurosis (flat tendon type) can be differentiated from the deep muscular fascia. Both are dense, regular CTs, but aponeuroses have the collagen fibre bundles in a single direction and deep fasciae have a multilayered structure with collagen fibres disposed in a variety of directions (see Chapter 3). These tissues have dissimilar functions: aponeuroses connect muscles to bone and fasciae connect muscles to one another.

● Dense CT connecting muscles to one another: these are referred to as deep fasciae (see Chapter 3) (Fig. 1.19)
● Dense CT connecting muscle to fascia: referred to as 'myofascial expansions' and have their collagen fibres parallel to each other. Some expansions are flat (e.g. the lacertus fibrosus that is the expansion of the biceps brachii into the medial region of the antebrachial fascia (Fig. 1.20). Other expansions could be tubular (like a tendon, e.g. the expansion of the gracilis, sartorius and semitendinosus into the crural fascia). The elastic fibres are scarce in this type of CT.

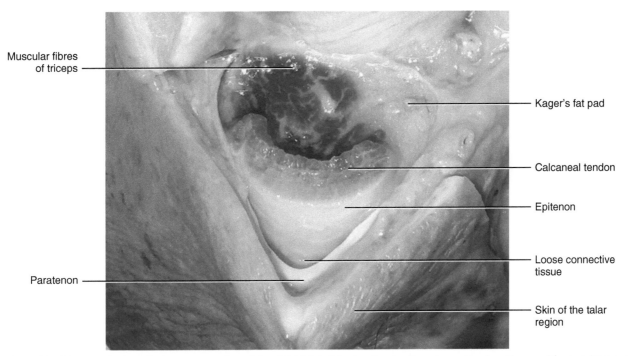

Muscular fibres of triceps

Kager's fat pad

Calcaneal tendon

Epitenon

Loose connective tissue

Paratenon

Skin of the talar region

FIGURE 1.17 Macroscopic view of a transverse section of the distal third of the leg showing the calcaneal tendon. The crural fascia splits around the tendon to form the paratenon. The paratenon envelops both the calcaneal tendon and Kager's fat pad. At this level some muscular fibres of the triceps are present. The tendon is formed by closely packed, parallel collagen fibres.

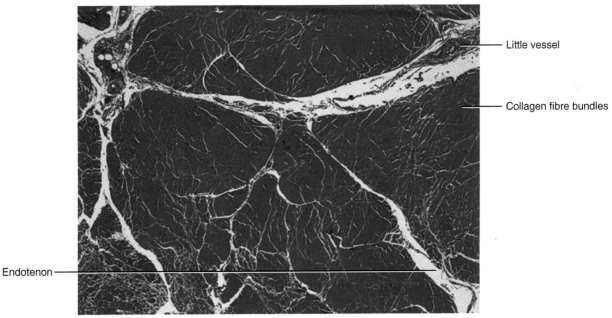

Little vessel

Collagen fibre bundles

Endotenon

FIGURE 1.18 Histology of the tendon. The fibres are typically arranged in bundles all parallel to each other, bound by the endotenon and rich in hyaluronan. The blood vessels penetrate into the tendon following the septa of the endotenon. The only cell type present is the fibroblasts and they are scarce. Only small amounts of ground substance are present. Mallory–Azan stain, enlargement 50×.

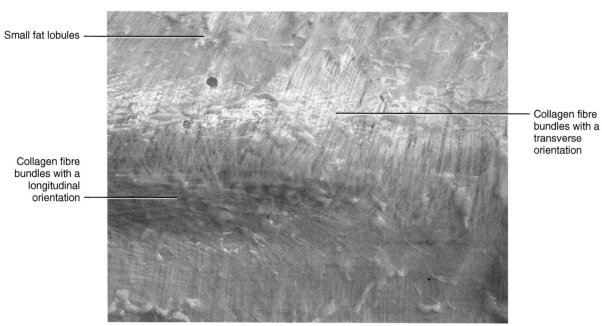

Small fat lobules —

Collagen fibre
bundles with a
transverse
orientation

Collagen fibre
bundles with a
longitudinal
orientation —

FIGURE 1.19 Macroscopic view of the fascia lata. The fascia lata is a dense CT formed by packed collagen fibre bundles with different orientations.

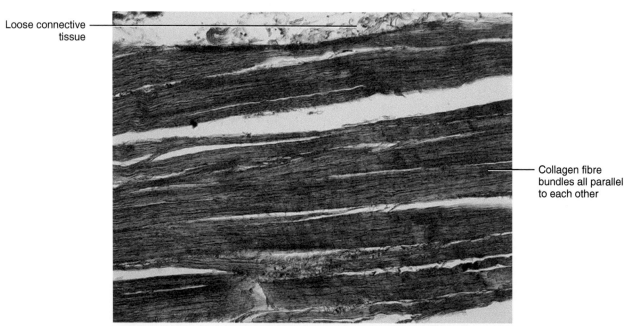

Loose connective —
tissue

Collagen fibre
bundles all parallel
to each other

FIGURE 1.20 Histology of the lacertus fibrosus (myofascial expansion of the biceps brachii muscle into the medial portion of the antebrachial fascia). The collagen fibres are all positioned parallel to each other and form a fibrous layer. Mallory–Azan stain, enlargement 50×.

References

Abbott, R.D., Koptiuch, C., Iatridis, J.C., Howe, A.K., Badger, G.J., Langevin, H.M., 2013. Stress and matrix-responsive cytoskeletal remodeling in fibroblasts. J. Cell. Physiol. 228 (1), 50–57.

Adhikari, A.S., Chai, J., Dunn, A.R., 2011. Mechanical load induces a 100-fold increase in the rate of collagen proteolysis by MMP-1. J. Am. Chem. Soc. 133 (6), 1686–1689.

Bartness, T.J., Vaughan, C.H., Song, C.K., 2010. Sympathetic and sensory innervation of brown adipose tissue. Int. J. Obes. 34 (Suppl. 1), S36–S42.

Benetazzo, L., Bizzego, A., De Caro, R., Frigo, G., Guidolin, D., Stecco, C., 2011. 3D reconstruction of the crural and thoracolumbar fasciae. Surg. Radiol. Anat. 33 (10), 855–862.

Carano, A., Siciliani, G., 1996. Effects of continuous and intermittent forces on human fibroblasts in vitro. Eur. J. Orthod. 18 (1), 19–26.

Clayton, H.A., Cressman, E.K., Henriques, D.Y., 2013. Proprioceptive sensitivity in Ehlers–Danlos syndrome patients. Exp. Brain Res. 230 (3), 311–321.

Hinz, B., Phan, S.H., Thannickal, V.J., et al., 2012. Recent developments in myofibroblast biology: paradigms for connective tissue remodeling. Am. J. Pathol. 180 (4), 1340–1355.

Huijing, P.A., Baan, G.C., 2003. Myofascial force transmission: muscle relative position and length determine agonist and synergist muscle force. J. Appl. Physiol. 94 (3), 1092–1107.

Hukinsa, D.W.L., Aspden, R.M., 1985. Composition and properties of connective tissues. Trends Biochem. Sci. 10 (7), 260–264.

Ito, T., Tanuma, Y., Yamada, M., Yamamoto, M., 1991. Morphological studies on brown adipose tissue in the bat and in humans of various ages. Arch. Histol. Cytol. 54 (1), 1–39.

Jaroszyk, F., Marzec, E., 1993. Dielectric properties of BAT collagen in the temperature range of thermal denaturation. Ber. Bunsenges Phys. Chem. 97 (7), 868–871.

Kaux, J.F., Drion, P., Libertiaux, V., et al., 2013. Eccentric training improves tendon biomechanical properties: a rat model. J. Orthop. Res. 31 (1), 119–124.

Loghmani, M.T., Warden, S.J., 2009. Instrument-assisted cross-fiber massage accelerates knee ligament healing. J. Orthop. Sports Phys. Ther. 39 (7), 506–514.

Loghmani, M.T., Warden, S.J., 2013. Instrument-assisted cross fiber massage increases tissue perfusion and alters microvascular morphology in the vicinity of healing knee ligaments. Complement. Altern. Med. 28 (13), 240.

Purslow, P.P., 2010. Muscle fascia and force transmission. J. Bodywork Mov. Ther. 14 (4), 411–417.

Sbarbati, A., Accorsi, D., Benati, D., et al., 2010. Subcutaneous adipose tissue classification. Eur. J. Histochem. 54 (4), e48.

Schleip, R., Naylor, I.L., Ursu, D., et al., 2006. Passive muscle stiffness may be influenced by active contractility of intramuscular connective tissue. Med. Hypotheses 66 (1), 66–71.

Smorlesi, A., Frontini, A., Giordano, A., Cinti, S., 2012. The adipose organ: white–brown adipocyte plasticity and metabolic inflammation. Obes. Rev. Suppl. 2, 83–96.

Standring, S., 2008. Gray's Anatomy, fortieth ed. Churchill Livingstone, London, pp. 156–163.

Sudi, K.M., Gallistl, S., Tafeit, E., Möller, R., Borkenstein, M.H., 2000. The relationship between different subcutaneous adipose tissue layers, fat mass and leptin in obese children and adolescents. J. Pediatr. Endocrinol. Metab. 13 (5), 505–512.

Testut, J.L., Jacob, O., 1905. Précis d'anatomietopographique avec applications medico-chirurgicales, vol. III. Gaston Doinet Cie, Paris, p. 302.

Yang, G., Im, H.J., Wang, J.H., 2005. Repetitive mechanical stretching modulates IL-1beta induced COX-2, MMP-1 expression, and PGE2 production in human patellar tendon fibroblasts. Gene 19 (363), 166–172.

Bibliography

Benjamin, M., 2009. The fascia of the limbs and back – a review. J. Anat. 214 (1), 1–18.

Cannon, B., Nedergaard, J., 2004. Brown adipose tissue: function and physiological significance. Physiol. Rev. 84 (1), 277–359.

Gao, Y., Kostrominova, T.Y., Faulkner, J.A., Wineman, A.S., 2008. Age-related changes in the mechanical properties of the epimysium in skeletal muscles of rats. J. Biomech. 41 (2), 465–469.

Gil, A., Olza, J., Gil-Campos, M., Gomez-Llorente, C., Aguilera, C.M., 2011. Is adipose tissue metabolically different at different sites? Int. J. Pediatr. Obes. Suppl. 1, 13–20.

Himms-Hagen, J., 1995. Role of brown adipose tissue thermogenesis in control of thermoregulatory feeding in rats: A new hypothesis that links thermostatic and glucostatic hypotheses for control of food intake. Proc. Soc. Exp. Biol. Med. 208 (2), 159–169.

Huijing, P.A., 2009. Epimuscularmyofascial force transmission: A historical review and implications for new research. J. Biomech. 42 (1), 9–21.

Huijing, P.A., Jaspers, R.T., 2005. Adaptation of muscle size and myofascial force transmission: a review and some new experimental results. Scand. J. Med. Sci. Sports 15 (6), 349–380.

Huijing, P.A., Van De Langenberg, R.W., Meesters, J.J., Baan, G.C., 2007. Extramuscular myofascial force transmission also occurs between synergistic muscles and antagonistic muscles. J. Electromyogr. Kinesiol. 17 (6), 680–689.

Järvinen, T.A., Józsa, L., Kannus, P., Järvinen, T.L., Järvinen, M., 2002. Organization and distribution of intramuscular connective tissue in normal and immobilized skeletal muscles. An immunohistochemical, polarization and scanning electron microscopic study. J. Muscle Res. Cell Motil. 23 (3), 245–254.

Marquart-Elbaz, C., Varnaison, E., Sick, H., Grosshans, E., Cribier, B., 2001. Cellular subcutaneous tissue. Anatomic observations. (Article in French). Ann. Dermatol. Venereol. 128 (11), 1207–1213.

McCombe, D., Brown, T., Slavin, J., Morrison, W.A., 2001. The histochemical structure of the deep fascia and its structural response to surgery. J. Hand Surg. 26 (2), 89–97.

Metcalfe, D.D., Baram, D., Mekori, Y.A., 1997. Mast cells. Physiol. Rev. 77 (4), 1033–1079.

Nishimura, T., Hattori, A., Takahashi, K., 1996. Arrangement and identification of proteoglycans in basement membrane and intramuscular connective tissue of bovine semitendinosus muscle. Acta. Anatomica. 155 (4), 257–265.

Passerieux, E., Rossignol, R., Chopard, A., et al., 2006. Structural organization of the perimysium in bovine skeletal muscle: Junctional plates and associated intracellular subdomains. J. Struct. Biol. 154 (2), 206–216.

Passerieux, E., Rossignol, R., Letellier, T., Delage, J.P., 2007. Physical continuity of the perimysium from myofibers to tendons: involvement in lateral force transmission in skeletal muscle. J. Struct. Biol. 159 (1), 19–28.

Purslow, P.P., 1989. Strain-induced reorientation of an intramuscular connective tissue network: implications for passive muscle elasticity. J. Biomech. 22 (1), 21–31.

Rowe, R.W., 1981. Morphology of perimysial and endomysial connective tissue in skeletal muscle. Tissue Cell 13 (4), 681–690.

Sakamoto, Y., 1996. Histological features of endomysium, perimysium and epimysium in rat lateral pterygoid muscle. J. Morphol. 227 (1), 113–119.

Smahel, J., 1986. Adipose tissue in plastic surgery. Ann. Plast. Surg. 16 (5), 444–453.

Stecco, A., Macchi, V., Masiero, S., et al., 2009. Pectoral and femoral fasciae: common aspects and regional specializations. Surg. Radiol. Anat. 31 (1), 35–42.

Stecco, C., Gagey, O., Macchi, V., et al., 2007. Anatomical study of myofascial continuity in the anterior region of the upper limb. Tendinous muscular insertions onto the deep fascia of the upper limb. First part: anatomical study. Morphologie 91 (292), 29–37.

Trotter, J.A., 1990. Interfiber tension transmission in series-fibered muscles of the cat hindlimb. J. Morphol. 206 (3), 351–361.

Trotter, J.A., 1993. Functional morphology of force transmission in skeletal muscle. A brief review. Acta. Anatomica. 146 (4), 205–222.

Trotter, J.A., Eberhard, S., Samora, A., 1983. Structural domains of the muscle-tendon junction. 1. The internal lamina and the connecting domain. Anat. Rec. 207 (4), 573–591.

Trotter, J.A., Purslow, P.P., 1992. Functional morphology of the endomysium in series fibered muscles. J. Morphol. 212 (2), 109–122.

Young, B., et al., 2008. Wheater – Histology and microscopic anatomy, fifth ed. Elsevier Masson, pp. 65–80.

Yucesoy, C.A., Baan, G., Huijing, P.A., 2008. Epimuscular myofascial force transmission occurs in the rat between the deep flexor muscles and their antagonistic muscles. J. Electromyogr. Kinesiol. 20 (1), 118–126.

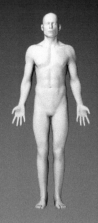

2

Subcutaneous Tissue and Superficial Fascia

History

The superficial fascia is still a subject area for debate. While some authors admit the existence of a membranous layer separating the subcutaneous tissue into two sublayers, others exclude it, and still others describe multiple such layers (Wendell-Smith 1997). The ancient anatomists (Fabrici, Casseri, Spiegel, Bartholin and Veslin, etc.), following the teachings of Vesalius (1543), described the subcutis as having an adipose and a carnosus layer. They knew that cutaneous musculature was present throughout the body in animals, but in humans it was limited to the neck, forehead, occiput and a few other regions. Under these layers they recognized the 'membrane muscolorum communis': membrane related to muscles. The term 'superficial fascia' appeared only at the end of the nineteenth century, when Camper (1801), Colles (1811) and Scarpa (1808 and 1819), studying the formation of inguinal hernias, described a fibrous layer inside the hypodermis of the abdominal and pelvic regions. This layer was designated as the 'superficial fascia', something separate from the term 'deep fascia'. In 1825, Velpau affirmed that 'the superficial fascia is a fibrous layer present throughout the body, not just in the abdomen and pelvis'. Unfortunately, no one continued the research of the superficial fascia and its relation to the panniculus carnosus as described in the ancient anatomical textbooks. Thus, the confusion about the terminology and organization of the subcutis remained. According to the French school, guided by Testut, the subcutis is formed by two fibrous sublayers: the first is just under the dermis and the second is near the deep fascia, and both separated by a thin layer of loose connective tissue. Adipose tissue is present between the two fibrous layers. But according to the Italian and German schools, the superficial fascia is a fibrous layer that divides the subcutis into a superficial and deep adipose layer that is loosely organized. Velpau agreed with this second version of the subcutis and described a superficial layer (the 'couche areolaire'), and a deep layer (the 'couche lamellare'), but his description was abandoned on behalf of Testut's idea.

It is interesting to note that the meanings of the terms 'panniculus adiposus' and 'superficial fascia' differ in English, French and German-speaking countries. For example, the fibrous lamina dividing the subcutis is named 'textus connectives compactus' by the Federative Committee on Anatomic Nomenclature (FACT), 'fascia superficialis' by Italian and French anatomists, 'membranous layer' by English anatomists, 'straffen Bindegewebe' by German authors, and 'subcutaneous fascia' or 'tela subcutanea' by Wendell-Smith (1997). Today many authors suggest simply using the term 'hypodermis' or 'subcutis' without further elaboration, and even the Nomina Anatomica of 1997 uses the general term 'hypodermis' instead of 'superficial fascia'.

Current Evidence

To understand the organization of the subcutis and the eventual presence of the superficial fascia, we must consider the whole human body and think that a common organization must exist, probably with some local differences. Therefore, dissections, layer by layer, were performed on the entire human body. These dissections of fresh cadavers revealed that the subcutis is divided by a fibrous lamina into sublayers, each with distinct features (Fig. 2.1). The superficial sublayer is referred to as 'superficial adipose tissue' (SAT), the deep one as 'deep adipose tissue' (DAT) and the fibrous lamina in the middle as 'superficial fascia' (Figs 2.2 and 2.3). This text uses the term 'superficial fascia', following the description by Professor Sterzi (1910). The Terminologia Anatomica defines 'fascia' as a sheath, a sheet, or any number of other dissectible aggregations of connective tissue. Consequently, according to our dissections, the superficial fascia is to all intents and purposes a true fascia.

The superficial fascia is connected to the skin (retinaculum cutis superficialis) and to the deep fascia (retinaculum cutis profundus) by fibrous septa, which impart specific mechanical proprieties to the subcutis (Nash et al 2004). Some septa are very oblique and analysis of a small portion of these areas would reveal, what appear to be, multiple fibrous laminae, but if larger areas are dissected it is found that these laminae do not merge into a distinctive structure. These conclusions were confirmed by imaging and histological examination. It is evident that the subcutis is uniformly structured, with specific features that differ according to the region of the body. In some parts the fibrous component is prevalent, in others the adipose component is prevalent. This defines the mechanical and biological features of the subcutis. Sometimes the

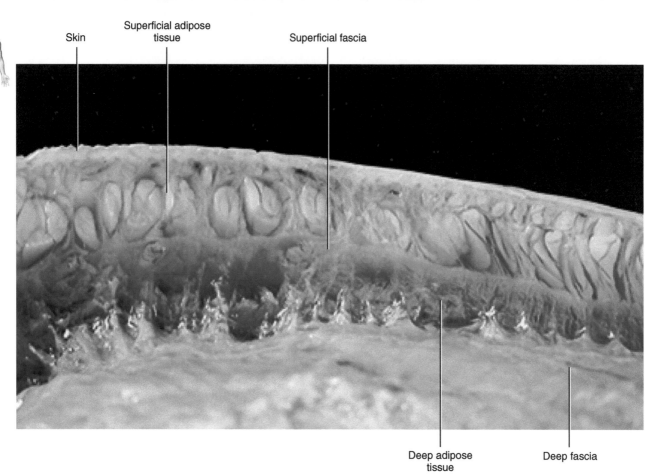

Skin | Superficial adipose tissue | Superficial fascia

Deep adipose tissue | Deep fascia

FIGURE 2.1 Section of the subcutis of the thigh. Layers of the subcutis are shown. The superficial fascia divides the SAT from the DAT. The SAT has a distinct structure, with fibrous septa that are vertically orientated with fat lobules situated between them. The DAT is formed by loose connective tissue, there are few fat cells and the septa are thinner and less fibrous. This structure permits a plane of gliding between the superficial and deep fascia.

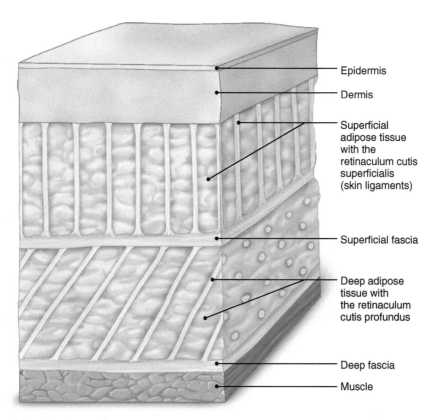

Epidermis

Dermis

Superficial adipose tissue with the retinaculum cutis superficialis (skin ligaments)

Superficial fascia

Deep adipose tissue with the retinaculum cutis profundus

Deep fascia

Muscle

FIGURE 2.2 Organization of the subcutaneous tissue.

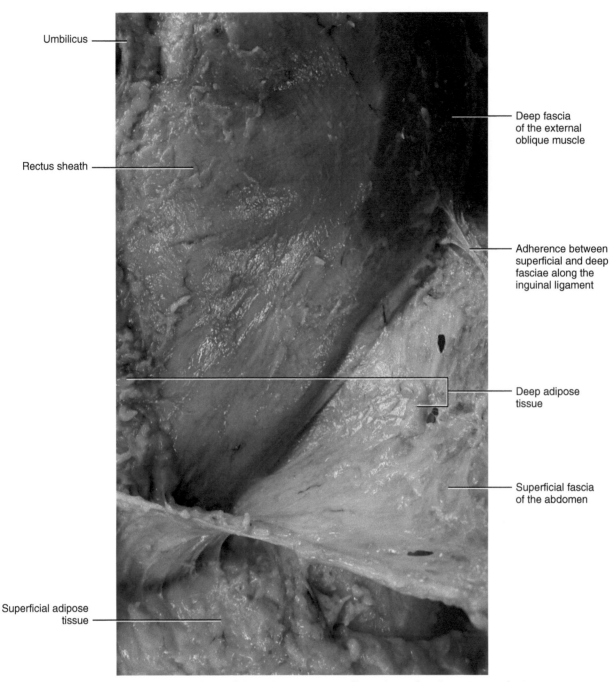

Umbilicus

Rectus sheath

Deep fascia
of the external
oblique muscle

Adherence between
superficial and deep
fasciae along the
inguinal ligament

Deep adipose
tissue

Superficial fascia
of the abdomen

Superficial adipose
tissue

FIGURE 2.3 Macroscopic view of the superficial fascia of the abdomen. It is a very fibrous layer referred to as Scarpa's fascia.

superficial fascia splits to envelop vessels, nerves or fat cells, and it seems that the fascia is composed of more than one layer.

The features of the subcutaneous tissue vary throughout the body, in particular the SAT and DAT differ in thickness, form, and disposition of the adipose lobes and fibrous septa. The retinacula cutis superficialis (or 'skin ligaments' in English textbooks) are usually almost perpendicular (Fig. 2.4). The retinacula cutis profundus is usually more oblique and thinner than the superficial septa, and creates a clear separation of the superficial fascia from the deep fascia. Where the superficial and deep retinacula cutis insert into the

superficial fascia, they typically often show a large area of attachment, similar to a fan or a cone. In these areas the superficial fascia appears thicker. It is probable that the arrangement of these septa have contributed to the great variability in the fascial thickness values reported in the literature.

The superficial fascia and the retinacula cutis form a three-dimensional network between the fat lobules of the hypodermis, and this network provides a dynamic anchor of the skin to underlying tissues. This arrangement permits a flexible and yet resistant mechanism of transmission of mechanical loads from multidirectional forces. According to Li and Ahn (2011) the

23

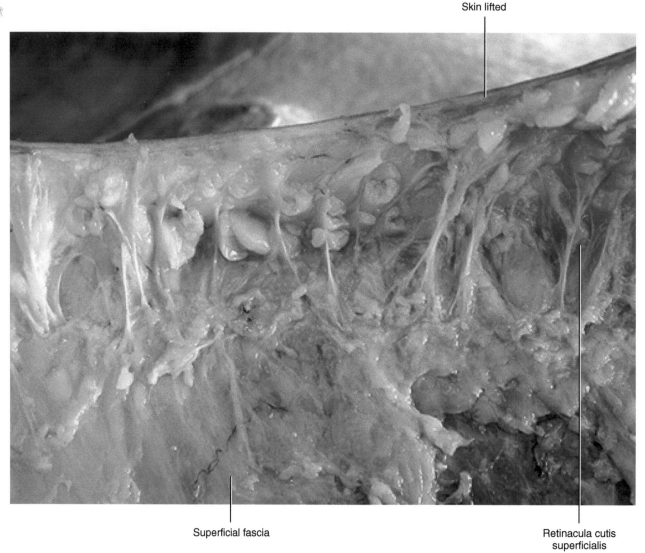

Skin lifted

Superficial fascia

Retinacula cutis
superficialis

FIGURE 2.4 The skin of the abdomen has been cut and lifted. In this way the superficial retinacula cutis are stretched to provide greater visual definition.

superficial and deep retinacula cutis and superficial fascia (which they collectively name as 'subcutaneous fascial bands') could be considered as structural bridges that mechanically link the skin, subcutaneous layer and deeper muscle layer. Their quantity and morphological characteristics vary according to the region of the body. For example, the area occupied by the retinacula cutis, with respect to the subcutaneous tissue, is thicker in the thigh and calf than in the arm. These areas are unrelated to hypodermis thickness. The thigh has the highest average number of retinacula cutis, while the greatest average retinacula cutis thickness is seen in the calf. Regional variations determine the differences in mobility of the skin with respect to underlying tissues and may reflect the composite mechanical forces experienced by the body part. For example, in the eyelids, penis and scrotum the adipose tissue and the retinacula cutis are absent, and so the skin shows an increased mobility with respect to the underlying planes. Other examples are the palm of the hand and

the plantar surface of the foot where the DAT is absent. In these areas, the superficial fascia adheres to the deep fascia, and in SAT the skin ligaments are very thick and densely packed, strongly connecting the skin with the underlying planes.

Superficial Adipose Tissue

The SAT is composed of large fat lobules encased between fibrous septa (Fig. 2.5). The fat lobules are almost circular and the septa (retinacula cutis superficialis or skin ligaments) are well defined and generally orientated perpendicular to the surface, anchoring the dermis to the deeper planes. The fat lobules are organized in single or multiple layers: depending on the fat content and the thickness of the SAT in the subject (Fig. 2.6).

The thickness of the SAT is quite uniform throughout the trunk and generally shows less variation by region than the DAT. In the extremities, the SAT is thicker in

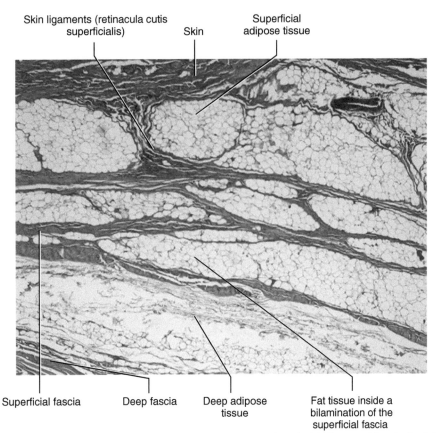

Skin ligaments (retinacula cutis superficialis)   Skin   Superficial adipose tissue

Superficial fascia   Deep fascia   Deep adipose tissue   Fat tissue inside a bilamination of the superficial fascia

FIGURE 2.5 Histology of the subcutaneous tissue of the thigh. The skin ligaments and the fat lobules are evident in the SAT, while in the DAT the loose connective tissue is prevalent. The superficial fascia (SF) is formed by multiple layers of fibrous tissue and fat tissue. These sublayers are well defined in a histological study, while in macroscopic studies the superficial fascia appears as a unique layer.

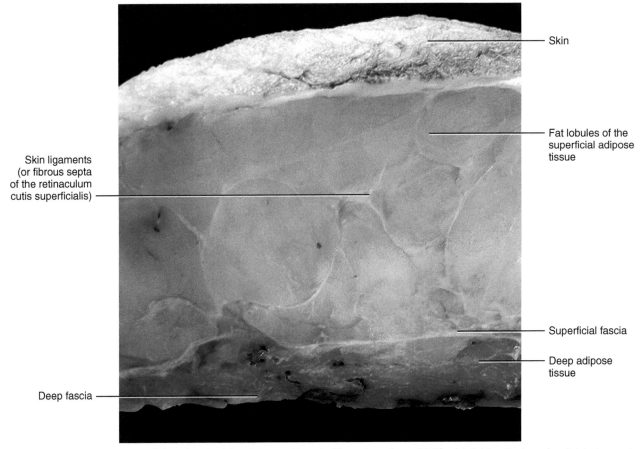

Skin

Fat lobules of the superficial adipose tissue

Skin ligaments (or fibrous septa of the retinaculum cutis superficialis)

Superficial fascia

Deep adipose tissue

Deep fascia

FIGURE 2.6 Macroscopic aspect of the subcutis of the abdomen. Note the fibrous layer (superficial fascia) dividing the hypodermis into two parts: the SAT and the DAT.

the lower limbs than in the upper limbs. The SAT in the palm of the hand and the plantar region of the foot is thin and contains more and stronger vertical retinacula cutis. Therefore, the skin in these areas adheres strongly to the deeper planes. In the dorsum of the hand, a different fascial anatomy permits more movement of the skin with respect to the underlying planes because the superficial retinacula cutis is thin.

The SAT thickness varies by subject. In obese subjects, the SAT of the trunk has a mean thickness of 17.2 mm (range 6–35 mm), and in normal-weight subjects the mean thickness is 3.7 mm (range 1–10 mm). In obese subjects, the SAT thickness increases significantly and progressively from T10 to the femoral head, and in slim subjects the SAT is uniform. The thickness of the retinacula cutis superficialis also changes by region of the body and subject. For example, in the trunk the retinacula cutis superficialis is thicker and stronger in the back, giving the SAT of the dorsum a greater resistance compared to the SAT of the abdomen. Sterzi (1910) found that the skin ligaments of a labourer's hand presented a double or triple thickness compared to the septa of a sedentary subject's hand. Sterzi also describes sexual differences in the SAT: females have more fat cells in the SAT, the skin ligaments are thinner and the fat lobules are arranged in multiple layers. These features probably explain why cellulite (herniation of subcutaneous fat within fibrous connective tissue that manifests topographically as skin dimpling and nodularity) is more frequent in females. In the elderly, the fat lobules of the SAT are less swollen and the retinacula are less vertical, and thereby connect the skin to the superficial fascia with decreased strength. Both of these elements are responsible for flaccidity of the superficial tissue with increased age.

The secretory portion of the sweat glands, hair follicles and Pacini's corpuscles are in the SAT. Usually these structures are near the retinacula cutis superficialis (skin ligaments) that offer protection from stretching and mechanical loads.

Superficial Fascia (Fascia Superficialis)

The superficial fascia is a fibrous layer of connective tissue, formed by loosely packed interwoven collagen fibres mixed with abundant elastic fibres (Fig. 2.7). It is homologous with the cutaneous muscle layer (panniculus carnosus) found in many lower mammals, where a thin sheet of striated muscle could be found within or just beneath the superficial fascia, and serving to produce local movement of the skin. For example, a grazing animal may twitch the panniculus carnosus to frustrate the attempts of a bird to perch on its back. This muscular layer is rare in humans and when found assumes a precise muscular structural arrangement primarily in the neck (platysma muscle) (Fig. 2.8), in

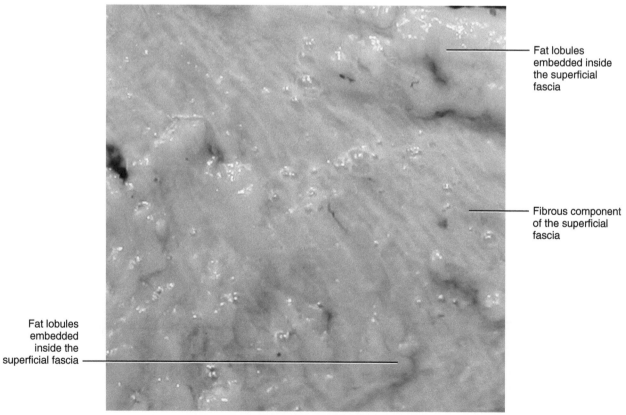

Fat lobules embedded inside the superficial fascia

Fibrous component of the superficial fascia

Fat lobules embedded inside the superficial fascia

FIGURE 2.7 Macroscopic aspect of the superficial fascia of the back. The fibrous component (white) and the fat lobules intermingle in the superficial fascia.

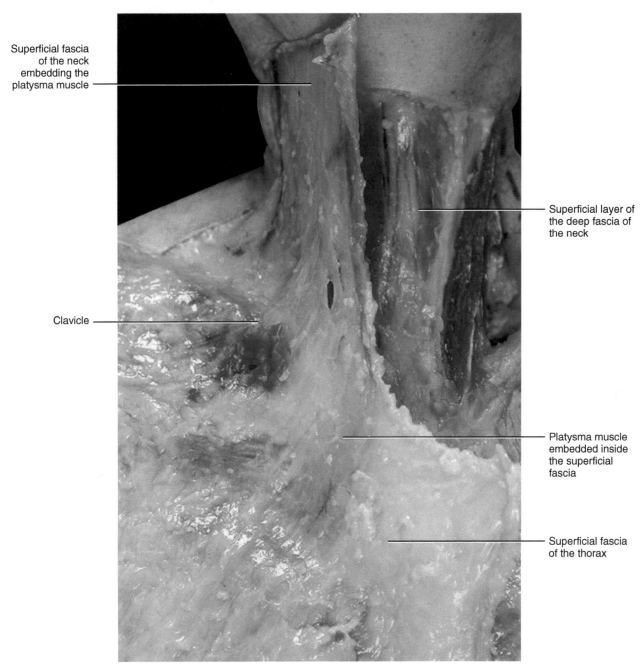

Superficial fascia of the neck embedding the platysma muscle

Clavicle

Superficial layer of the deep fascia of the neck

Platysma muscle embedded inside the superficial fascia

Superficial fascia of the thorax

FIGURE 2.8 Platysma muscle inside the superficial fascia. Note that the superficial fascia of the neck continues into the superficial fascia of the thorax. Also the platysma muscle does not stop at the neck, but continues into the thorax.

the face (the SMAS or superficial muscular aponeurotic system), in the anal region (external anal sphincter), and in the scrotum (the dartos muscle). Isolated muscle fibres can be found in all superficial fasciae.

The superficial fascia is present throughout the body, and according to Abu-Hijleh et al (2006) its arrangement and thickness vary according to body region, body surface, and gender. In the abdomen, the superficial fascia has a mean thickness of 847.4 ± 295 μm and increases in a proximocaudal direction, with a mean value of 551 μm in the epigastrium and 1045 μm in the hypogastrium (Lancerotto et al 2011). It is thicker

in the lower than in the upper extremities and on the posterior rather than the anterior aspect of the body. Abu-Hijleh et al (2006) found that the mean thickness of the superficial fascia on the dorsal aspect of the foot, the anterior aspect of the thigh and periphery of the breast is significantly higher in females than in males. On the other hand, the mean thickness of the superficial fascia on the dorsal aspect of the hand and arm and on the anterior aspect of the leg is significantly higher in males than in females. In the obese, the superficial fascia is usually stuffed with fat cells and shows a thickness increase of 50%. Sterzi (1910)

27

describes the superficial fascia as thicker and more resistant in sturdy individuals with well-developed muscles. In humans, the superficial fascia becomes very thin at the distal ends of the limbs, and it is impossible to separate it out as a distinct fibrous layer; however, it is always possible to distinguish between the SAT and DAT. In mammals, like the rabbit for example, the panniculus carnosus is absent in the distal portion of the limbs, and only a thin fibrous layer continues just until the carpus and tarsus. This explains why it is so easy to skin these animals, except for the paws, tail, ears and around the muzzle.

Histologically, the superficial fascia is formed by a net of collagen and elastic fibres arranged irregularly (Fig. 2.9). Macroscopically, the superficial fascia appears and can be isolated as a well-defined membrane, but microscopically its structure is better described as multilamellar, or like a tightly packed honeycomb. The various sublayers have a mean thickness of 66.6 ± 18.6 µm and many points of interconnection between the sublayers can be distinguished. Irregular islands of fat cells (mean thickness 83.87 ± 72.3 µm) may be deposited between sublayers of collagen fibres.

In the young, the superficial fascia is very elastic permitting the subcutis to adapt to stress in all directions and then spring back to its original state. With age, the superficial fascia and retinacula cutis lose their elasticity. This could explain the eventual ptosis of the skin, formation of wrinkles and the general hypotonicity of the subcutis.

On bony prominences and at some ligamentous folds, the superficial fascia adheres to the deep fascia. Inside the superficial fascia, many nerve fibres are observed and in some regions the superficial fascia splits, forming special compartments. This occurs particularly around major subcutaneous veins (Caggiati 1999) and lymphatic vessels. Fibrous septa extend out from the tunica externa of the vessel walls to the superficial fascia.

Functionally, the superficial fascia plays a role in the integrity of the skin and supports subcutaneous structures, particularly the veins, ensuring their patency. The superficial fascia together with the retinacula cutis support and help organize the position of fat tissue. Finally, the superficial fascia separates the skin from the musculoskeletal system allowing normal sliding of the muscles and skin upon each other.

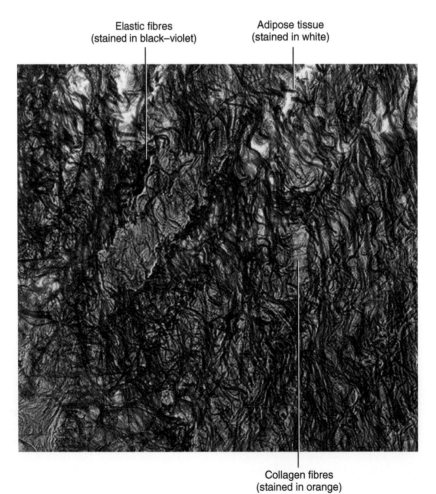

Elastic fibres
(stained in black–violet)

Adipose tissue
(stained in white)

Collagen fibres
(stained in orange)

FIGURE 2.9 Histology of the superficial fascia of the abdomen, van Gieson's stain, to highlight the elastic fibres (stained in black–violet). Enlargement 200×. Note the richness in elastic fibres. The superficial fascia could be defined as a very elastic tissue.

Deep Adipose Tissue

By comparison with the SAT, the DAT is generally formed by relatively loose, less organized and more obliquely arranged fibrous septa (retinaculum cutis profundus) (Fig. 2.10). The fat lobules are more oval and have a tendency towards displacement (Fig. 2.11). The elastic properties of DAT are good. These elements may explain how the superficial fascia slides over the deep fascia. According to Markman and Barton (1987), the DAT varies significantly in thickness and fat content across different regions of the body. Generally, the DAT tends to be thinner in the anterior region of the trunk and presents the maximum thickness posterolaterally at the level of the flanks, where a 'fat accumulation pouch' is present. In some regions, such as in the flank, the DAT can contain even more adipose tissue than the SAT. Under the mimetic muscles, only loose connective tissue containing very few adipocytes is present. DAT thickness varies according to the subject. In the obese subject, DAT of the trunk has a mean thickness of 18.5 mm (range 10–35 mm), and in normal-weight subjects it is 3.14 mm (range 0.5–8 mm). In both the slim and obese, DAT thickness increases substantially from T10 to the femoral head.

In some regions the DAT is either absent or very thin, while the septa of the retinaculum cutis profondus become thicker. Thus the superficial fascia anchors to the deep fascia. These points of adhesion are constant and can be mapped. The adhesions may be organized in two ways to form horizontal and vertical lines. These lines of adhesions are similar to the belts described by Ida Rolf (Schultz and Feitis, 1996). Mapping all the adhesions in the body reveals well-defined compartments inside deep adipose tissue referred to as 'quadrants'. These quadrants seem to correspond to the

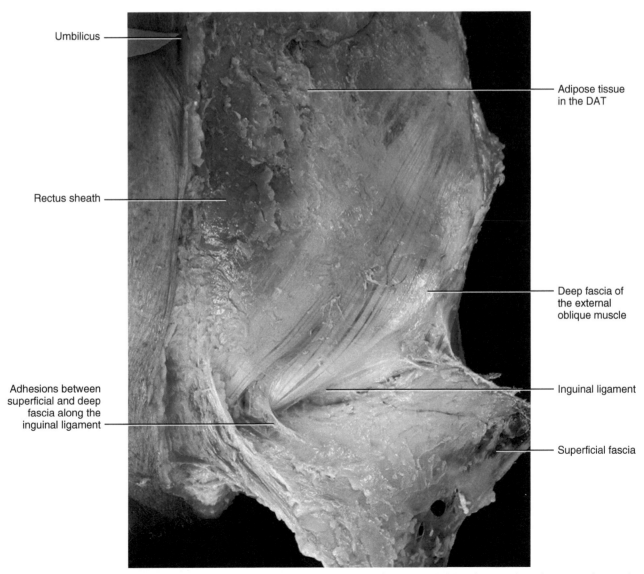

Umbilicus

Rectus sheath

Adhesions between superficial and deep fascia along the inguinal ligament

Adipose tissue in the DAT

Deep fascia of the external oblique muscle

Inguinal ligament

Superficial fascia

FIGURE 2.10 Dissection of the abdominal region. The superficial fascia was detached from the underlying planes to show the DAT. In the anterior region of the abdomen the DAT is scarce and with fewer and thinner retinacula cutis. This permits a perfect plane of gliding between the superficial and deep fasciae.

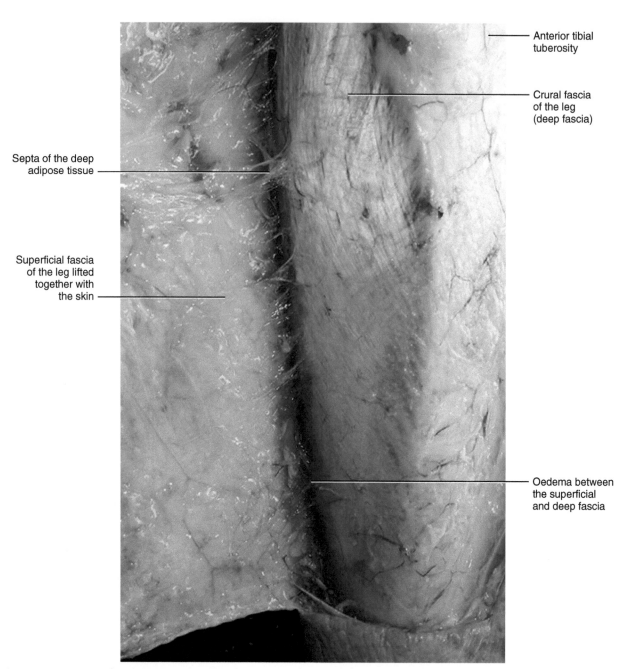

Anterior tibial
tuberosity

Crural fascia
of the leg
(deep fascia)

Septa of the deep
adipose tissue

Superficial fascia
of the leg lifted
together with
the skin

Oedema between
the superficial
and deep fascia

FIGURE 2.11 Dissection of the leg to show the septa of the retinacula cutis profundus. In this subject, an oedema is evident. It involves, above all, the superficial fascia and the DAT, causing their fibrosis.

distribution of the superficial vessels and nerves and also to lymphatic drainage. This suggests a precise organization of the subcutis that defines the distribution of the vessels and nerves. Both subcutaneous bursae and lymph glands are found in the DAT.

Transverse and Longitudinal Lines of Adhesions

In some areas of the human body the SAT and DAT are absent. In these areas adhesion between the superficial and deep fascia (Fig. 2.12), and sometimes also between skin and superficial fascia, occurs. Bichat (1799) demonstrated that when subcutaneous emphysema

is created, air can not move across the midline of the body due to these adhesions that create specific subcutaneous compartments. These points of adhesion are especially evident in obese people because in areas where there is no SAT or DAT there is no accumulation of fatty tissue. In the obese subjects, the bony processes at the level of the spine, iliac crests, wrists and ankles are always easily palpable due to the lack of fat in these areas. The points of adhesion among the different subcutaneous planes can be mapped and are always present in the same locations in all humans. There are adhesions in longitudinal and transverse planes. Considering all the adhesion lines of the body, the subcutaneous tissue could be divided into quadrants

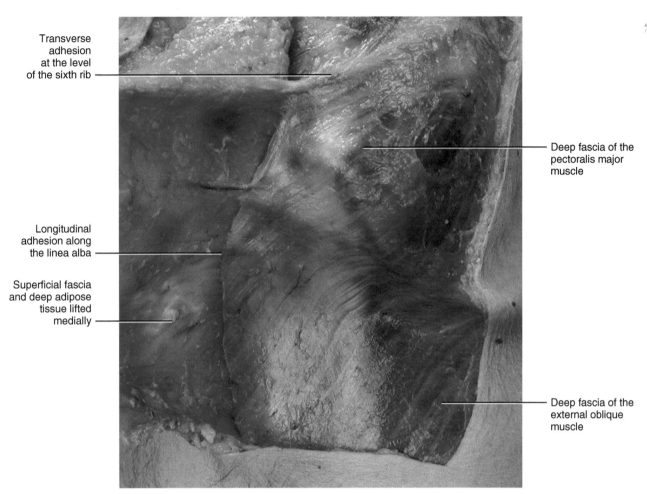

Transverse adhesion at the level of the sixth rib

Longitudinal adhesion along the linea alba

Superficial fascia and deep adipose tissue lifted medially

Deep fascia of the pectoralis major muscle

Deep fascia of the external oblique muscle

FIGURE 2.12 Dissection of the anterior region of the trunk. The superficial fascia was detached from the underlying planes together with the DAT. Along the mid-line a strong adhesion between superficial and deep fascia is present called the abdominal linea alba. In this dissection a transverse adhesion is seen at the sixth rib.

CLINICAL PEARL 2.1 LIPOSUCTION RELATED TO THE ANATOMY OF SUBCUTANEOUS FAT

Understanding the topographic anatomy of the subcutaneous layers may help explain body contour deformities and provide the anatomical basis for surgical correction. According to Markman and Barton (1987), the thickness of the SAT in each individual is relatively constant throughout the body. The deep adipose tissue, however, varies significantly according to the anatomical region. They suggested that the thickness of the SAT correlates with the 'pinch test' that is commonly used to clinically gauge the depth of cannula insertion when performing liposuction. According to Chopra et al (2011), the surgeon should stay beneath the superficial fascia to avoid postoperative skin dimpling, waviness, over

resection and other irregularities in suction lipolysis. Suction-assisted body contouring should aim to remove the deep layer of subcutaneous tissue without disturbing the SAT and superficial fascia.

According to Joseph and Remus (2009) the preservation of superficial fascia is important in abdominoplasty of the lower abdomen. After resection of the soft tissue, tension is placed on the superficial fascia that allows the skin to be closed with relatively little tension and without vascular compromise. The preservation of the superficial fascia could be seen as a way of lowering complications associated with conventional abdominoplasty.

(Fig. 2.13). These quadrants organize the subcutaneous tissue and probably define the distribution of the superficial vessels, nerves, and lymphatic drainage.

Longitudinal Adhesions

The main longitudinal adhesions are along the midline in the front and in the back of the trunk. The most

important and well-known line of fusion is the linea alba of the abdomen where the three layers of the deep fascia and the superficial fascia fuse. Along this line, the skin adheres to the deeper planes creating a complete division between the two sides. A similar line of fusion is the cervical linea alba found in the neck and caudal to the hyoid bone. In the neck, however,

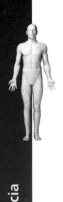

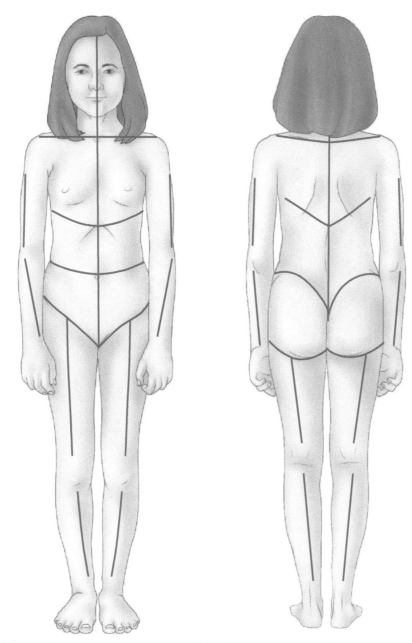

FIGURE 2.13 Diagram of the main lines of adhesion between superficial and deep fascia. If we consider all these adhesions, it is evident that they divide the subcutis into various quadrants. The longitudinal lines of adhesions are along the sternum and linea alba, spinous processes, middle line of the anterior and posterior region of the thigh, tibial crest, middle line of the posterior region of the leg, and intermuscular septa of the upper limbs. The transverse lines of adhesions are along the angle of the mandible, the occipital tuberosities, at the level of the sixth rib, over the inguinal ligament, along the inferior border of the trapezius muscle, along the iliac crest, along the inferior border of the gluteus maximus muscle and around all the joints of the upper and lower limbs.

this connection is not as strong as in the abdomen and the superficial fascia can be detached from the deep fascia by careful dissection. The cervical and abdominal linea alba are joined in the thorax by another line of adhesion, less evident, over the sternum. The pectoral fascia, over the sternum, partially adheres to the periosteum and to the superficial fascia.

Similar longitudinal adhesion can be traced in the back along the spine. Over the spine, the deep fascia inserts along the spine via many strong septa, except caudally to L4, where the thoracolumbar fascia crosses the midline connecting the two sides. Along the spine, the DAT is absent so the superficial fascia adheres to the deep fascia. Strong retinacula cutis in the SAT connects the skin to the deeper planes. In the thoracic area, these septa are numerous and separated by less than a millimeter from one another; in the lumbar region these septa are less numerous. In the parascapular region, the superficial fascia crosses the midline to connect the two sides.

In the skull, the galea capitis (superficial fascia) adheres to the epicranial fascia (deep fascia) along the midline. Anteriorly, this adhesion continues along the nose, the nasolabial sulcus and the mental protuberance. Posteriorly, the adhesion continues along the nuchal ligament. In the other parts of the head, the two fascial layers are separated by loose connective tissue.

The longitudinal adhesions are also present along the limbs. There is an adhesion in the thigh along the course of the lateral femoral cutaneous nerve. This nerve runs along a tract through a fibroadipose compartment formed by the fusion of the superficial and deep fascia. Other longitudinal adhesions in the lower limbs are along the tibial crest and over the septum between the two heads of the gastrocnemius muscle. The short saphenous vein runs inside the superficial fascia between the two heads of this muscle, but here the superficial fascia is directly connected to the deep fascia due to the absence of DAT. A specific compartment for the short saphenous vein is created between the two fascial layers. Along this line of adhesion in the calf, the deep fascia is connected to the deeper planes by an intermuscular septum. This prevents displacement of the short saphenous vein.

In the plantar region of the foot and in the palm of the hand, the plantar and palmar aponeurosis are formed by the fusion of the superficial with the deep fasciae, as the DAT is completely absent. In addition, the SAT is scarce and its retinaculum cutis is short, strong and contains vertical septa, which firmly connect the skin to the deeper planes.

Transverse Adhesions

The transverse adhesions are located around all the joints especially in the flexor sections. The DAT is absent and the deep and superficial fasciae adhere to each other. The deep fascia always adheres (completely or partially) to the joint capsule and bony prominences. The SAT is usually thin around the joints (Fig. 2.14), and so the skin is strongly anchored to the deeper planes. This organization of the subcutis permits the skin to follow the joint movement without interference. In the extension surface of the joints, a subcutaneous bursa is often present between the superficial and deep fasciae to facilitate gliding.

Additional transverse adhesions are located over the occipital protuberances, in front of the tragus of the ears, along the inferior border of the trapezius muscles, along the sixth ribs, along the iliac crests, over the inguinal ligaments (Fig. 2.15), and along the inferior border of the gluteus maximus muscles (Fig. 2.16).

Subcutaneous Vessels

If we consider skin and subcutis vascularization, it is possible to recognize specific vascular territories called angiosomes, which are supplied by a source artery and its accompanying vein(s). The connective tissue framework of the subcutis has developed an intimate relationship with the vascular system of the body. This framework furnishes mechanical support and protection for the vessels.

Arteries

The subcutis contains arteries of both small and medium calibre. Most commonly, the arteries cross the hypodermis in two ways: perpendicularly and longitudinally. The perpendicular course crosses the fascial layers and the subcutis to reach the skin (perforantes arteries) (Fig. 2.17). In the longitudinal course (long arteries), they cross the subcutis with a very oblique course following the superficial fascia for extensive lengths. In the subcutis, vessels follow the retinacula to go from the deeper planes to the skin. The retinacula provide protection to these vessels and prevent vessel displacement when the skin is tractioned. Around the retinacula the vessels have a tortuous route with many curves. Thus, when the skin is lifted the vessels can stretch out without damage. The greater elasticity of the retinacula cutis is thus able to substitute for the lesser elasticity of the vessels. Li and Ahn (2011) propose that the cohesive network of vessels and retinacula cutis may indirectly mediate blood flow.

The long arteries are usually connected by long anastomoses, which form tidy arches in the DAT of the subcutis. From these oblique arteries all the capillaries of the fat lobules originate. Schaverien et al (2009) have demonstrated that the subcutaneous tissue is arranged in anatomical units or compartments, and each anatomical compartment is associated with an identifiable artery and vein. We hypothesize that these compartments could correspond to the quadrants, and that the specific organization of the superficial fascia and retinacula cutis defines the subcutaneous compartments and the vessel distribution.

All the subcutaneous arteries participate in the formation of two subcutaneous plexuses: the subpapillary plexus, just under the papillary dermis, and the deep plexus, inside the superficial fascia (Fig. 2.18). The two plexuses freely communicate. Only one-fifth of the capillaries are necessary for skin vascularization while all the others function for thermoregulation. The arteries of the deep plexus present many arteriovenous links that provide shunts that control blood flow to the skin and consequently regulate the body temperature. The dilating and narrowing of the subcutaneous arteries determines the skin temperature and colour in light-skinned races. Marked pallor of the skin, which is seen in acute shock, results from vasoconstriction of the arterial plexus in the hypodermis. It can be hypothesized that a fibrotic superficial fascia could choke the arteries inside it, thereby causing a change in skin colour or even chronic ischaemia of the skin. According to Distler et al (2007), chronic ischaemia can increase the fibrosis of the subcutis, creating a vicious circle. If the arteriovenous shunts become deficient, an alteration of thermoregulation may occur, resulting in sensations of excessively hot or cold skin.

Text continued on p. 38

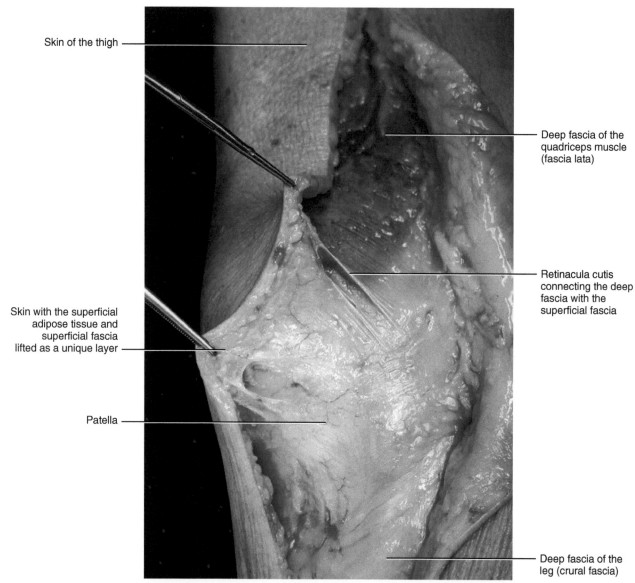

Skin of the thigh

Deep fascia of the quadriceps muscle (fascia lata)

Retinacula cutis connecting the deep fascia with the superficial fascia

Skin with the superficial adipose tissue and superficial fascia lifted as a unique layer

Patella

Deep fascia of the leg (crural fascia)

FIGURE 2.14 Dissection of the anterior region of the knee. The skin and the subcutaneous tissue were detached from the deeper layers. The separation is easy in the thigh and in the leg, where the DAT forms a plane of gliding between the superficial and deep fasciae, but it is impossible over the knee, where strong retinacula cutis connect the two fasciae. These retinacula also define the anterior knee bursa.

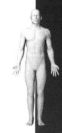

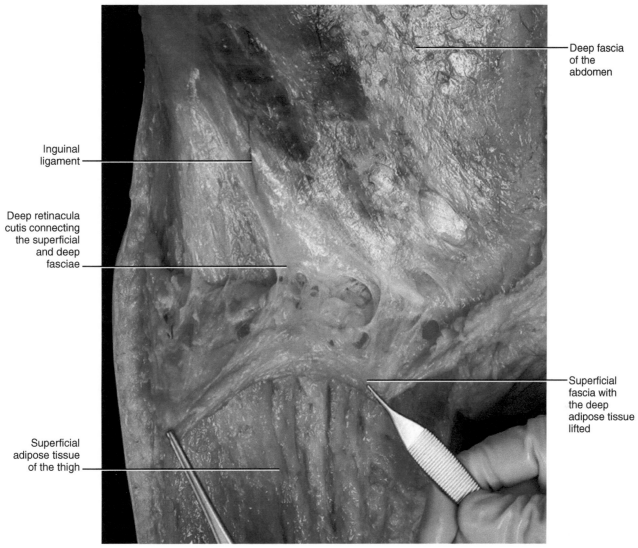

Deep fascia of the abdomen

Inguinal ligament

Deep retinacula cutis connecting the superficial and deep fasciae

Superficial fascia with the deep adipose tissue lifted

Superficial adipose tissue of the thigh

FIGURE 2.15 Inguinal region. Transverse adhesion of the superficial fascia to the deep fascia. In this region the DAT disappears and the septa of the retinaculum cutis profondus become thick, vertical, short and strong. This adhesion divides the subcutaneous tissue of the abdomen from that of the thigh.

Deep fascia of the gluteus maximus muscle

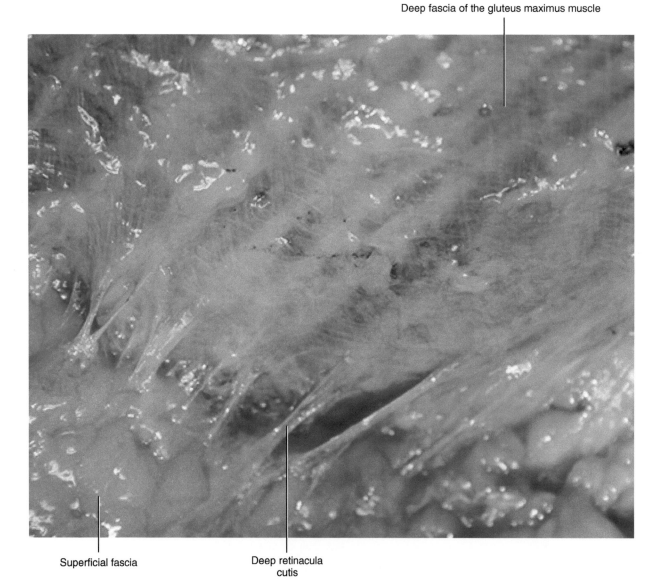

Superficial fascia

Deep retinacula cutis

FIGURE 2.16 Dissection of the gluteal region. Transverse adhesions between the superficial and deep fascia at the gluteal fold. At this level, the skin adheres to the deeper planes. As the skin is stretched, the tension is transmitted to the underlying muscles, thanks to the adhesion of the superficial fascia with the underlying planes.

Superficial
adipose tissue

Superficial fascia

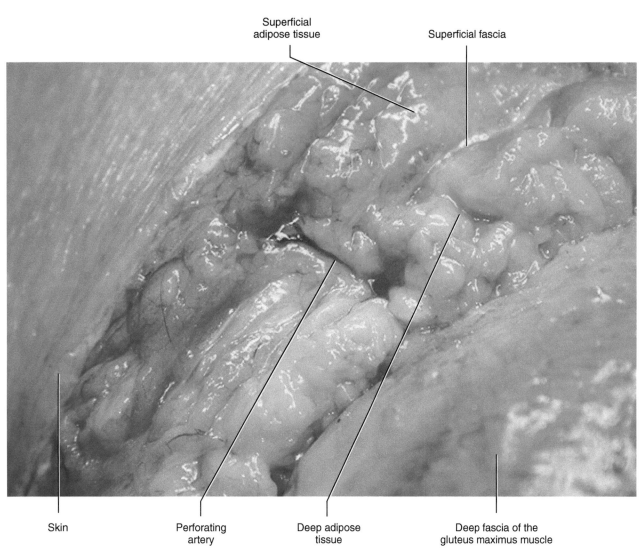

Skin

Perforating
artery

Deep adipose
tissue

Deep fascia of the
gluteus maximus muscle

FIGURE 2.17 Perforating vessel in the subcutis of the gluteal region.

Small artery   Superficial fascia

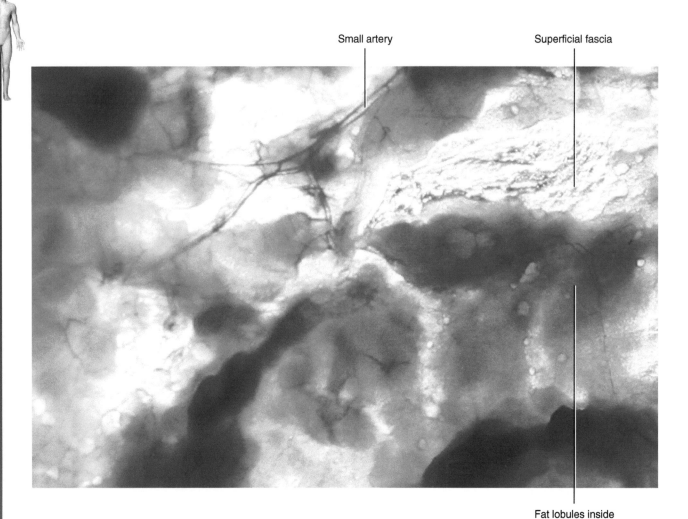

Fat lobules inside
the superficial fascia

FIGURE 2.18 The superficial fascia was isolated and a light was placed behind it to show the small artery inside this fascia.

Veins

The veins are generally classified by their relationship to the deep fascia based on whether they are located near the surface or in the deeper areas of the deep fascia. The perforating veins connect these two areas crossing the deep fascia in an almost perpendicular direction. Communicating veins connect veins within the same system (i.e. deep to deep, superficial to superficial). The superficial veins drain the cutaneous microcirculation and the deep veins drain the muscles. The superficial veins are arranged in two plexuses similar to the superficial arteries.

The superficial venous system includes the reticular veins and the larger epifascial[1] veins (such as the saphenous veins and the cephalic veins). The reticular veins form a network of veins in the SAT parallel to the

---

[1]The medical dictionary refers to 'epifascial' as on the surface of the fascia, meaning the deep fascia. Indeed these veins are superficial with respect to the deep fascia, but embedded in the superficial fascia.

skin surface (Figs 2.19 and 2.20). Caggiati (1999) asserts that the lack of any fascial support around these veins could be a contributing cause of varicose veins, which most frequently occur above the level of the superficial fascia.

The larger superficial veins flow inside the superficial fascia. Indeed the superficial fascia splits into two sublayers to envelop these veins. From their adventitia thin ligaments originate, connecting the walls of these veins to the superficial fascia. It is these connections that permit the walls of the superficial veins to remain open.

The perforating veins are commonly located in the intramuscular septa. They vary in number and dimension; Thomson (1979) found an average number of 64 in the lower limb. The perforating veins have valves that direct the flow from the superficial to the deep veins.

Lymphatic Vessels

Mascagni (1755–1815) was the first to describe the lymphatic vessels in the subcutaneous adipose tissue. Hoggan in 1884 affirmed that in humans two

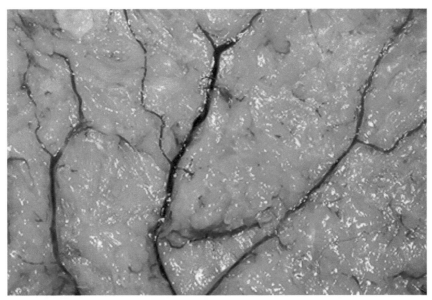

FIGURE 2.19 Dissection of the subcutis of the abdomen. The vessels (paraumbilical veins) were injected with resin to better show their flow. These veins are inside the superficial fascia so that their position is maintained during the movement of the trunk.

types of superficial lymphatic vessels are present: the dermal vessels and hypodermal vessels. A lymphatic plexus lies just under the dermis and from it small vessels originate. Lymphatic vessels cross the subcutaneous tissue along the retinacula cutis superficialis. Often these vessels are completely enveloped by the fibrous septa that provide good support to their very thin walls. Along their course they receive the small lymphatic vessels from the adipose lobules and, at the level of the superficial fascia, an anastomotic web[2] is formed among all these vessels. They then join the large lymphatic vessels localized in the deep adipose tissue.

All of the superficial lymph glands are in the DAT (Fig. 2.21). Generally they are separated from the superficial and deep fascia by loose connective tissue. The superficial lymph glands could be palpated as soft and mobile and are usually less than 1 cm in size. During inflammation or cancer infiltration they adhere to the surrounding tissues and become fixed.

Subcutaneous Nerves

In the subcutaneous tissue, the nerves are usually very thin and follow the retinacula cutis to reach the skin. Just under the dermis they form a nerve plexus, in the same manner as the subdermal vascular plexus of Spalteholz (1893) and the subdermal lymphatic plexus of Unna (1908).

As the nerves penetrate more deeply into the tissue, the more mobile superficial fascia provides a pathway for long tracts of larger nerves and protects the larger nerves from excessive stretching (Figs 2.22 and 2.23). The nerves are also protected from excessive movement because they usually cross the various fascial planes in an oblique direction. Inside the SAT and the superficial fascia some Ruffini's and Pacini's corpuscles are present. Ruffini's capsules are embedded in the fascial tissue allowing them to perceive the stretching of the superficial fascia. Pacini's corpuscles are sensitive

---

[2]The presence of another lymphatic plexus in the subcutis was described for the first time by Bartels in 1909 and then confirmed by Sterzi in 1910.

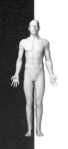

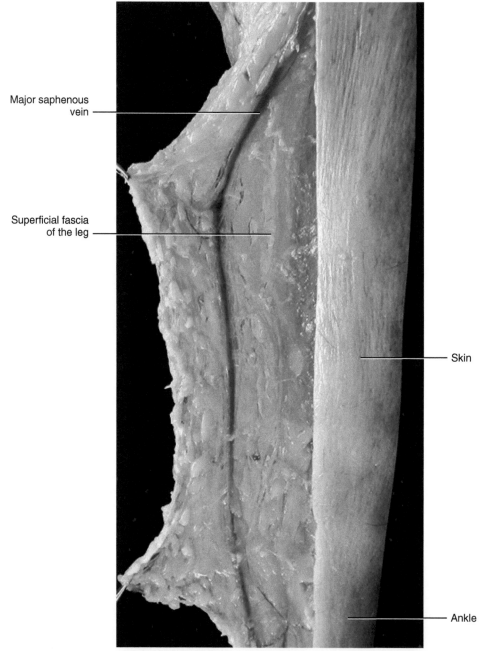

Major saphenous
vein

Superficial fascia
of the leg

Skin

Ankle

FIGURE 2.20 Saphenous vein inside the superficial fascia of the leg. The superficial fascia of the leg was isolated from the SAT and DAT and lifted. The saphenous vein was injected with resin to keep the walls open and thus to show more clearly the relationship of the vein to the superficial fascia. The specific relationship of the adventitia of the vein and the collagen fibres of the superficial fascia maintains the opening of the lumen of the vessel.

CLINICAL PEARL 2.3 LYMPHOEDEMA

Hauck (1992) demonstrated the existence of a 'low-resistance pathway' along the connective tissue fibres for the transinterstitial fluid movement from the capillaries to the lymphatic vessels. We suggest that the disposition of the collagen and elastic fibres inside the superficial fascia could guide the lymphatic flux in the correct direction. If superficial fascia is altered, then lymphatic drainage will be compromised.

In clinical practice the superficial fascia and DAT are often involved in lymphoedema. According to Tassenoy et al (2009), in the case of lymphoedema the DAT has a honeycomb picture on MRI and corresponds to fluid bound to fibrotic tissue. In particular, the retinaculum cutis profondus septa increase in thickness and the outer boundary of the fat cells significantly increases (P <0.05) with fluid noted near the muscle fascia. Marotel et al (1998), using computerized tomography (CT) scanning in patients with lymphoedema, found the following in order of frequency: skin thickening, an increase of the subcutaneous tissue area, muscular fascia thickening, fat infiltration, lines parallel and perpendicular to the skin (corresponding to fibrous retinacula cutis), and oedematous areas along deep fascia.

to compression and the SAT is a highly modifiable tissue. Their position relative to the skin may help these corpuscles to discriminate between light and heavy pressures. The more superficial Pacini's corpuscles may perceive the light pressure and the deeper corpuscles the heavy pressure. The superficial fascia and SAT have to be considered together with the skin for their involvement in exteroception.

In the DAT very few nerve receptors are present. We suggest that the DAT may be considered the watershed between the exteroceptive system (formed by skin, superficial adipose tissue and superficial fascia) and the proprioceptive system (placed in the muscles and deep fasciae). Where the DAT disappears and the superficial and deep fasciae fuse (as in the palm of the hand and in the plantar part of the foot), the exteroceptive and proprioceptive systems are combined. This facilitates the perception of form, volume, surfaces of various objects and consequent movement, guaranteeing the adaptation of the foot and hand to variable contact surfaces. In scars, where pathological fibrous tissue results in fusion between skin, superficial and deep fasciae, the stretching of the deep fascia could affect also the superficial fascia, and vice versa. In this type of situation even normal muscular contraction or skin stretching could result in overstimulation of the exteroceptive and proprioceptive receptors.

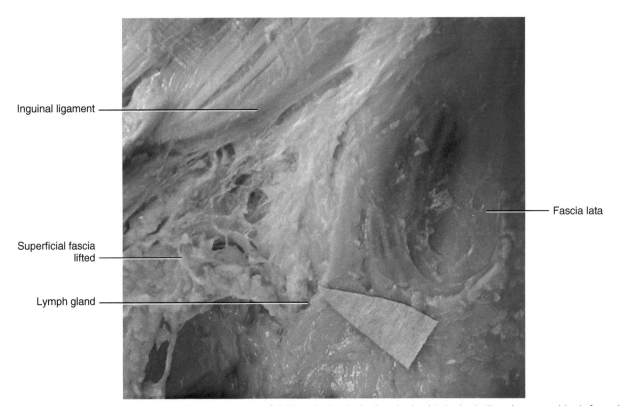

FIGURE 2.21 Dissection of the left inguinal region and superficial lymph gland. The lymph gland is in the DAT, and separated both from the superficial fascia and deep fascia.

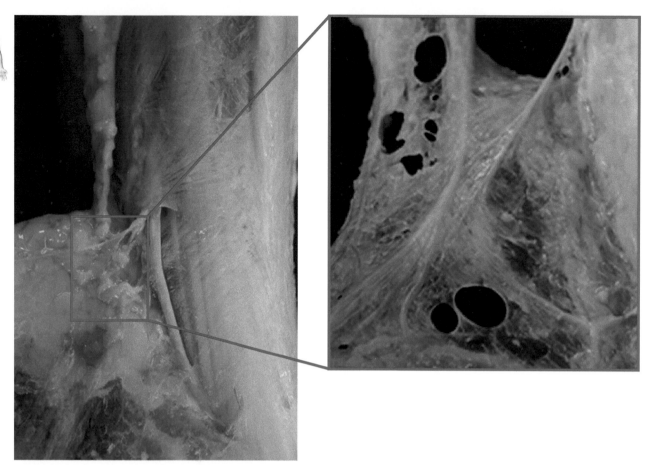

FIGURE 2.22 Dissection of the lateral region of the ankle and enlargement of the superficial fascia to show the superficial peroneal nerve. To become superficial this nerve has to cross the deep fascia and then run along a tract into the superficial fascia where it divides into many branches. A frequent site of compression of this nerve is at the level of the hole in the deep fascia, but sometimes a fibrotic superficial fascia can alter the nerve transmission.

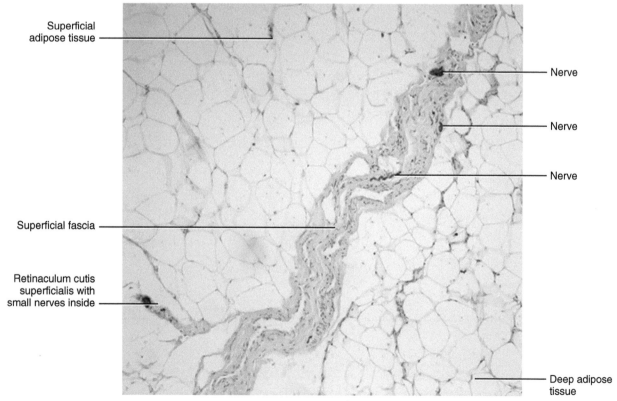

Superficial adipose tissue

Nerve

Nerve

Nerve

Superficial fascia

Retinaculum cutis superficialis with small nerves inside

Deep adipose tissue

FIGURE 2.23 Small nerves inside the superficial fascia of the thigh. Anti-S100 immunohistochemical stain allows only visibility of the myelinated fibres.

Subcutaneous Bursa

The subcutaneous bursae are usually in the deep adipose tissue. They are formed by the fusion of the superficial and deep fasciae (Fig. 2.24) which forms a virtual space. Some bursae are found inside the superficial fascia or between the skin and the superficial

fascia. The function of a bursa is to facilitate movement and reduce friction between moving parts. Canoso et al (1983) demonstrated that a true synovial lining is not recognizable in the subcutaneous bursa. Therefore, subcutaneous bursa could be considered as a fascial specialization instead of a specific anatomical entity. The synovial fluid is probably produced by the fasciacytes, which are commonly present inside fasciae (see Chapter 3) and produce hyaluronan (HA). In areas subjected to friction, fasciacytes probably become more organized and produce more HA to facilitate gliding between the various fascial layers.

Development of the Superficial Fascia

According to Sterzi (1910), a fetus has a uniform layer of connective tissue present under the skin. In the fifth fetal month, little lobules of adipose tissue appear and in the middle, a fibrous layer rich in cells divides the subcutis into two layers. In the sixth fetal month, the superficial fascia is clearly evident, and at eight months

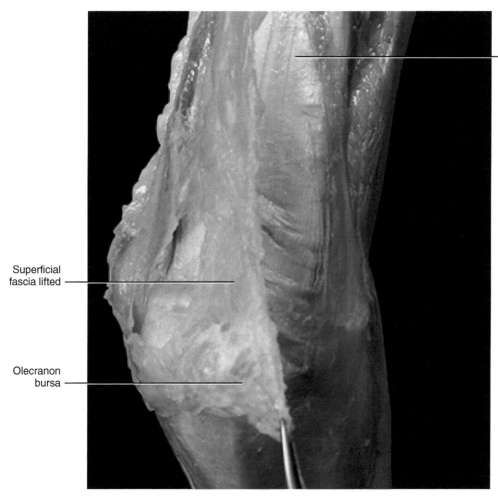

Deep fascia of the triceps brachii muscle

Superficial fascia lifted

Olecranon bursa

FIGURE 2.24 Dissection of the elbow. The olecranon bursa was injected with resin before the dissection to better evaluate the borders and relation with the surrounding structures. The deep retinacula cutis were cut to remove the superfcial fascia. The olecranon bursa was also detached from the underlying planes. The bursa is in the DAT but strongly adherent to the superficial fascia.

the adipose lobules form a continuus single layer in the SAT, and some fat lobules also appear in the deep adipose tissue. Thick retinacula cutis also appear, more evident in the SAT, and divide fat into little lobules and anchor the skin to the superficial fascia. Retinacula are thicker than in adults, but less resistant to traction. This is probably due to the absence of a mechanical load.

In the newborn the SAT is rich in fat, but this adipose tissue is more white than the adult fat. The fat cells are arranged in a single layer and have an oval form, with the main axis perpendicular to the skin. According to Sterzi, the superficial fascia is present throughout the body.

From 20 weeks after birth, the superficial fascia is the main location of the brown adipose tissue (BAT). In the newborn, the BAT is essential for ensuring effective adaptation to the extra uterine environment. Its growth during gestation is largely dependent on glucose supply from the mother to the fetus. The amount, location and type of adipose tissue depots can also determine fetal glucose homeostasis (Symonds et al 2012). During postnatal life some, but not all depots are replaced by white fat.

Mechanical Behaviour

The superficial fascia is a fibroelastic layer that may be easily stretched in various directions and then returns to its initial state. The mechanical behaviour of the superficial fascia cannot be understood without considering the superficial and deep retinacula cutis, because they are strongly connected with the superficial fascia to form a three-dimensional network. This structure of the subcutis supports the fatty tissue and anchors the skin to the deep anatomical planes. At the same time it permits some independent movement of the skin and muscles. During skin movement the subcutaneous tissue also moves, but the SAT moves more than the DAT because both the retinacula cutis and superficial fascia are elastic and they progressively mitigate the shifting. If the SAT retinacula are short, strong and vertical, they provide a strong connection between the skin and the underlying planes, allowing stress to the skin to be more directly transmitted to deeper planes. If the retinacula are thin, long and oblique, they have a greater capacity for muting mechanical stresses applied to the deep fascia by way of the skin (Fig. 2.25). This is also important for the protection of nerves and vessels that cross the deep fascia. Notably, this shifting assures that the receptors inside the deep fascia will not be activated during normal stretching of the skin.

In addition to muting skin stresses to subcutaneous tissues, the superficial fascia and retinacula also help prevent the harmful effects of muscular contraction to the skin. Normally, when muscles contract they slide easily under the subcutaneous tissue and the skin is not involved. This occurs because while muscle movement always stretches specific portions of the deep

fascia (see Chapter 3), their action into the skin is mitigated by the DAT and by the mutual movement of the superficial fascia with respect to the deep fascia. According to Nakajima et al (2004), the two adipose layers of the subcutis differ in mechanical and functional aspects. The superficial layer (SAT) forms a solid structure together with skin and superficial fascia and is understood to protect against external forces. The deep layer (DAT) forms a mobile layer and is understood to isolate musculoskeletal movement.

Scar tissue analysis reveals that scars have lost the ability to mute stress as the entire subcutis is transformed into fibrous tissue that creates a rigid connection between skin and deep fascia. Every time mechanical stress is applied to scar tissue the deep fascia is also stressed causing activation of its receptors. Whenever a muscle is activated, the deep fascia receptors in this area will be activated along with the receptors within the locally stretched skin. This may explain why stressing scars can result in confusion of afferentation and probable overstimulation of certain receptors resulting in over sensitive and painful scar tissue areas.

The mechanical behaviour of the retinacula cutis and superficial fascia supports the skin and subcutaneous fat. Tsukahara et al (2012) show a relationship between the depth of facial wrinkles and the density of the retinacula cutis in the subcutaneous tissue of the skin. In particular, these authors demonstrate that facial wrinkles seem to develop above the sites of reduced retinacula cutis density. As wrinkles increase, the density of the retinacula cutis decreases even more.

Ahn and Kaptchuk (2011) demonstrated, with ultrasound imaging, the spatial anisotropy[3] of subcutaneous tissues. In particular, the calf was significantly associated with greater anisotropy compared with the thigh and arm. Anisotropy was significantly increased with longitudinally orientated probe images compared with transversely orientated images. Maximum peaks in spatial anisotropy were frequently observed when the longitudinally orientated ultrasound probe was swept across the extremity, suggesting that longitudinal channels with greater tension exist in the subcutaneous layer. These results suggest that subcutaneous biomechanical tension is mediated by collagenous/echogenic bands; these are greater in the calf than in the thigh and arm. The tension is increased in thinner individuals and is maximal along longitudinal trajectories parallel to the underlying muscle. Spatial anisotropy analysis of ultrasound images has yielded meaningful patterns, and may be an effective means to understanding the biomechanical strain patterns within the subcutaneous tissue of the extremities. Isolated superficial fascia shows strong anisotropy and great

---

[3]Anisotropy is the property of a material for being directionally dependent with regard to its physical or mechanical features.

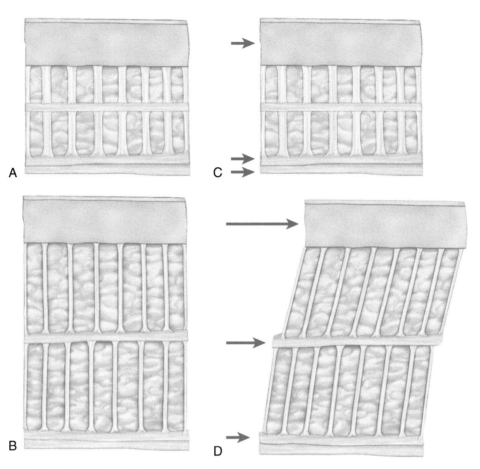

FIGURE 2.25 Illustration of the role of the superficial and deep retinacula cutis as they allow mobility of the skin against the underlying planes. The blue arrows indicate the strain developed in the various layers as a consequence of skin stretching. (**A** and **C**) the retinacula are short and thicker. Retinacula like these transmit every stress to the skin onto the deeper planes (**C**). (**B** and **D**) retinacula are longer and thinner. This type absorbs mechanical stress, so the cutaneous strains are not transmitted to the deep fascia (**D**). Similarly, muscular contraction does not affect the skin.

CLINICAL PEARL 2.5 SUPERFICIAL OR DEEP MASSAGE?

A frequent question for practitioners who use manual therapy is whether a superficial or a deep manual load is necessary. At present there is no firm answer as to which method to use. There are practitioners who affirm that a more superficial load will have an equal effect on the deep tissues and others who prefer a heavier manual load. Knowledge of the anatomy and physiology of fascia derived from this text may aid in arriving at an answer. The superficial fascia is more involved in alterations of thermoregulation, lymphatic flow, venous circulation and in skin perception, while the deep fascia is more involved in proprioception and peripheral motor coordination (see next chapter).

The structural organization of the subcutis and the mechanical behaviour of the superficial fascia and retinacula cutis in the different regions of the body may influence the modality of manual treatment of the superficial and deep fascia. It is evident that in areas with loose and thin retinacula cutis, superficial massage to the skin will be unlikely to affect the deep fascia (except for possible indirect effects). To mechanically affect the deep fascia, the subcutaneous fatty tissue must be displaced, so it is necessary to use a small-surface localized contact and to point directly into the deeper planes. There are also areas where the two fascial layers fuse and interact, where clearly treatment focused on one layer will automatically affect the other layer.

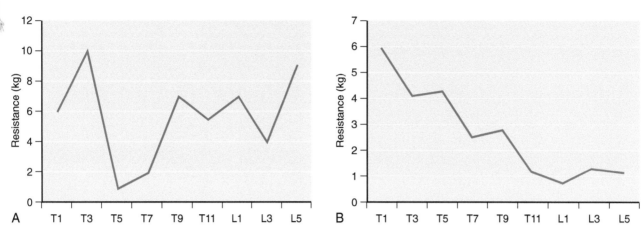

FIGURE 2.26 Resistance to traction of the superficial fascia of the back at the different levels. **(A)** The resistance is applied in a transverse direction. **(B)** The resistance is applied in a longitudinal direction. It is evident that the superficial fascia is not a homogeneous tissue and its resistance changes, going from a maximum of 10 kg to a minimum of 0.5 kg.

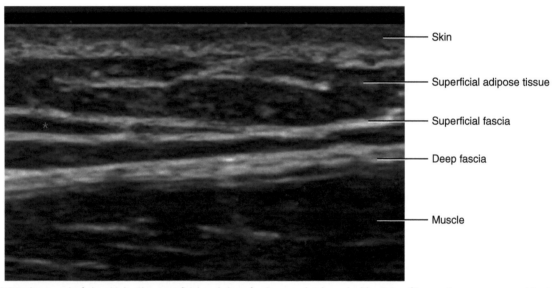

FIGURE 2.27 Ultrasound of the thigh. The superficial and deep fasciae are clearly evaluable. Being fibrous, they appear as white layers. The superficial fascia splits into two sublayers, enveloping some fat tissue (*).

variation of its mechanical proprieties depending on the different regions analysed (Fig. 2.26). It is possible that spatial anisotropy can be an effective surrogate for the summative tensile forces experienced by subcutaneous tissues.

Imaging of the Superficial Fascia

The superficial fascia and all the skin ligaments can easily be observed with CT, nuclear magnetic resonance (NMR) (particularly in T1-weighted sequences) and ultrasound (Figs 2.27–2.29). In CT images the superficial fascia appears as a relatively hyperdense tortuous line between hypodense superficial adipose tissue and hypodense deep adipose tissue. In NMR the superficial fascia appears as a thin continuous line: hypointense

in T1- and T2-weighted sequences. No significant differences are apparent in the thickness of the superficial fascia between CT and NMR.

Using ultrasonography, fibrous connective tissue layers appear as echogenic and echolucent bands. Ultrasonography has the great advantage of permitting evaluation of the sliding between the different fascial layers in real time and allows accurate measurement of their thickness. There are, however, two major limitations: experience of the operator and limitations of the scanned area. This could cause a misunderstanding of the fascial anatomy, especially of the superficial fascia that can split around anatomical structures. For example, it is difficult to distinguish the fascia from the retinacula cutis because sometimes they are almost parallel to the superficial fascia, giving the impression of a double layer of superficial fascia.

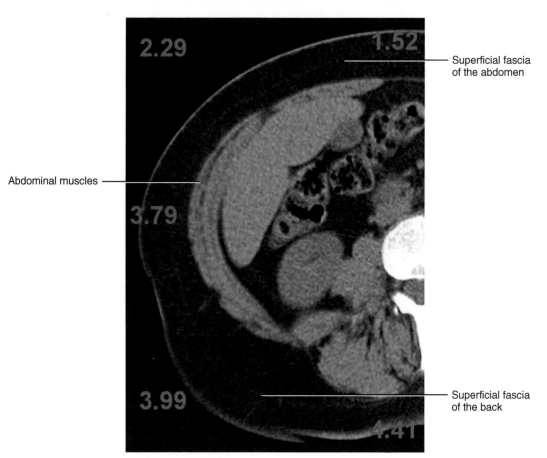

FIGURE 2.28 CT scan of the abdomen. The superficial fascia is clearly visible in the middle of the hypodermis. It is possible to evaluate the continuity between the superficial fascia of the abdomen and the back. It is also possible to measure the thickness of the superficial fascia, the SAT and DAT at the various levels. The numbers refer to the superficial fascia thickness (mm).

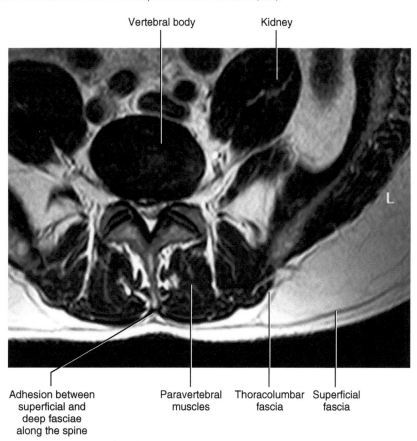

FIGURE 2.29 MR of the lumbar region. The superficial fascia is clearly visible as a fibrous layer (black) in the middle of the subcutaneous adipose tissue (white). It is difficult to visualize the thoracolumbar fascia due to the diminished amount of loose connective tissue between it and the underlying muscles.

47

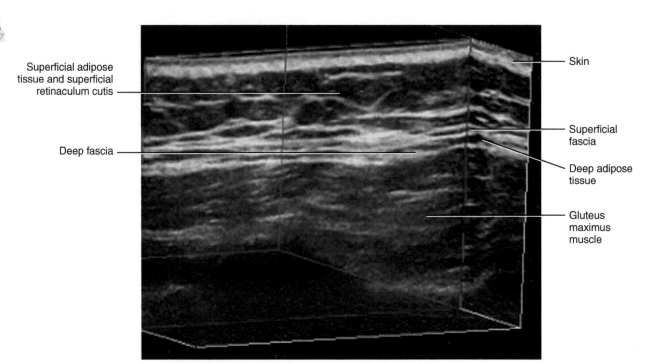

Superficial adipose tissue and superficial retinaculum cutis

Deep fascia

Skin

Superficial fascia

Deep adipose tissue

Gluteus maximus muscle

FIGURE 2.30 Three-dimensional ultrasonography of the superficial fascia of the gluteal region. Note the honeycomb structure of the superficial fascia due to the presence of adipose tissue (in black) among its fibrous sublayers (white). The deep fascia is very thin and adherent to the muscle. The DAT is scarce. (*With the permission of Jouko Heiskanen, Finland*)

Two recent additions are elastography, which could have a role in the study of the superficial fascia (especially by enabling us to evaluate tissue stiffness), and three-dimensional ultrasonography, which also permits the three-dimensional visualization the superficial fascia and retinacula cutis network (Fig. 2.30)

References

Abu-Hijleh, M.F., Roshier, A.L., Al-Shboul, Q., Dharap, A.S., Harris, P.F., 2006. The membranous layer of superficial fascia: evidence for its widespread distribution in the body. Surg. Radiol. Anat. 28 (6), 606–619.

Ahn, A.C., Kaptchuk, T.J., 2011. Spatial anisotropy analyses of subcutaneous tissue layer: potential insights into its biomechanical characteristics. J. Anat. 219 (4), 515–524.

Bichat, M.F.X., 1799. Traité sur les membranes (Treatise on Membranes). Richard, Caille, Ravier, Paris, pp. 121–139.

Caggiati, A., 1999. The saphenous venous compartments. Surg. Radiol. Anat. 21 (1), 29–34.

Camper, P., 1801. Icones herniarum. Editae S.T. Soemmering. Varrentrappet Wenner, Frankfurt am Main, pp. 1–16.

Canoso, J.J., Stack, M.T., Brandt, K.D., 1983. Hyaluronic acid content of deep and subcutaneous bursae of man. Ann. Rheum. Dis. 42 (2), 171–175.

Chopra, J., Rani, A., Rani, A., Srivastava, A.K., Sharma, P.K., 2011. Re-evaluation of superficial fascia of anterior abdominal wall: a computed tomographic study. Surg. Radiol. Anat. 33 (10), 843–849.

Colles, A., 1811. A treatise on surgical anatomy. Gilbert & Hodges, Dublin, p. 185.

Distler, J.H., Jüngel, A., Pileckyte, M., et al., 2007. Hypoxia-induced increase in the production of extracellular matrix proteins in systemic sclerosis. Arthritis Rheum. 56 (12), 4203–4215.

Hauck, G., Castenholz, A., 1992. Contribution of prelymphatic structures to lymph drainage. Z. Lymphol. 16 (1), 6–9. (Review, German).

Hoggan, G., 1884. On multiple lymphatic nævi of the skin, and their relation to some kindred Diseases of the Lymphatics. J. Anat. Physiol. 18 (3), 304–326.

Hunstad, J.P., Repta, R., 2009. Atlas of Abdominoplasty. In: Anatomic considerations in abdominal contouring, first ed. Elsevier Health Sciences, Philadelphia, pp. 5–15.

Krnić, A., Vucić, N., Sucić, Z., 2005. Correlation of perforating vein incompetence with extent of great saphenous insufficiency: cross sectional study. Croat. Med. J. 46 (2), 245–251.

Lancerotto, L., Stecco, C., Macchi, V., Porzionato, A., Stecco, A., De Caro, R., 2011. Layers of the abdominal wall: anatomical investigation of subcutaneous tissue and superficial fascia. Surg. Radiol. Anat. 33 (10), 835–842.

Li, W., Ahn, A.C., 2011. Subcutaneous fascial bands: A qualitative and morphometric analysis. PLoS ONE 6 (9): e23987.

Ludbrook, J., 1966. The musculovenous pumps of the human lower limb. Am. Heart J. 71 (5), 635–641.

Markman, B., Barton, F.E., Jr., 1987. Anatomy of the subcutaneous tissue of the trunk and lower extremity. Plast. Reconstr. Surg. 80 (2), 248–254.

Marotel, M., Cluzan, R., Ghabboun, S., Pascot, M., Alliot, F., Lasry, J.L., 1998. Transaxial computer tomography of lower extremity lymphedema. Lymphology 31 (4), 180–185.

Nakajima, H., Imanishi, N., Minabe, T., Kishi, K., Aiso, S., 2004. Anatomical study of subcutaneous adipofascial tissue: a concept of the protective adipofascial system (PAFS) and lubricant adipofascial system (LAFS). Scand. J. Plast. Reconstr. Surg. Hand Surg. 38 (5), 261–266.

Nash, L.G., Phillips, M.N., Nicholson, H., Barnett, R., Zhang, M., 2004. Skin ligaments: regional distribution and variation in morphology. Clin. Anat. 17 (4), 287–293.

Scarpa, A., 1809. Sull'ernie. Memorie anatomo-chirurgiche, first ed. Reale Stamperia, Milano, pp. 7–15.

Scarpa, A., 1819. Sull'ernie. Memorie anatomo-chirurgiche, second ed. Stamperia Fusi e Compagno, Pavia, pp. 9–15.

Schaverien, M.V., Pessa, J.E., Rohrich, R.J., 2009. Vascularized membranes determine the anatomical boundaries of the subcutaneous fat compartments. Plast. Reconstr. Surg. 123 (2), 695–700.

Schultz, R.L., Feitis, R., 1996. The endless web. Fascial anatomy and physical reality. North Atlantic Books, Berkeley, California, p. 54.

Spalteholz, W., 1893. Die vertheilung der blutgefasse in der haut. Arch. Anat. Physiol. 1, 54 (B).

Sterzi, G., 1910. Il tessuto sottocutaneo (tela subcutanea). Luigi Niccolai, Firenze, pp. 1–50.

Symonds, M.E., Pope, M., Sharkey, D., Budge, H., 2012. Adipose tissue and fetal programming. Diabetologia 55 (6), 1597–1606.

Tassenoy, A., De Mey, J., Stadnik, T., et al., 2009. Histological findings compared with magnetic resonance and ultrasonographic imaging in irreversible postmastectomy lymphedema: a case study. Lymphat Res Biol. 7 (3), 145–51.

Thomson, H., 1979. The surgical anatomy of the superficial and perforating veins of the lower limb. Ann. R. Coll. Surg. Engl. 61 (3), 198–205.

Tsukahara, K., Tamatsu, Y., Sugawara, Y., Shimada, K., 2012. Relationship between the depth of facial wrinkles and the density of the retinacula cutis. Arch. Dermatol. 148 (1), 39–46.

Unna, P., 1908. Untersuchungen über die Lymph- und Blutgefässe der äusseren Haut mit besonderer Berücksichtigung der Haarfollikel. Arch. Mikroskop Anat. 72, 161–208.

Vesalius, A., 1543. De Humani corporis fabrica (On the Structure of the Human Body) Ex officina Joannis Oporini, Basileae, Basel.

Wendell-Smith, C.P., 1997. Fascia: an illustrative problem in international terminology. Surg. Radiol. Anat. 19 (5), 273–277.

Bibliography

Federative Committee on Anatomical Termi, 1998. Terminologia Anatomica: International Anatomical Terminology. Thieme, Stuttgart, p. 33.

Gasperoni, C., Salgarello, M., 1995. Rationale of subdermal superficial liposuction related to the anatomy of subcutaneous fat and the superficial fascial system. Aesthetic Plast. Surg. 19 (1), 13–20.

Mascagni, P., 1787. Vasorum Lymphaticorum Corporis Humani Historia et Iconographia (History and images of lymphatic vessels of human body). Carlied, Siena.

Meissner, M.H., 2005. Lower Extremity Venous Anatomy Semin Intervent Radiol. 22 (3), 147–156.

Prost-Squarcioni, C., 2006. Histologie de la peauet des folliculespileux. Med. Sci. 22 (2), 131–137.

Testut, L., 1899. Traité d'Anatomie Humaine. Gaston Doin and Cie, Paris.

Velpeau, A.L.M., 1825. Traité d'Anatomie chirurgicale, ou Anatomie des régions, considérée dans ses rapports avec la Chirurgie. Crevot, Paris.

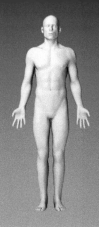

3
Deep Fasciae

Introduction

In this chapter the main features of the deep fasciae and their classifications are presented. The fasciae will be described from a macroscopic, microscopic and mechanical point of view. Particular attention will be devoted to the discussion of their possible role in motor control, proprioception and peripheral motor coordination. Finally, the various modalities used to study fasciae in vivo will be discussed.

Definition

The term 'deep fascia' refers to all the well-organized, dense, fibrous layers that interact with the muscles. The deep fasciae connect different elements of the musculoskeletal system and transmit muscular force over a distance. Based on thickness and relationship with underlying muscles, there are two main types of deep muscular fasciae, the aponeurotic fasciae and the epimysial fasciae (Fig. 3.1).

The term 'aponeurotic fasciae' refers to all the 'well-defined fibrous sheaths that cover, and keep in place, a group of muscles or serve for the insertion of a broad muscle' (*Stedman's Medical Dictionary* 1995). The thoracolumbar fascia, the rectus sheath and all the deep fasciae of the limbs are common examples of aponeurotic fasciae (Fig. 3.2).

The term 'epimysial fasciae' refers to all the thin but well-organized collagen layers that are strongly connected with muscles (Fig. 3.3). Typical of this kind of fascia is the deep fascia of trunk muscles, such as the pectoralis major, latissimus dorsi and deltoid muscles. The epimysia of the muscles of the limbs are also included in this definition. Epimysial fascia is a concise fibrous structure that transmits forces between adjacent synergistic muscular fibre bundles, including some that may not be related to the same motor unit.

The epimysial fasciae are specific for each muscle and define their form and volume. The aponeurotic fasciae envelop various muscles and connect them, forming the various compartments of the limbs.

The muscles in the trunk are generally only enveloped by epimysial fascia, while in the limbs a double envelope is present: the epimysial fascia (called also epimysium), firmly adherent to each muscle, with the aponeurotic fascia located externally. In the trunk there are three separate musculofascial layers: the superficial layer, the intermediate layer and the deep layer. In the abdomen, for example, the external oblique (superficial layer), the internal oblique muscle (intermediate layer) and the transversus abdominis (deep layer) are all enveloped by their own epimysial fascia. The three musculofascial layers of the trunk are generally free to glide with respect to each other due to the loose connective tissue between the layers. But at some points the laminae (layers) fuse, for example, over the spinous processes, the linea alba, lateral to the rectus sheath and at the lateral raphe. This layered organization of the trunk muscles is absent in the limbs. In the limbs, the muscles are each enveloped by their own epimysium with only one aponeurotic fascia covering that connects adjoining muscles.

There are instances where epimysial fasciae connect to aponeurotic fasciae. For example, the epimysial fascia of the trunk (pectoralis major) has myofascial expansions to the brachial fascia (aponeurotic fascia of the upper limb). A trunk muscle, the external oblique muscle (covered by epimysial fascia) continues on to form the rectus sheath (aponeurotic fascia). It then, by myofascial expansions, joins the fascia lata, which is an aponeurotic fascia of the lower limbs. These connections between the fasciae of the trunk and the limbs follow a precise spatial organization that permits accurate transmission of myofascial forces from the trunk to the limbs (see p. 67 Myofascial expansions).

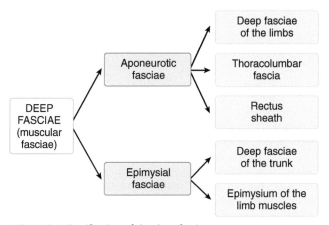

FIGURE 3.1 Classification of the deep fasciae.

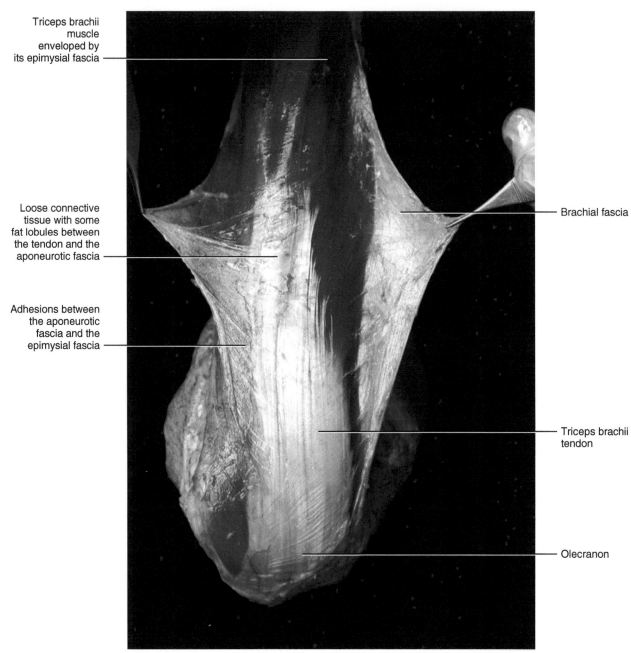

Triceps brachii muscle enveloped by its epimysial fascia

Loose connective tissue with some fat lobules between the tendon and the aponeurotic fascia

Adhesions between the aponeurotic fascia and the epimysial fascia

Brachial fascia

Triceps brachii tendon

Olecranon

FIGURE 3.2 Aponeurotic fascia of the posterior region of the arm (brachial fascia). This fascia appears as a well-defined fibrous layer, easy to detach from the underlying muscles. The triceps brachii is enveloped by its epimysial fascia (or epimysium), which define the form of the muscular belly and assures autonomy of contraction. Loose connective tissue lies between the aponeurotic and epimysial fasciae and over the tendon.

Aponeurotic Fascia

The aponeurotic fascia consists of a well-defined fibrous sheath (Figs 3.4 and 3.5) with a mean thickness of 1 mm (590–1453 μm). It is separated from the underlying muscles and able to transmit muscular forces over a distance. The most notable aponeurotic fasciae are: fascia lata (deep fascia of the thigh), crural fascia (deep fascia of the leg), brachial fascia (deep fascia of the arm), antebrachial fascia (deep fascia of the forearm), thoracolumbar fascia (anterior and posterior layers) and the rectus sheath. Other aponeurotic fasciae exist and will be described in the following chapters.

Based on our morphometric analysis, the fascia lata presents a mean thickness of 944 μm (SD±156 μm), the crural fascia of 924 μm (±220 μm), while the brachial fascia is thinner (0.7 mm). The deep fascia of the thigh is thinner in the proximal region, and thicker near the knee. The anterior and posterior layers of the thoracolumbar fascia (TLF) have a mean thickness of 0.65 mm.

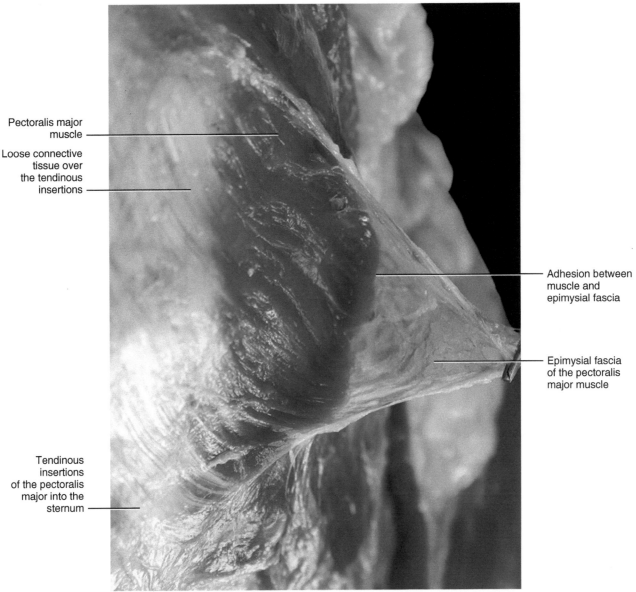

Pectoralis major
muscle

Loose connective
tissue over
the tendinous
insertions

Adhesion between
muscle and
epimysial fascia

Epimysial fascia
of the pectoralis
major muscle

Tendinous
insertions
of the pectoralis
major into the
sternum

FIGURE 3.3 The epimysial fascia of the pectoralis major muscle is a well-defined, thin, fibrous layer adherent to the underlying muscle belly. The loose connective tissue is absent between the epimysial fascia and the pectoral belly. It is only present over the tendinous insertions where the pectoralis major muscle inserts into the sternum. This allows the pectoralis major fascia to glide over the sternum and connect with the epimysial fascia on the contralateral side.

Although the aponeurotic fasciae of the limbs and trunk have the same macroscopic and histological features (Fig. 3.6), from a biomechanical point of view they are completely different. The aponeurotic fasciae of the limbs are connected to the underlying muscles only by myofascial expansions, particularly evident around the joints. Under these aponeurotic fasciae, the muscles are free to slide because of the loose connective tissue between it and the epimysium (Fig. 3.7). This loose connective tissue appears as a pliable gelatinous substance rich in hyaluronan (HA) and containing widely dispersed fibroblasts, along with collagen and elastic fibres, to form an irregular mesh. The aponeurotic fasciae of the limbs,

therefore, work in parallel with respect to the underlying muscles. In the trunk the aponeurotic fasciae (thoracolumbar and rectus sheath) function as a flat tendon for the adjoining muscles; the large muscular laminae of the trunk insert completely into these aponeurotic fasciae. A 'digastric' arrangement exists (two muscle bellies separated by a common central tendon) where the aponeurotic fasciae of the trunk are in sequence with the connecting flat muscles of the trunk (Fig. 3.8).

The aponeurotic fasciae continue with the periosteum, the paratenon (the fibrous sheath around the tendons), the neurovascular sheath and the fibrous capsules of the joints. These elements can thus be

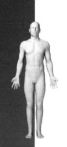

Fascia lata

Quadriceps
muscle in
transparence

Iliotibial tract

Oblique fascial
expansions of
the iliotibial tract
under the patella

Longitudinal fascial
expansion of the
iliotibial tract

Crural fascia

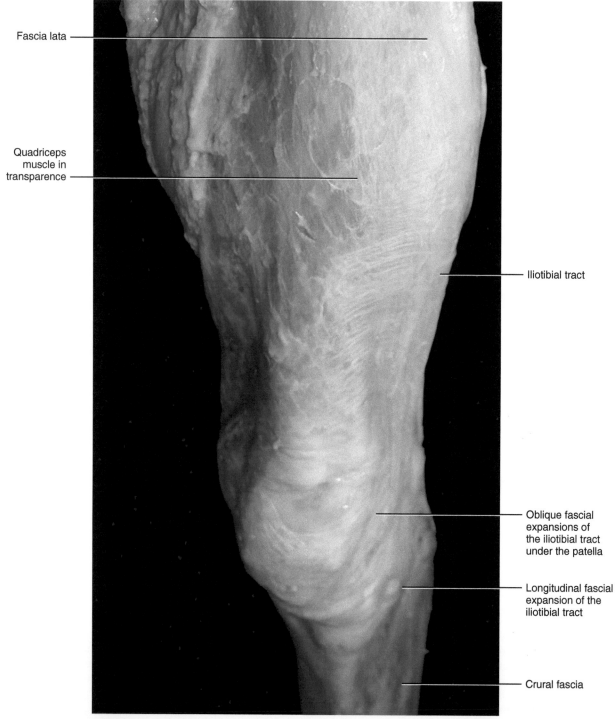

FIGURE 3.4 The aponeurotic fascia of the thigh (fascia lata) appears as a white sheet of connective tissue that covers the muscles of the thigh and continues over the knee with the crural fascia.

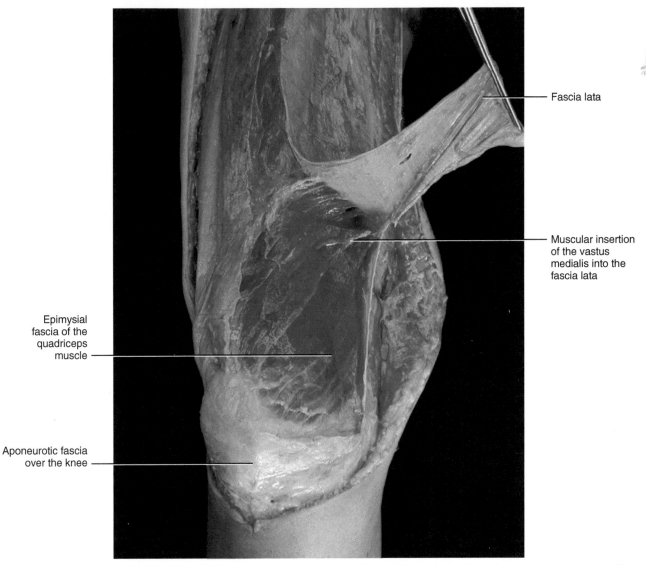

Fascia lata

Muscular insertion of the vastus medialis into the fascia lata

Epimysial fascia of the quadriceps muscle

Aponeurotic fascia over the knee

FIGURE 3.5 Right thigh: anteromedial view. The fascia lata (aponeurotic fascia of the thigh) is detached from the quadriceps muscle and lifted medially. The epimysium of the quadriceps muscle is found beneath the aponeurotic fascia. The aponeurotic fascia is easily separated from the underlying muscle due to the loose connective tissue present between this fascia and the epimysium of the muscle. An adherence exists at some points due to the presence of muscular insertions of the vastus medialis into the inner aspect of the fascia lata.

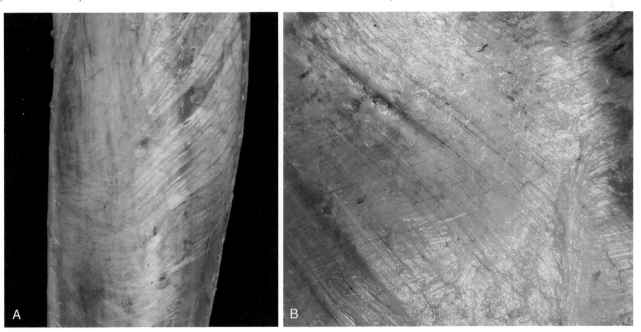

A

B

FIGURE 3.6 (A) Crural fascia of the posterior region of the leg. **(B)** Rectus sheath. Since these two fasciae have the same macroscopic characteristics they can both be considered as aponeurotic fasciae. Note the almost regular disposition of the collagen fibres.

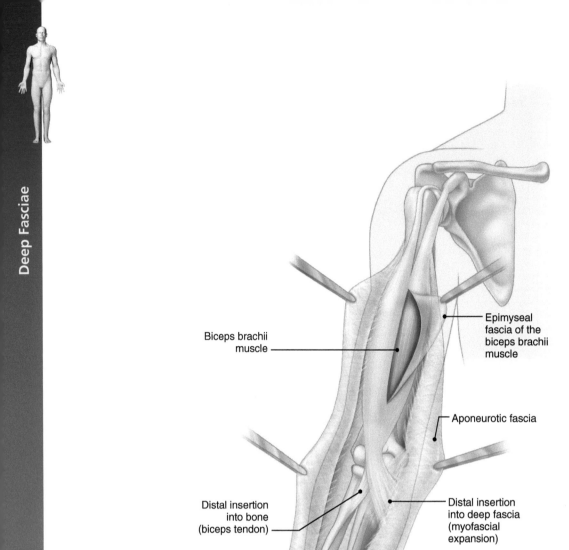

Biceps brachii
muscle

Epimyseal
fascia of the
biceps brachii
muscle

Aponeurotic fascia

Distal insertion
into bone
(biceps tendon)

Distal insertion
into deep fascia
(myofascial
expansion)

FIGURE 3.7 The limbs have a parallel arrangement of aponeurotic and epimysial fasciae. The aponeurotic fascia covers all the muscles of the upper limb. The biceps brachii muscle is enveloped by epimysium (or epimysial fascia) that adheres to the muscle. Between the aponeurotic and epimysial fascia there is loose connective tissue that allows autonomy of the two fasciae. These two fasciae join only at the myofascial insertions of the muscles. For example, the biceps brachii muscle inserts distally into the radius (biceps brachii tendon) and into the antebrachial fascia by a smaller, flat tendon (myofascial expansion called lacertus fibrosus).

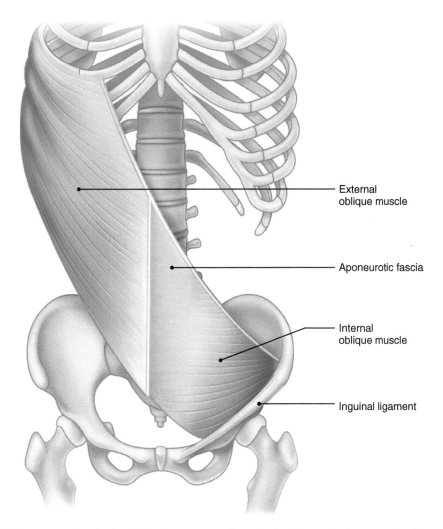

External
oblique muscle

Aponeurotic fascia

Internal
oblique muscle

Inguinal ligament

FIGURE 3.8 In the trunk, the aponeurotic and epimysial fasciae are arranged in series. In this example, the rectus sheath (aponeurotic fascia) inserts into the external oblique and the internal oblique muscles. These two muscles are enveloped by their epimysial fascia that continue into the rectus sheath. The external and internal contralateral oblique muscles may therefore be considered as a digastric type muscle connecting to the middle aponeurotic fascia.

considered as specializations of the deep fascia, not only because they are continuous with it, but also because they have the same histological features (Fig. 3.9).

Microscopic Anatomy of Aponeurotic Fasciae

The aponeurotic fasciae are formed essentially by collagen type I (Fig. 3.10) and, in some areas, it is also possible to recognize fibres of collagen types III and II (Fig. 3.11). Inside the aponeurotic fasciae, many fibrous bundles running in different directions are macroscopically visible. For this reason, the aponeurotic fasciae were formerly classified as irregular, dense connective tissues. But recent works (Benetazzo et al 2011, Stecco et al 2009b, Tesarz et al 2011) have demonstrated that the aponeurotic fasciae consist of two or three layers of parallel collagen fibre bundles, with

each layer having a mean thickness of 277 μm (± SD 86.1 μm).

These layers are composed of parallel collagen fibre bundles presenting a wave-like arrangement. Moreover, the collagen fibres of adjacent layers are orientated along different directions forming angles of 75–80° (Fig. 3.12). This description was also confirmed by the three-dimensional reconstruction of the crural and thoracolumbar fasciae. It is apparent that this tissue cannot be classified as 'irregular'. We therefore suggest that aponeurotic fasciae should be classified as dense regular connective tissue. Aponeurotic fasciae can be compared to plywood with its light, thin structure withstanding a strong resistance to traction in all directions. The multilayered structure of aponeurotic fasciae differentiates it from aponeurosis (or flat tendon) that contains unidirectional collagen fibres. Each fascial layer is separated by thin layers of loose connective tissue (mean thickness 43±12 μm) that

Splitting of the
crural fascia

Crural fascia

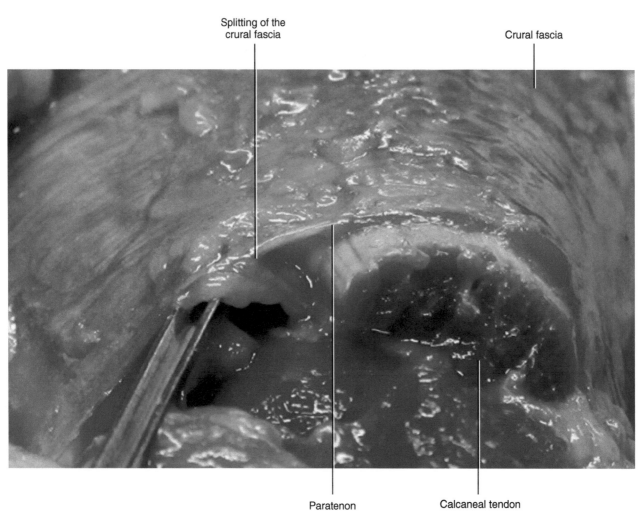

Paratenon

Calcaneal tendon

FIGURE 3.9 Splitting of the crural fascia around the calcaneal tendon. The paratenon is a specialization of the deep fascia.

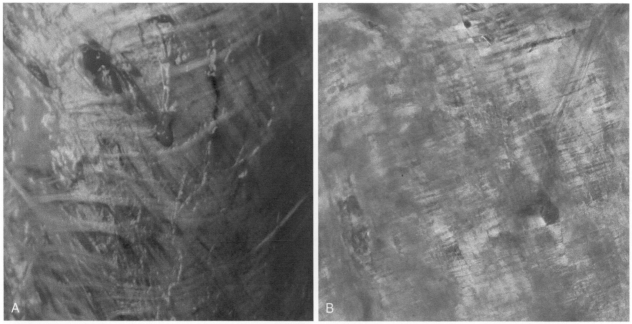

FIGURE 3.10 (A) Macroscopic aspect of the crural fascia. Note the fibre bundles disposed in different directions. **(B)** Crural fascia (polarized light). The collagen fibre bundles are clearly visible, with each layer forming an angle of between 75° and 80°.

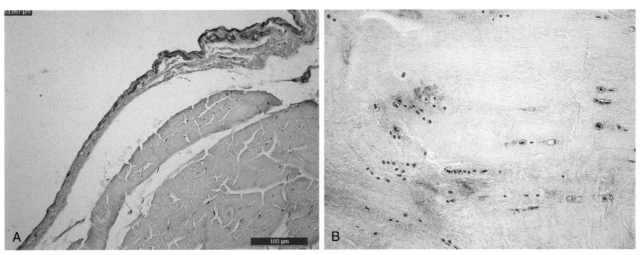

FIGURE 3.11 Immunohistochemical stain of plantar fascia samples, enlargement 200×. **(A)** Brown highlights collagen type III. It is present only along the margin of the plantar fascia, not in the body. **(B)** The stain shows the collagen type II fibres. This sample is taken near the heel insertion. Collagen type II is evident in the extracellular matrix and around some large cells (chondrocytes).

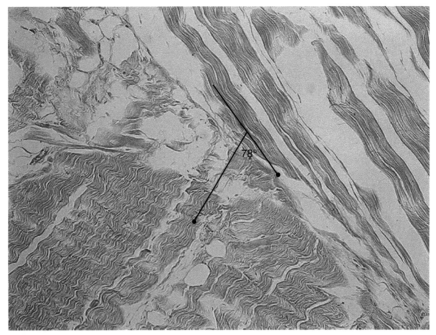

FIGURE 3.12 Direction of the collagen fibres in the aponeurotic fasciae. Note the crimping conformation (undulation) of the various collagen bundles.

permit the sliding of adjacent fascial layers. From a mechanical point of view, due to these layers of loose connective tissue, each fibrous layer may be considered to have a specific influence on the functionality of the tissue.

The elastic fibre content of aponeurotic fasciae is less than 1% and is almost absent in their fibrous sublayers. The elastic fibres are present mostly in the loose connective tissue between the different fibrous layers (Fig. 3.13). Three-dimensional reconstruction confirms a volume fraction for the elastic component within a range of 0.3–1.5%, which is the total value of the elastic fibres in the fascia, not just in the loose connective tissue.

In some subjects, well-defined bundles of muscular fibres are inside the aponeurotic fasciae. These are probably the myofascial expansions of the underlying muscles.

The dominant cells in fascia are the fibroblasts. According to Langevin et al (2005, 2006) and Benjamin (2009), the resident fibroblasts inside the fascia are integral to mechanotransduction. They communicate with each other via gap junctions and respond to tissue stretch by shape changes mediated by their cytoskeleton. In stretched tissue the cells become sheet like and exhibit larger cell bodies. In unstretched tissue they are smaller, dendritic in shape and have numerous attenuated cell processes (Langevin et al 2005). The cell

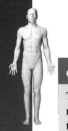

The capacity of the aponeurotic fasciae to transmit muscular force at a distance, similar to a tendon, is due to the collagen fibre content. The aponeurotic fasciae contain collagen fibre bundles aligned mainly along the main axis of the limbs. Consequently, in longitudinal and oblique directions the aponeurotic fasciae function like a tendon allowing force transmission along the limbs. Another important characteristic of aponeurotic fasciae is their ability to adapt to the volume variations of the underlying muscles during contraction. In the transverse direction collagen fibre bundles are less compact, and due to the presence of loose connective tissue, can be easily separated from each other. This motion of the collagen fibre bundles allows the aponeurotic fasciae to adapt to the volume variations of the underlying muscles and enables aponeurotic fasciae to be flexible despite having few elastic fibres. It is apparent that the adaptability of the aponeurotic fascia is based on its unique relationship with loose connective tissue. The loose connective tissue is an important reservoir of water and salts for its surrounding tissues, and it can also accumulate a variety of waste products. An abnormal accumulation of water, ions and other substances may alter the biomechanical properties of loose connective tissue. Specifically, the normal glide of the collagen layers over one another may be hampered. Failure of loose connective tissue gliding occurs in cases of overuse syndrome, trauma and surgery. It is possible that an abnormal accumulation may be related to myofascial pathology (along with HA, see below).

shape changes may also influence tension within the connective tissue itself. Some myofibroblasts are also present (Schleip et al 2005) and these can be considered a pathological response of the fibroblasts to excessive mechanical loading. Fibroblasts, if adequately stimulated, can accumulate actin stress fibres, and thus the contraction of the actin fibres of the myofibroblasts may increase the basal tone of the fasciae, causing pathologies such as frozen shoulder, Dupuytren's disease, etc. Where deep fascia is subject to significant levels of compression (e.g. in certain retinacula or in parts of the plantar fascia) some chondrocytes may be present (Benjamin & Ralphs 1998, Kumai & Benjamin 2002) (Fig. 3.11B).

HYALURONAN

HA-secreting cells have been identified in the inner layer of the deep fascia and they are apparently the source of the lubricant HA. We have termed these fascia-associated, HA-secreting cells 'fasciacytes' (Stecco et al 2011) (Figs 3.14 and 3.15). These fibroblast-like cells may be of monocyte/macrophage origin, similar to the HA-secreting cells of joints and eyes. In joints these are termed synoviocytes and secrete the HA of the synovial fluid. In the eye, they are called hyalocytes and are responsible for the HA of the vitreous fluid.

HA is present between the sublayers of aponeurotic fascia and between the deep fascia and the underlying muscles. In skeletal muscles HA is present in the epimysium, perimysium and endomysium (Piehl-Aulin et al 1991; Laurent et al 1991; Mc Combe et al 2001). Perivascular and perineural fascia also contain high levels of HA. HA occurs both as individual molecules, and as macromolecular complexes that contribute to the structural and mechanical properties of fascia. HA is a lubricant that allows normal gliding of joint and connective tissues. It is likely that these gliding interactions are influenced by the composition and efficacy of the HA-rich instructional matrix. Changes in this

Although they are commonly viewed as a composite of independent chemical subsystems, cells have recently been described as a unitary organization of integrated mechanical components (Ingber 2003). The changes in cell shape and the changes in force distribution among the cells constitutes a kind of rapid information propagation that can, in principle, support a mechanically based regulation and coordination of the cell's processes (Turvey 2007).

It is known that the fibroblasts inside deep fascia are all connected by gap junctions. It is probable that variations in the shape of one cell could be transmitted to the surrounding cells. We hypothesize that the deep fascia could map the fibroblasts and their connections. This allows mechanical stress in a specific region of the deep fascia to be transmitted over a distance. The change in force distribution among the fibroblasts of the deep fascia may represent a rapid form of information propagation to facilitate a mechanically-based distribution of pain and peripheral motor coordination. Neurological (electrochemical) transmission is slower, localized, and context independent. Coordination by mechanical force distribution is faster, both locally and globally, and above all occurs in a context-sensitive manner (Chen 2008).

HA-rich matrix contribute to pain, inflammation and loss of function, and may in fact be critical to these changes in pathology (Lee & Spicer 2000). The HA-rich layer between aponeurotic fascia and muscle seems to function to protect the muscle, to support recovery from injury and to stimulate satellite cell proliferation following loss of muscle fibres. This layer also plays a role in the inflammatory process and HA is prevalent

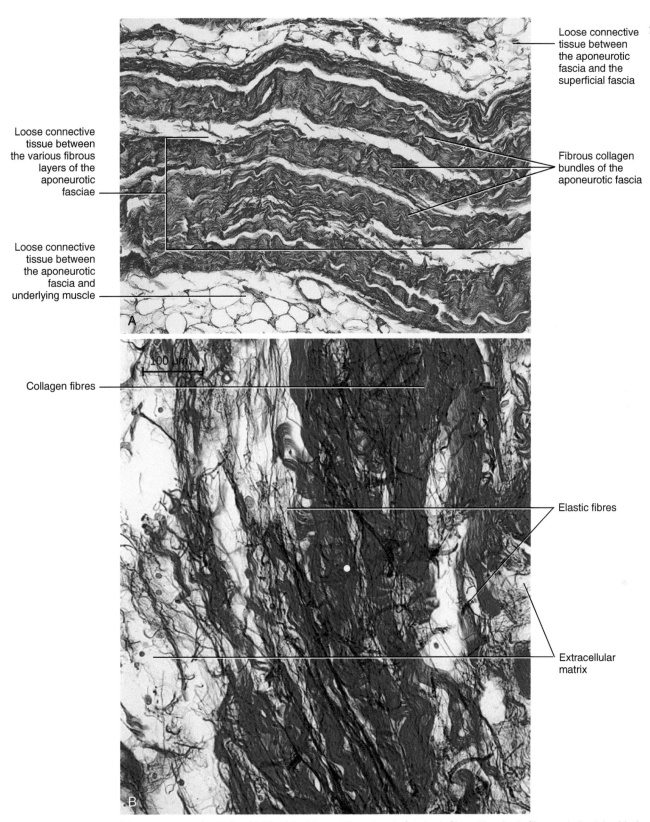

Loose connective tissue between the aponeurotic fascia and the superficial fascia

Loose connective tissue between the various fibrous layers of the aponeurotic fasciae

Fibrous collagen bundles of the aponeurotic fascia

Loose connective tissue between the aponeurotic fascia and underlying muscle

A

Collagen fibres

100 μm

Elastic fibres

Extracellular matrix

B

FIGURE 3.13 Histology of the aponeurotic fascia (brachial fascia) with van Gieson's stain for elastic fibres. The elastic fibres stain in violet–black, the collagen fibres in red–orange. **(A)** The aponeurotic fascia is slightly amplified. Note there are relatively few elastic fibres and the collagen fibres are layered. **(B)** Greater magnification shows the loose connective tissue between the sublayers. Note the increased amounts of elastic fibres and the collagen fibres disposed in an irregular way and embedded in the extracellular matrix (white).

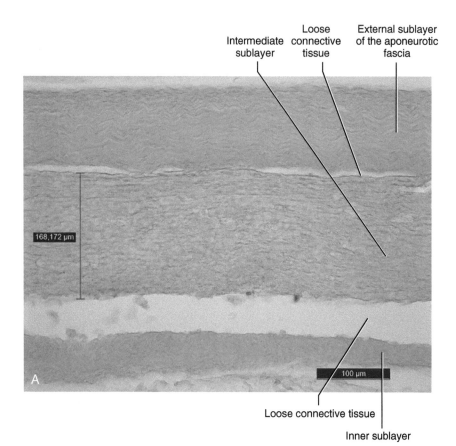

Intermediate sublayer

Loose connective tissue

External sublayer of the aponeurotic fascia

168,172 µm

100 µm

A

Loose connective tissue

Inner sublayer

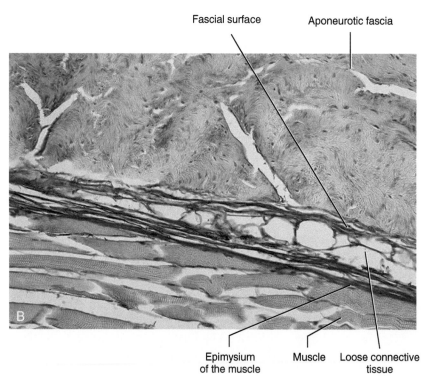

Fascial surface

Aponeurotic fascia

B

Epimysium of the muscle

Muscle

Loose connective tissue

FIGURE 3.14 (A) Alcian blue stain of the fascia lata. This fascia stains particularly well in blue, indicating a high concentration of proteoglycans. **(B)** Immunohistochemical stain of antiprotein binding HA. The HA stains in brown. The HA is located between the epimysium of the muscle and the overlying fascia.

Fasciacytes

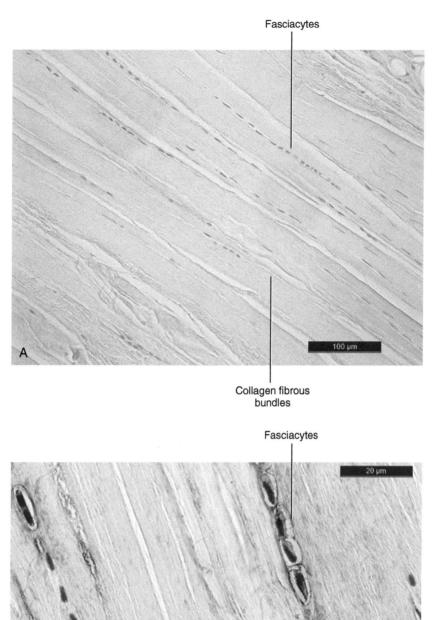

Collagen fibrous
bundles

Fasciacytes

Fibroblast

FIGURE 3.15 Fasciacytes inside the aponeurotic fascia. **(A)** Alcian blue stain: the HA stains in blue. **(B)** Immunohistochemical stain: anti-HA-binding protein, the HA stains in brown.

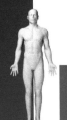
during the earliest stages of wound healing, by open-
ing up tissue spaces through which cells can travel. By
binding to cell receptors and interacting with the cytoskeleton, HA confers motility to the cells. HA is particularly prominent during embryogenesis in tissues
undergoing rapid growth and during repair and regeneration (Spicer & Tien 2004, West et al 1985). Depending on its chain length, HA has a wide range of biological functions and sometimes opposing ones. Its high
molecular weight form is found in normal, quiescent
tissues, while fragmented HA indicates tissues under
stress exhibiting highly angiogenic, inflammatory and
immunostimulatory influences.

Vascularization of the Aponeurotic Fasciae

Information on the structural details of deep fascia
remains inadequate. Originally it was described as
relatively avascular with a predominantly protective
function. Wavreille et al (2010) demonstrated that the
aponeurotic fasciae are in fact well vascularized. They
found in the brachial fascia a rich vascular network located between the deep and superficial sublayers of
the fascia. The internal diameter of these small arteries was between 0.3 and 0.5 mm. These authors also
found many anastomoses between the various arterioles and an abundant venous network. Battacharya
et al (2010) described a subfascial and suprafascial
vascular network connected by extensive vascular arcades traversing the fascial planes. The deep fascia also
contains well-developed lymphatic channels with a
high rate of flow of lymphatic fluid (Bhattacharya et al
2005).

Innervation of the Aponeurotic Fasciae

Several studies demonstrate that the aponeurotic fascia is richly innervated (mean volume fraction: 1.2%).
Abundant free and encapsulated nerve endings (including Ruffini and Pacinian corpuscles) have been found
in the thoracolumbar fascia, the bicipital aponeurosis
and various retinacula (Palmieri et al 1986, Sanchis-
Alfonso & Rosello-Sastre 2000, Stecco et al 2007a, Stilwell 1957, Tanaka & Ito 1977, Yahia et al 1992). Nerve
fibres, particularly numerous around vessels, are distributed throughout the fibrous components of fascia
(Fig. 3.16). The capsules of the corpuscles and free
nerve endings (mechanoreceptors) are closely connected to the surrounding collagen fibres and fibrous
stroma that make up the fascia (Fig. 3.17). This finding
is substantiated by embryogenetic studies that show
how the fibrous capsules of all mechanoreceptors are
derived from the surrounding connective tissue. Deising et al (2012) found a dense neuronal innervation
with nonpeptidergic nerve fibre endings and encapsulated mechanoreceptors in the muscle fascia; Stecco
et al (2007a) have also demonstrated the presence of
autonomic nerve fibres in the deep fasciae.

The innervation of the fascia is not homogeneous.
Spatial analysis indicates that nerves are more numerous in the superficial and intermediate sublayers and
rather scarce or absent in the deep layers. These results
were confirmed by Tesarz et al (2011) for the posterior
layer of the TLF where nonpeptidergic nerve fibre endings were found mostly in the superficial sublayer. Due
to its dense sensory innervation, including presumably
nociceptive fibres, these authors considered the TLF
an important link in unspecified low-back pain. Mense
(2011) found that 90% of the free nerve endings were
located very superficially, and he also found postgan-
glionic sympathetic fibres that may relate to blood vessel constriction and ischaemic pain. There are local
differences in the density of innervation and the particular type of nerve. For example, myofascial expansions, such as the lacertus fibrosus, are less innervated
than retinacula, which are the most innervated fascial
structure. Pacinian and Ruffini corpuscles are located
in large numbers in the retinacula (around the joints),
while in the other portions of the aponeurotic fasciae
they are less numerous. These differences in innervation may be related to tissue function. The principle
function of myofascial expansions is mechanical transmission. This requires a minimal proprioceptive role
compared to that of the retinacula surrounding joints,
which receive many muscular insertions. Similar to
myofascial expansions, aponeurotic fascia situated between two joints also requires scant innervation, since
its main function is to allow a directional continuity
along a particular myokinetic chain.

Deising et al (2012) injected nerve growth factor into
the fascia of the erector spinae muscles, at the lumbar level, and observed a long-lasting sensitization to
mechanical pressure and to chemical stimulation with
acidic solution. Sensitization was confined to deeper
tissues and did not reach the skin. This suggests that

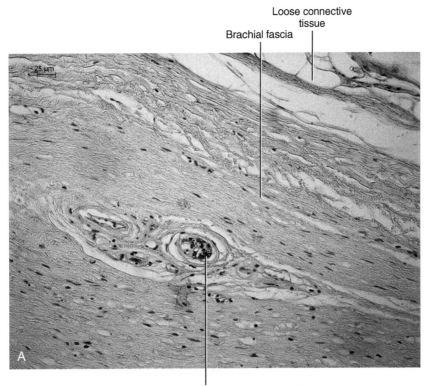

Loose connective tissue

Brachial fascia

Small nerve (diameter: 25μ) inside the fascia. Note the concentric disposition of the connective tissue creating a telescopic mechanism to protect the nerve

The nerve courses in the loose connective tissue along the surface of the plantar fascia

Plantar fascia

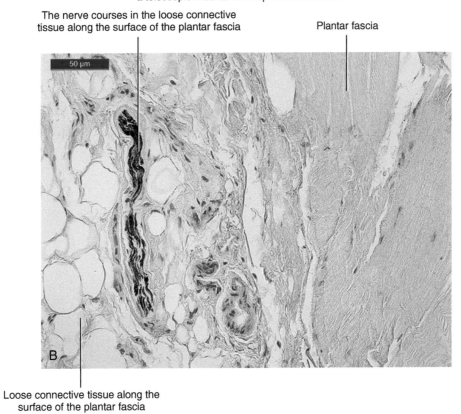

Loose connective tissue along the surface of the plantar fascia

FIGURE 3.16 (A, B) Innervation of the aponeurotic fascia. Stained in brown (immunohistochemical stain: anti-S100) are usually in the loose connective tissue or protected by multiple concentric layers of loose and dense connective tissue. These layers form a structure similar to a telescopic tube.

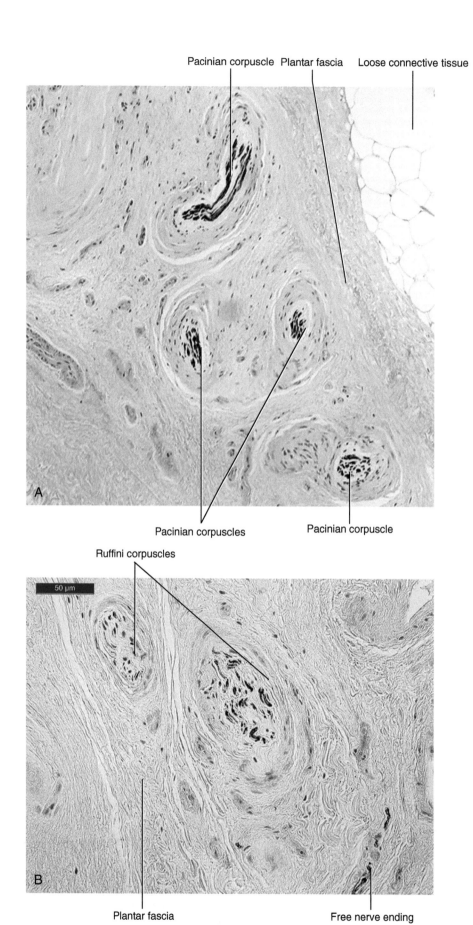

FIGURE 3.17 (A, B) Pacini's and Ruffini's corpuscles inside the plantar fascia.

the sensitization of fascial nociceptors to mechanical and chemical stimuli may contribute to the pathophysiology of chronic musculoskeletal pain. These authors also demonstrated that the sensitized free nerve endings, within the muscle fascia, are further stimulated when the fascia is 'prestretched' by muscle contraction. We hypothesize that due to the close relationship between muscles and deep fascia, muscle activity must necessarily stretch the fascia and activate its embedded mechanoreceptors. It is possible that since free nerve endings are orientated perpendicularly to the fascial collagen fibres, they would be more inclined to be stimulated when the fascia is stretched. It is also possible that increased viscoelasticity of the fascia may modify the activation of the free nerve endings within the fascia.

Changes in innervation can occur pathologically in fascia. Sanchis-Alfonso and Rosello-Sastre (2000) report the ingrowth of nociceptive fibres and immunoreaction to substance P in the lateral knee retinaculum of patients with patellofemoral malignment problems. Bednar et al (1995) found an alteration in both the histological structure (inflammation and microcalcifications) and the degree of innervation of the TLF in patients with chronic lumbalgia, indicating a possible role of the fascia in lumbar pain. In particular, these authors found a loss of nerve fibres in the TLF of back pain patients.

Larger nerves are usually surrounded by layers of dense and loose connective tissues (epineurium and paraneurium) that protect them from excessive nerve traction. Loss of normal fascial extensibility and increased levels of abnormal HA molecules in the perivascular and perineural fasciae are possible causes of compression syndromes (Fig. 3.18).

Myofascial Expansions

The term 'myofascial expansion' indicates each connection that originates from a skeletal muscle, or from its tendon, tendon that inserts into the aponeurotic fascia. The most well-known expansion is the lacertus fibrosus, an aponeurosis that originates from the biceps brachii tendon and then merges with the antebrachial fascia (Fig. 3.19). Many researchers have found that almost all muscles have fascial insertions (Chiarugi 1904, Huijing & Baan 2001, Platzer 1978, Standring et al 2008, Stecco et al 2007b, Testut & Jacob 1905), but their role was unknown. These expansions were usually considered anatomical variations, but they have been found to be constant and present a precise organization (Stecco et al 2010). Eames et al (2007) suggested that these expansions might stabilize the tendons and thereby reduce movement near their entheses, thus helping to reduce stress at the bony insertions. Luigi Stecco (1990) states that these expansions permit selective stretching of the fascia during movement. When muscles contract, not only do they move bones but, due to these fascial expansions, they stretch the deep fascia. The repetitive selective stretching of specific portions of the deep fascia stimulates the alignment of collagen fibres along these lines of force. Marshall (2001) suggests that a map of these thickenings of the deep fascia provides an excellent illustration of how myofascial insertions attach to the

Sciatic nerve

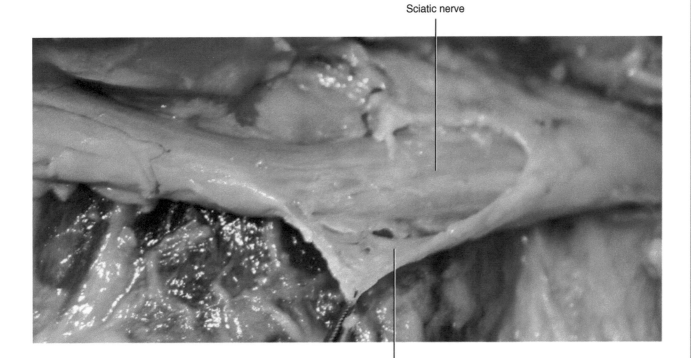

Paraneurium

FIGURE 3.18 Paraneurium of the sciatic nerve.

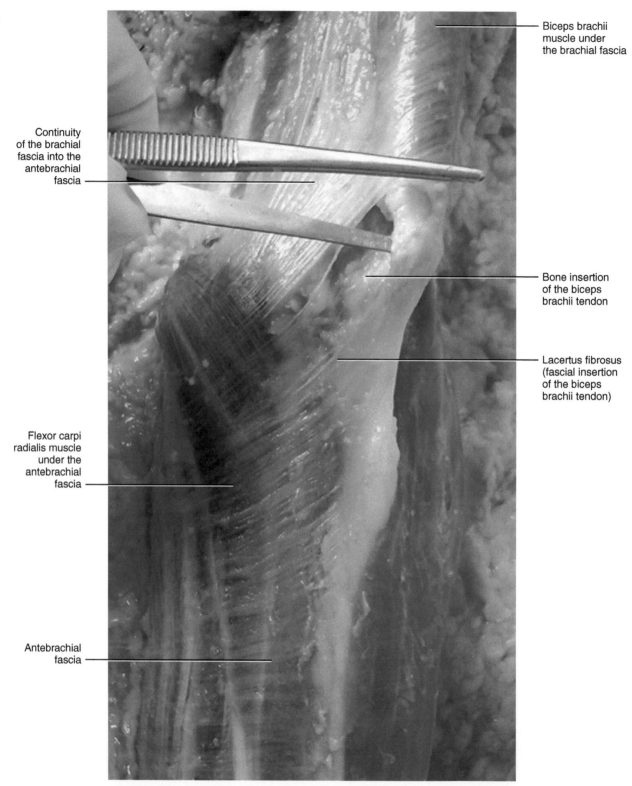

Biceps brachii muscle under the brachial fascia

Continuity of the brachial fascia into the antebrachial fascia

Bone insertion of the biceps brachii tendon

Lacertus fibrosus (fascial insertion of the biceps brachii tendon)

Flexor carpi radialis muscle under the antebrachial fascia

Antebrachial fascia

FIGURE 3.19 Anterior view of the elbow. The lacertus fibrosus originates from the tendon of the biceps brachii and inserts into the medial aspect of the antebrachial fascia.

fasciae and are a precise mirror of the forces generated by muscular action into deep fascia.

Different types of myofascial connections can be recognized:

- muscle fibres that originate directly from fascia (Fig. 3.20)
- muscle fibres that insert into fascia (Fig. 3.21)
- tendinous expansions that originate from fascia (Fig. 3.22).
- tendinous expansions that insert into fascia (Fig. 3.19).

Some examples of muscle–fascia connections include the quadriceps muscle that inserts into the tibia by way of the quadriceps tendon. This tendon has a fascial expansion that passes anterior to the patella and joins the anterior knee retinaculum (Toumi et al 2006). In a similar manner, the Achilles tendon not only attaches to the posterior aspect of the calcaneus, but maintains a fascial continuity with the plantar fascia over the back of the heel (Snow et al 1995, Milz et al 2002, Wood 1944) and with the fibrous septa of the heel fat pad (Benjamin 2009). Both the pes anserinus and iliotibial tract have fascial connections. Dissections of the shoulder region of unembalmed cadavers (Stecco et al 2007b, 2008) have shown the constant presence of specific myofascial expansions originating from pectoralis major, latissimus dorsi and deltoid muscles that merge into the brachial fascia (Figs 3.23 and 3.24).

These myofascial expansions have a precise orientation: apparently correlated to the spatial planes and to the different actions performed by the muscles. The specific distribution of the myofascial expansions suggests their particular functional role. When muscles contract to activate a movement, they simultaneously stretch the related fascial expansions. It becomes apparent, therefore, that for almost all of our movements, specific muscles are activated and selective portions of the deep fascia are stretched by way of specific myofascial expansions. Myofascial expansions permit a reciprocal feedback between fascia and muscles. Fascia can perceive stretch produced by a muscle due to its expansions and transmit this tension over a distance. Thus, the distal muscle is informed about the state of contraction of the proximal muscle, possibly via fascial muscle spindle activation (see below). For example,

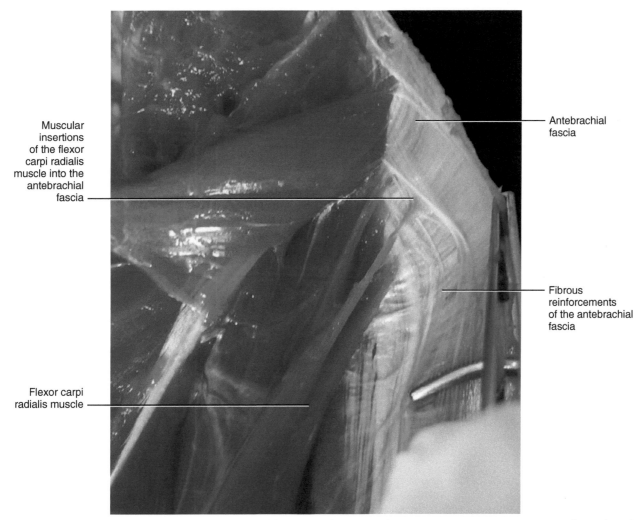

Muscular insertions of the flexor carpi radialis muscle into the antebrachial fascia

Antebrachial fascia

Fibrous reinforcements of the antebrachial fascia

Flexor carpi radialis muscle

FIGURE 3.20 Dissection of the left forearm. The antebrachial fascia is tilted laterally to show the muscular insertions in its inner surface. Where the muscle inserts, the fascia presents some fibrous reinforcements lying along the direction of the muscular traction.

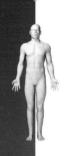

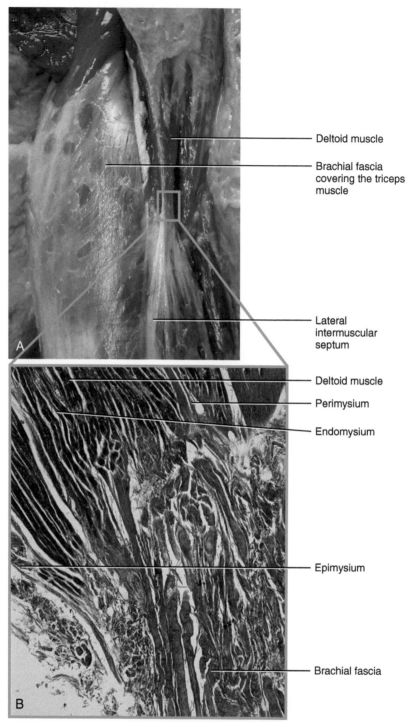

Deltoid muscle

Brachial fascia
covering the triceps
muscle

Lateral
intermuscular
septum

A

Deltoid muscle

Perimysium

Endomysium

Epimysium

Brachial fascia

B

FIGURE 3.21 (A) Insertion of the deltoid muscle into the brachial fascia at the level of the lateral intermuscular septum. **(B)** Histological view of the area highlighted in green. Azan-Mallory stain: the muscle stains in red/violet, the collagen tissue in blue. The continuity of the perimysium and epimysium (epimysial fascia) into the brachial fascia (aponeurotic fascia) is evident. This view affirms that the aponeurotic fasciae of the limbs originate from the fusion of numerous epimysial fasciae of the trunk that converge into the limbs.

during forward movement of the entire upper limb the contraction of the clavicular fibres of pectoralis major will stretch the anterior region of the brachial fascia due to its myofascial expansion (Figs 3.23 and 3.24). At the same time, there will be a simultaneous contraction of the biceps muscle that stretches the anterior region of the antebrachial fascia by way of the lacertus fibrosus. This sequence of tension continues on to the flexor carpi radialis and palmaris longus. These in turn pull on the wrist flexor retinaculum,

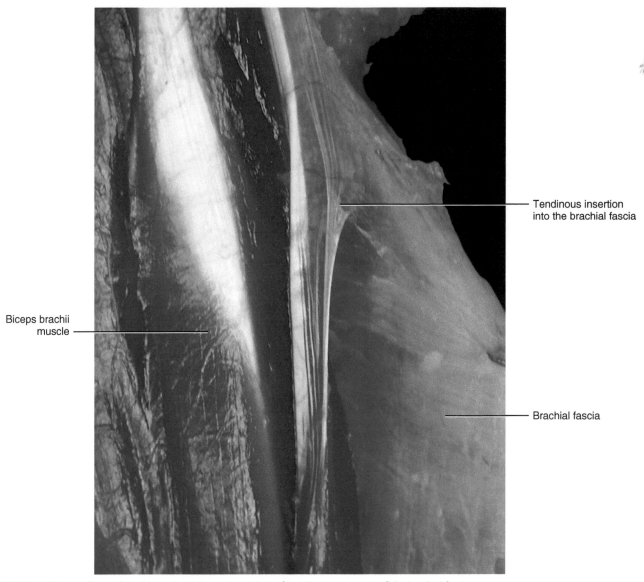

Biceps brachii muscle

Tendinous insertion into the brachial fascia

Brachial fascia

FIGURE 3.22 Some fibres of the biceps brachii muscle originate from the inner aspect of the brachial fascia.

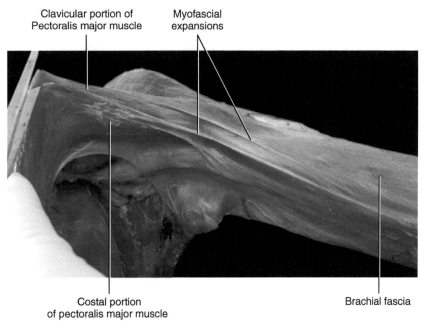

Clavicular portion of Pectoralis major muscle

Myofascial expansions

Costal portion of pectoralis major muscle

Brachial fascia

FIGURE 3.23 Myofascial expansions of the pectoralis major muscle (PM) into the brachial fascia. The pectoralis major muscle is lifted, by forceps, to highlight the myofascial expansions of the costal and clavicular parts into the medial and anterior portions of the brachial fascia.

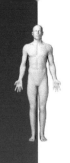
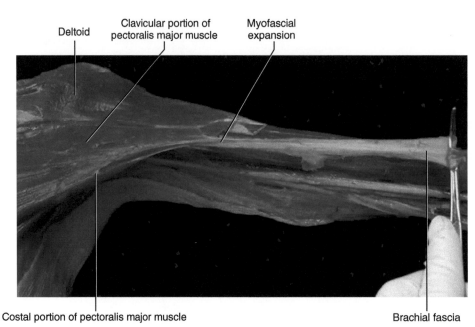

Deltoid — Clavicular portion of pectoralis major muscle — Myofascial expansion

Costal portion of pectoralis major muscle — Brachial fascia

FIGURE 3.24 The medial portion of the brachial fascia is detached and stretched distally, by forceps, to show the tension that could develop inside the deep fascia and along the myofascial expansion to the costal portion of the pectoralis major muscle (PM).

palmar aponeurosis and thenar fascia (Stecco et al 2007b)(Fig. 3.25). Thus, the deep fascia assures an anatomical continuity between specific muscles and their associated fascial proprioceptive elements. This myofascial association underlines the peripheral coordination among the various muscles involved in the movement and perception of correct motor direction. This organization suggests that the aponeurotic fasciae could act as a transmission belt between two adjacent joints and synergistic muscle groups, coordinating the synergic activation of particular muscles. Benninghoff and Goerttler (1978) have, for example, demonstrated that during the movement of crouching, the angles of the hip, knee and ankle, although not the same, maintained a reciprocal constancy. We believe that it is the aponeurotic fascia that coordinates this synchrony, e.g. if there is ankle damage causing a limited angle, then compensatory angular change would occur in the proximal joints based on the stress perceived by the proximal aponeurotic fascia.

Considering all the myotendinous expansions into the fasciae, it becomes evident that the aponeurotic fascia is the recipient of the convergence of all these expansions. The aponeurotic fascia may, therefore, be considered as a large, flat tendon receiving all of the traction of the associated muscles and then serving as a transmitter of their tension. For example, the fascia lata is formed by the confluence of the myofascial expansions of many muscles; 80% of the fibres of the gluteus maximus muscle insert into the fascia lata (Stecco et al 2013a). The tensor fasciae latae muscle continues as the iliotibial band, which acts as a lateral reinforcement for the fascia lata[1] (Fig. 3.26). The internal and external oblique muscles insert partially

into the inguinal ligament and then continue into the ipsilateral and contralateral fascia lata. Distally, the vastus medialis and lateralis partially insert into the inner aspect of the fascia lata (directly or by way of the medial and lateral intermuscular septa) and then their expansions form the retinacula of the knee. The tendons forming the pes anserinus partially insert onto the tibial bone and help reinforce the deep fascia of the medial region of the knee and leg. The fascia lata is, therefore, a composite of all these myotendinous expansions. Gerlach and Lierse (1990) stated that examination of this bone–fascia–tendon system allows us to understand the alignment of the collagen fibre bundles inside the fascia lata (Fig. 3.27).

Fascial Reinforcements: Retinacula

The term retinaculum is derived from the Latin 'retinere', to restrain, meaning a structure that retains an organ or tissue in place, or from the Latin 'rete', net, for the typical configuration of fibre bundles that form a cross pattern[2].

---

[1]The fascia lata is a fibrous sheath that encircles the thigh like a subcutaneous stocking and tightly binds its muscles. The tensor fasciae latae is a muscle of the hip that is considered a proper tensor of the iliotibial tract.

[2]The term retinaculum is never synonymous with ligament. The term ligament comes from the Latin ligare, to bind, and means a sheet or band of tough, fibrous tissue connecting bones or cartilages at a joint or supporting an organ.

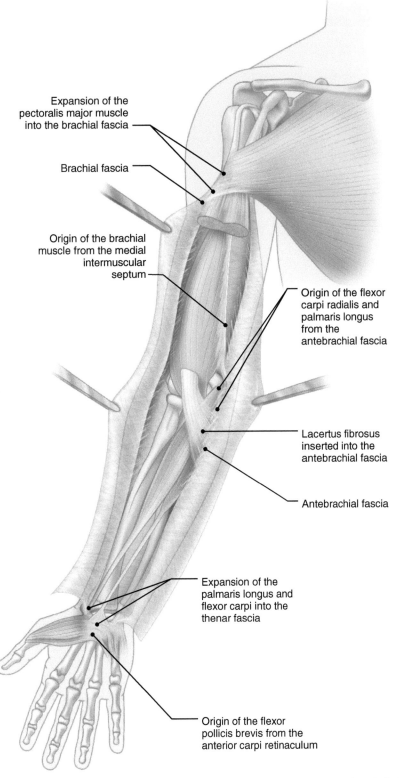

Expansion of the pectoralis major muscle into the brachial fascia

Brachial fascia

Origin of the brachial muscle from the medial intermuscular septum

Origin of the flexor carpi radialis and palmaris longus from the antebrachial fascia

Lacertus fibrosus inserted into the antebrachial fascia

Antebrachial fascia

Expansion of the palmaris longus and flexor carpi into the thenar fascia

Origin of the flexor pollicis brevis from the anterior carpi retinaculum

FIGURE 3.25 The origins and insertions of the muscles into the fascia delineates an anterior sagittal myofascial chain. Note the myofascial expansions of the clavicular fibres of pectoralis major, the origin of the brachial muscle from the intermuscular septa (that are connected with the brachial fascia), the lacertus fibrosus, the myofascial expansions into the flexor retinaculum and thenar eminence of the flexor carpi radialis and palmaris longus muscles. These myofascial connections form an anatomical continuity between the various muscular components involved in antepulsion* of the upper limb, stretching all the anterior portions of the brachial and antebrachial fascia.*The term 'antepulsion' is preferred to 'flexion' because it underlies the direction of movement.

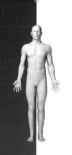

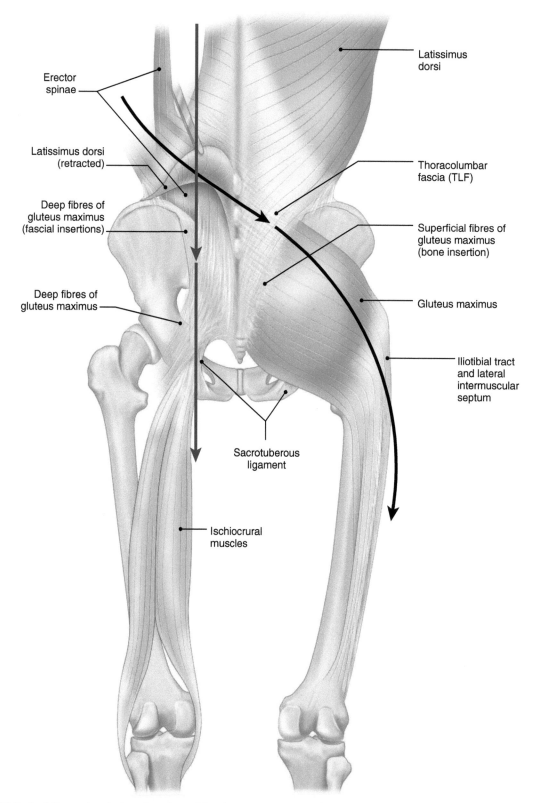

Erector
spinae

Latissimus dorsi
(retracted)

Deep fibres of
gluteus maximus
(fascial insertions)

Deep fibres of
gluteus maximus

Sacrotuberous
ligament

Ischiocrural
muscles

Latissimus
dorsi

Thoracolumbar
fascia (TLF)

Superficial fibres of
gluteus maximus
(bone insertion)

Gluteus maximus

Iliotibial tract
and lateral
intermuscular
septum

FIGURE 3.26 On the left note that the bony insertions of the gluteus maximus (deep fibres, red lines) connect to the erector spinae and ischiocrural muscles. In this way a longitudinal anatomical continuity is formed between the spine and lower limb. On the right, the fascial insertions of the superficial fibres of the gluteus maximus (black lines) insert proximally into the TLF and distally into the iliotibial tract and lateral intermuscular septum (both connected to the fascia lata). In this way a spiral continuity is formed between the lower limb of one side and the latissimus dorsi of the contralateral side.

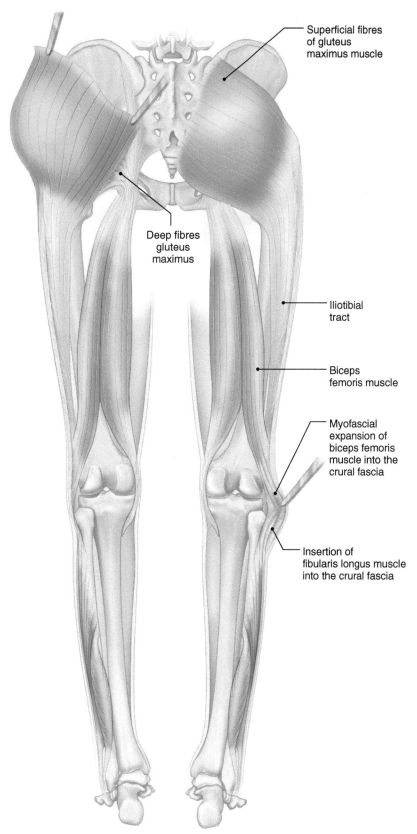

Superficial fibres
of gluteus
maximus muscle

Deep fibres
gluteus
maximus

Iliotibial
tract

Biceps
femoris muscle

Myofascial
expansion of
biceps femoris
muscle into the
crural fascia

Insertion of
fibularis longus muscle
into the crural fascia

FIGURE 3.27 The fascia lata is responsible for myofascial continuity along the lower limbs. The superficial fibres of the gluteus maximus muscle insert into the iliotibial tract and the lateral intermuscular septum that connects with the fascia lata. The deeper fibres of the gluteus maximus insert into the sacrotuberous ligament where the biceps femoris muscle originates. At the insertion of the iliotibial tract near the knee, some fibres of the biceps femoris muscle insert into the crural fascia. At this point some of the muscular fibres of the fibularis longus muscle originate. Therefore, contraction of the gluteus maximus will stretch the iliotibial tract that creates tension at the insertions of the fibularis longus muscle, causing activation of its spindles. (see p. 92 Role of the Muscle Spindles).

From a functional point of view, the retinacula have classically been considered as a pulley system, adhering the tendons to the underlying bones during joint movement (Vesalio 1543). This idea was supported by clinical evidence that showed, for example, that acute and chronic lesions of the retinacula may lead to subluxation of the tendons over their sharp edge (Geppert et al 1993, Sobel et al 1993, Tytherleigh-Strong et al 2000). The retinacula were also considered important ankle stabilizers that connected the bones of the ankle (Leardini & O'Connor 2002, Umidon 1963). However, Viladot et al (1984) found that because the retinacula are thin and flexible, they have a modest effect on the mechanical stability of the joint. They have a far more important role in proprioception. Pisani (2004) concluded that the histological features of the retinacula are more suggestive of a perceptive function, whereas the tendons and ligaments are structured for a mechanical role.

In many atlases the retinacula are considered to be isolated anatomical elements. Recent studies, however, have proven that they serve as reinforcements for the deep fasciae rather than as separate structures (Abu-Hijleh & Harris 2007, Stecco et al 2010a,b) (Figs 3.28 and 3.29). Thus, instead of considering retinacula as individual insertional structures, they can be perceived as a local thickening of the deep fasciae with broad insertions into bones, muscles and tendons. The well-known retinacula are those of the ankles and wrists, but there are retinacula around all the joints of the limbs: at the front (anterior retinaculum) and at the back (posterior retinaculum). In the trunk, the fibrous bundles crossing in front of the xiphoid process and the pubis are large retinacula. The aponeurotic fasciae of the trunk may also be considered as large retinacula that receive various muscular insertions and shunt the various lines of forces (Fig. 3.30).

A morphometrical analysis of retinacula shows a mean thickness of 1200 μm for the lower limbs and 780 μm for the upper limbs. The retinacula are composed of multiple layers (2–3) of parallel collagen fibre bundles as seen in the aponeurotic fasciae, but in the retinacula the fibrous bundles are packed more densely and there is less loose connective tissue (Fig. 3.31). Klein et al (1999) described three distinct layers in the wrist and ankle retinacula: the inner gliding layer containing hyaluronic acid-secreting cells; the thick middle layer containing collagen bundles, fibroblasts and interspersed elastin fibres; and the outer layer consisting of loose connective tissue containing vascular channels. According to Benjamin et al (1995), the inner layer of the retinacula may become fibrocartilaginous when there is significant compression between retinacula and underlying tendons.

The retinacula are the most highly innervated fascial tissues and are rich in free nerve endings, corpuscles (Ruffini, Pacinian and Golgi-Mazzoni) and rare spherical clubs. The retinacula cannot be considered merely as a passive stabilizer, but rather as a specialized proprioceptive organ to better perceive joint movements. Sanchis-Alfonso and Rosello-Sastre (2000) demonstrated an increase in free nerve endings and nerve ingrowth in the shortened/compressed lateral retinacula of patients with patellofemoral malalignment and anterior knee pain. Samples of lateral knee retinacula were excised at the time of proximal realignment or isolated lateral retinacular release. Their results support the clinical observation that the lateral retinaculum may have a key role in the origin of patellofemoral pain as a result of increased neural growth factor production. Neural growth factor production induces proliferation of nociceptive axons mainly in perivascular locations.

The retinacula can sense bone movement and muscular contraction due to their connections to specific muscular (Fig. 3.32) and bony areas. For example, the fibular retinacula bridging the fibula and the calcaneus may be stretched by supination of the foot. This occurs by separation of the bone insertions and stretching of the tendons that slide under the retinacula. During pronation the flexor retinaculum would also be stretched (Fig. 3.33). If a patient has an abnormal gait or if the anatomical alignment of the bones and muscles of the foot are altered (i.e. pes cavus, pes planus), there will be an atypical traction of the fasciae. As there is a strong relationship between mechanical function and molecular composition of the fibrous connective tissues (Milz et al 2005), a chronic anomalous traction of the foot fasciae and ankle retinacula may result in an alteration of the fibrous bundles of the retinacula. This may result in the formation of accessory fibrous bundles inside the aponeurotic fasciae.

A general conclusion may be drawn from the continuity of the retinacula within the fascial system. If a patient presents with ankle retinacula damage, there will be proprioceptive modifications at the level of the ankle and along the deep fascia of the leg. This can alter the activation of the muscle fibres that insert within the ankle retinaculum, eventually resulting in new retinacula/fascial bony insertions. This may result in a change in the distribution of forces within the deep fascia, affecting ankle joint function and even extending to the knee area, resulting in knee pain. Thus, involvement of a distant area, which initially was not pathological, may now become a compensatory painful site. The variability in size or number of retinacula (as described in literature about the ankle retinacula, for example) indicates that the retinacula is morphological evidence of the integrative role played by the fascial system. New increased bundles and anatomical variations of the retinacula (occurring in the distal ankle, for example), as described in the literature, indicates that the retinacula should be considered as morphological evidence of the integrative role played by the fascial system. This idea is confirmed by the work of Abu-Hijleh and Harris (2007), who found 'retinacular structures' in regions

Text continued on p. 82

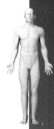

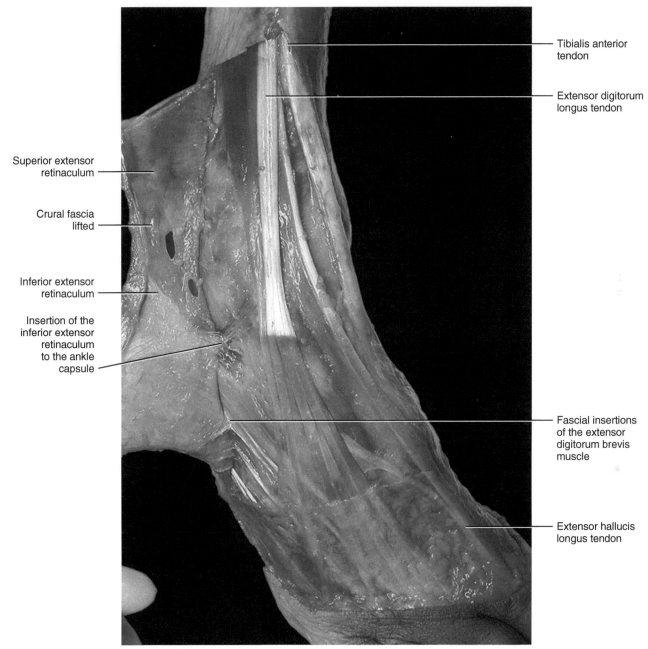

Tibialis anterior
tendon

Extensor digitorum
longus tendon

Superior extensor
retinaculum

Crural fascia
lifted

Inferior extensor
retinaculum

Insertion of the
inferior extensor
retinaculum
to the ankle
capsule

Fascial insertions
of the extensor
digitorum brevis
muscle

Extensor hallucis
longus tendon

FIGURE 3.28 Anterior view of the right ankle. The crural fascia is lifted. The superior and inferior extensor ankle retinacula are shown inside the crural fascia, appearing as reinforcements. The retinacula have bony and muscular insertions. Note the adhesions at the ankle capsule and the insertion of the muscular fibres of the digitorum brevis muscle into the inferior extensor retinaculum.

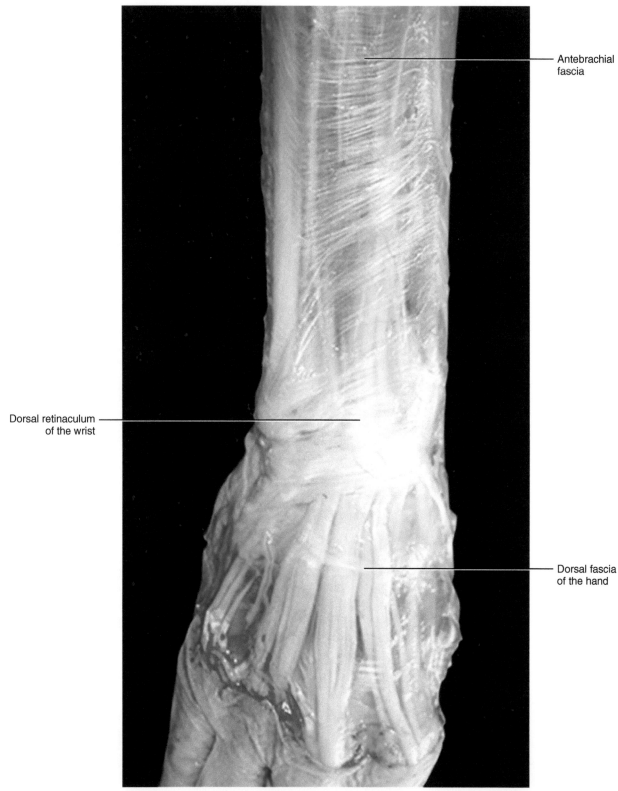

Antebrachial fascia

Dorsal retinaculum of the wrist

Dorsal fascia of the hand

FIGURE 3.29 Dissection of the dorsal region of the forearm and hand. The antebrachial fascia continues distally with the aponeurotic fascia of the hand. At the level of the wrist it is reinforced by the dorsal retinaculum of the wrist.

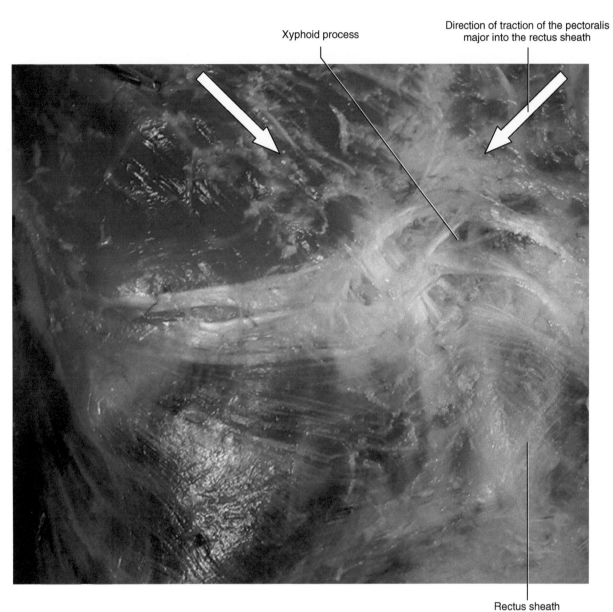

Xyphoid process

Direction of traction of the pectoralis major into the rectus sheath

Rectus sheath

FIGURE 3.30 Crossing of the collagen fibre bundles in front of the xiphoid process. This is, essentially, a large retinaculum connecting the muscles of the thorax and abdomen, and the right and left sides.

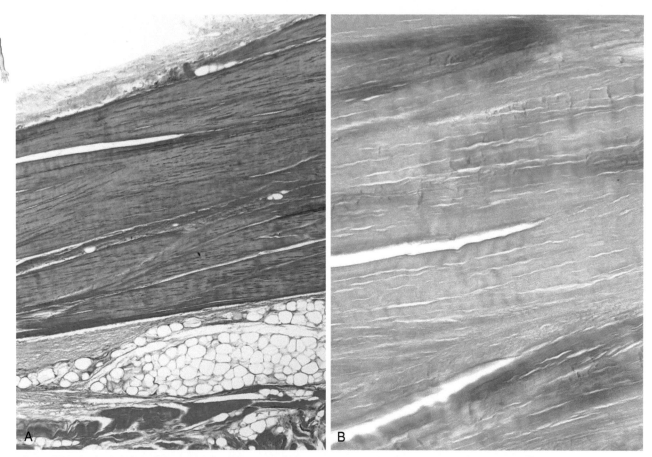

FIGURE 3.31 Histological view of the retinacula. **(A)** Azan-Mallory stain shows the fibrous component. The collagen fibres (stained in blue/violet) are compacted in bundles and the loose connective tissue (white) is scarce. **(B)** Van Gieson's stain shows the elastic component, usually coloured in black. In this picture, no colour black is shown due to the complete absence of elastic fibres. The collagen fibres stain in orange.

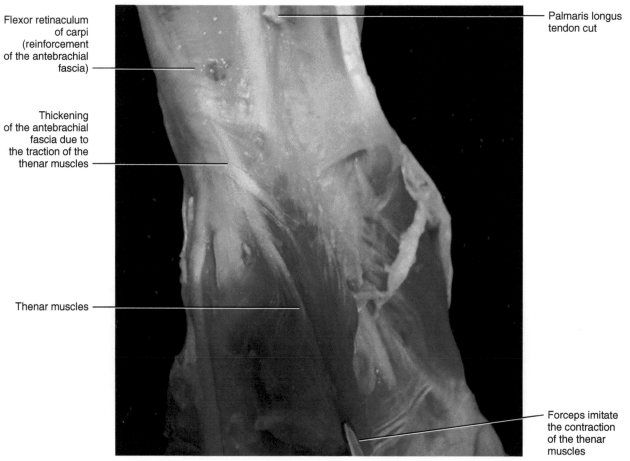

Flexor retinaculum of carpi (reinforcement of the antebrachial fascia)

Palmaris longus tendon cut

Thickening of the antebrachial fascia due to the traction of the thenar muscles

Thenar muscles

Forceps imitate the contraction of the thenar muscles

FIGURE 3.32 Insertion of the thenar muscles into the flexor retinaculum of carpi.

CLINICAL PEARL 3.4 ANKLE SPRAIN AND RETINACULA

Stecco et al (2011) used MRI to analyse the possible damage to ankle retinacula in patients with an ankle sprain. From a clinical point of view, all these patients had alterations of proprioception and functional ankle instability that were evaluated with static posturography. The MRI study of the ankle retinacula revealed new adherences between the retinacula and the subcutaneous tissues, formation of new fibrous bundles into the deep fasciae of the foot and interruption of the retinacula. The patients were divided in two groups: one with only ankle retinacula damage, and the another with both ankle retinacula damage and anterior talofibular ligament rupture or bone marrow oedema. Both groups underwent three treatments of deep connective tissue massage (fascial manipulation technique) directed at the retinacula. All the subjects improved, suggesting that the symptoms of the two groups were due more to changes in myofascial structure than to alterations in bones or ligaments. When a correct state of myofascial tension was restored the symptoms of ankle sprain decreased. Damage to the retinacula and their embedded proprioceptors result in inaccurate proprioceptive afferentation. This may result in poorly coordinated joint movement and eventual inflammation and activation of nociceptors. A treatment focused on restoring normal fascial tension may improve the outcome of ankle sprain.

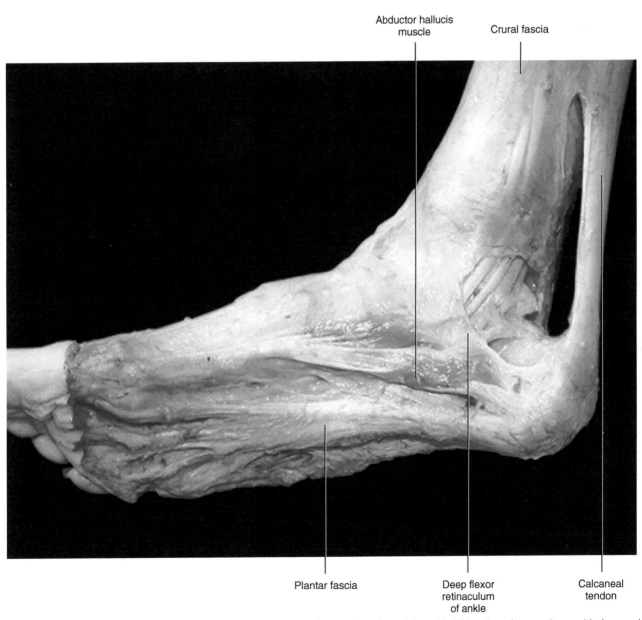

Abductor hallucis muscle

Crural fascia

Plantar fascia

Deep flexor retinaculum of ankle

Calcaneal tendon

FIGURE 3.33 Insertions of the abductor hallucis muscle into the deep flexor retinaculum of the ankle. This retinaculum continues with the crural fascia and serves as the roof of the tarsal tunnel.

of deep fascia, although they were not formally referred to as 'retinacula'.

In the trunk, the aponeurotic fasciae could be considered as large retinaculum. For example, the thoracolumbar fascia (TLF) could be considered one of the main insertion areas of the gluteus maximus, latissimus dorsi and large abdominal muscles. In this way the TLF could perceive the state of contraction of different muscles, could play a major role in coordinating movement and also play a role in the activation of single muscles. During flexion of the trunk, for example, activation of the abdominal muscles stretch the TLF along a particular direction, while activation of the gluteus maximus and latissimus dorsi stretch the TLF in another direction. It is the presence of various autonomous fibrous planes within the TLF that permit particular muscles to contract without opposition from other muscles that are inserted into the same fascia. If trauma, surgery, or an overuse syndrome alters the sliding system within an aponeurotic fascial plane, new lines of force inside this fascia may form. This could adversely affect other muscles, not directly related to the injured plane. This altered activity of muscles could be considered a compensation, and could be present also far from the original problem. The anatomical element that joins the old and new pain is the fascia.

Retinacula are not found in the fetus. Continuous mechanical load in the newborn stimulates the deposition of new collagen fibres along specific directions resulting in the formation of retinacula around joints. Retinacula can be compared to reinforcements in the sails of racing yachts (Fig. 3.34). The sails are not homogeneous structures, but provide specific reinforcement according to the force lines produced by the wind. In this way they could be at the same time a light but resistant structure. Similarly, the deep fascia has to be thin, adaptable and resistant to specific loads such as muscular contractions, tendon pressures and bony movements. The retinacula provide specific reinforcement where stresses frequently occur. Eventually, when all the bony insertions and muscular forces are identified, the true nature of the retinacula will be better understood.

Mechanical Behaviour[3]

The complex structural conformation of the aponeurotic fasciae is reflected in particular mechanical features discussed below:

- nonlinear mechanical response
- tensile strength to multiaxial loading
- anisotropy
- viscoelasticity
- multilayered mechanical response.

NONLINEAR MECHANICAL RESPONSE

Figure 3.35 shows the stress versus strain response of aponeurotic fascial tissue subjected to tensile stretch, from the unloaded to the failure state. One of the main characteristics affecting the mechanical response is the stiffness of the tissue, which is defined as the ratio of stress increment to strain increment. From a geometric point of view, this is the slope of a tangent to the curve. The opposite of stiffness is defined as compliance. For the same increment of stress, a tissue with high stiffness (low compliance) is subjected to less

---

[3]This section was written with the help of Piero Pavan, Associate Professor of Industrial Bioengineering at the Department of Industrial Engineering of the University of Padova, Italy.

CLINICAL PEARL 3.5 FASCIAL MEMORY

Chronic myofascial pain probably causes many alterations of the deep fascia, and the painful region is only one of the altered elements. To understand the origin of a fascial pain in patients and the evolution of fascial dysfunction, it is important to take a complete case history that includes past trauma or surgery. Indeed, past anomalous adhesions of the deep fasciae could have caused pathological lines of force inside the fasciae affecting the deep fascia at a distant location. This hypothesis may explain clinical results that occur when, for example, a chronic back problem is finally resolved after treating an old knee or ankle trauma of which the patient is no longer aware. Our clinical experience suggests that a persistent fascial densification/fibrosis will eventually become a compensation along a fascial continuity. In this way the original pain could disappear, but pathological lines of force are created inside the deep fasciae.

CLINICAL PEARL 3.6 FASCIAL LINES OF FORCE AND TAPING

Athletic taping is the process of applying tape directly to the skin in order to maintain a stable position of bones and muscles during athletic activity. The position of the tape often correspond to the fibrous bundles of the retinacula and the lines of force inside the deep fascia. We suggest that taping in a direction that stretches the deep fascia along the correct lines of force will aid in its rapid recovery. The proprioceptive role played by the retinacula may explain the anatomical basis for the early use of functional taping, e.g. after ankle sprains. Therapeutic taping may help to restore the original pretrauma tension of the retinacula. This would help to avoid the creation of anomalous fibrous bundles or muscular and bony adherences. Especially the use of kinesiotape could help in restoring original proprioceptive capacity.

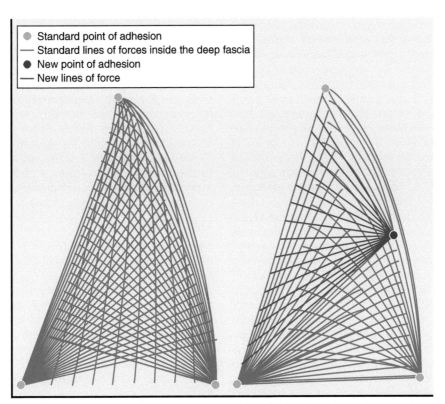

FIGURE 3.34 The aponeurotic fascia and the retinacula can be compared to the sails of racing yachts. Sails are not homogeneous structures, but provide specific reinforcements according to the force lines produced by the wind. This results in a light but resistant tissue. In the deep fascia, lines of forces are defined by muscular tractions and bony movements. Trauma or surgery may create new points of adhesion that can modify the lines of forces inside the fascia.

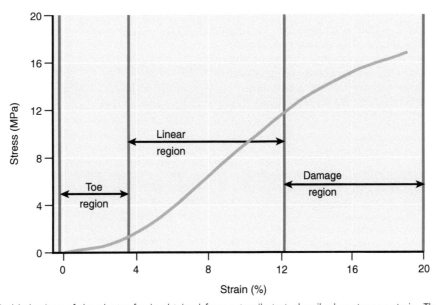

FIGURE 3.35 Mechanical behaviour of the plantar fascia obtained from a tensile test, described as stress vs strain. The so-called 'toe' region receives 0–4% of the strain, a range of linear response (4–12% of strain) and a range in which increasing damage occurs in the tissue (over 12% of strain).

strain than a tissue with low stiffness (high compliance). Similar to other connective tissues the stress–strain curve of aponeurotic fasciae shows a nonlinear response: a 'toe' region, a linear region and a failure region. The toe region is typically from small strains in the undeformed state. In this region the tissue has low stiffness, a mechanical characteristic that is related to the crimping conformation of the collagen fibres and the large compliance of elastin fibres. In experimental tests carried out on samples of aponeurotic fascia

(Stecco et al 2013), the toe region was found to extend up to 4% of strain. Over this value (linear region) the tissue shows a greater stiffness and an almost linear response. In this region, the stress increment is proportional to the strain increment. In some samples of aponeurotic tissue, a progressive failure was found at higher than 12% of strain. This failure is caused by damage in the collagen fibres and results in progressive reduction of the stiffness. The strength of the tissue is expressed by the maximum value of the stress shown by the stress–strain curve. The maximum strength of the tissue occurs in a region where damage phenomena occur (Fig. 3.35). The physiological range of strain is limited to a region free from damage phenomena. This means that the aponeurotic fasciae generally work with a safety factor based on their strength. Due to the anisotropic characteristic of aponeurotic fasciae, the stress–strain curves have been found to depend on the loading direction. Further, the mechanical response is different according to the compartment considered. For example, research (Stecco et al 2014a) demonstrates that samples taken from the anterior leg compartment are stiffer than samples removed from the posterior leg compartment, especially when stretched in a transverse direction. This data may explain why in clinical practice anterior compartment syndrome occurs more frequently than posterior compartment syndrome (Verleisdonk et al 2004).

TENSILE STRENGTH TO MULTIAXIAL LOADING

The aponeurotic fasciae show the capability of acting like tendons, transmitting part of the muscular contraction force from one segment to another. In this action, their strength appears to be related to muscle mass and to the maximum contraction force of the muscle (Stecco et al 2007b). For example, contraction of the gluteus maximus will stretch the fascia lata to which it inserts. The fascia lata will then transmit this force, in a longitudinal direction, along the iliotibial band extending the tension into the anterolateral portion of the crural fascia and the anterior knee retinaculum. This capability is due to the spatial orientation of the collagen fibre bundles, thus ensuring the ability of the fasciae to provide strength in the case of tensile forces applied in different directions (multiaxial loading). Thus, collagen fibre bundles play a strategic role. At low strains, only the collagen fibres that are initially aligned in the direction of the applied force contribute to the strength of the tissue; while at higher strains, more fibre bundles are progressively orientated along the loading direction (Fig. 3.36).

ANISOTROPY

Anisotropy can be attributed to a material that shows directionally dependent mechanical properties (basically, stiffness and strength). This characteristic is also due to the specific spatial orientation of the collagen fibres. Hurschler et al (1994) reported an average structural stiffness per unit width of the aponeurotic fascia of 50.9 ± 33 N/mm in the longitudinal direction and of 46.4 ± 16 N/mm in the transverse direction. Our studies (Stecco et al 2014a) confirm that aponeurotic fasciae are stiffer in the longitudinal rather than in the transverse direction, as shown in Fig. 3.37. The lower stiffness in a transverse direction could be associated with the capability of aponeurotic fascia to adapt to the effects of muscle fibre contraction. The higher stiffness in a longitudinal direction, as in a tendon, was described in the previous section. It could, therefore, be concluded that muscle contraction would be compromised if fascia were to lose this adaptability.

VISCOELASTICITY

Aponeurotic fascia, similar to other connective tissue, exhibits the property of viscoelasticity. Viscoelasticity

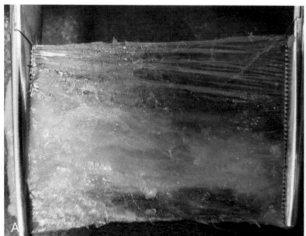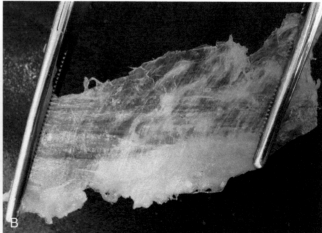

FIGURE 3.36 Aponeurotic fascia stretched along longitudinal direction **(A)** and oblique direction **(B).** When the aponeurotic fascia is stretched along a direction, the collagen fibre bundles are progressively aligned in the same direction and increase strength capability.

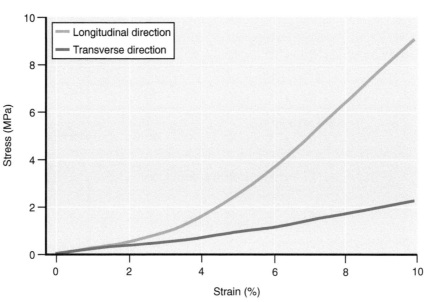

FIGURE 3.37 The crural fascia has a different mechanical behaviour when it is stretched along the main axis of a limb (longitudinal direction in the graph) or in a perpendicular direction (transverse direction). This confirms that fascia has anisotropic characteristics.

can be considered the macroscopic effect of internal rearrangement of the fibrous components of tissue and the migration of liquid phases over time. To understand the mechanics of viscoelastic materials it is necessary to start with the basic properties of elastic material. An ideal elastic material would deform instantaneously when subjected to stress, and return instantaneously to its original configuration once the stress is removed. The level of strain depends solely on the level of stress applied. Stiffness of the material is based on the ratio of stress and strain applied. In a viscoelastic material, the mechanical response is more complex because the rate of loading has to be taken into consideration. The principle phenomena expressed by viscoelastic material, as in aponeurotic fasciae or other connective tissues, are:

- Dependency of its stiffness on the rate of strain or stress applied: fascia stiffness, similar to tendons, increases when subjected to higher stress or strain rates. Even if not supported at the present time by quantitative data, it can be supposed that this behaviour has significant effects on the efficiency of a muscle in generating contraction forces.

- Creep: the continuous or viscous strain increasing in the fasciae in response to a maintained or constant load. Creep can be recovered at loading release apart the case in which excessive load can induce a damage of the tissue.

- Stress relaxation: a sort of dual behaviour of creep that consists of a decrease in stress over time when the tissue is subjected to constant strain. Despite the fact that the investigation of viscoelasticity is complicated by the strong anisotropy of aponeurotic fasciae, a recent study has made available some quantitative data

(Stecco et al 2014a). For example, experimental tests on the anterior compartment of the leg demonstrated a stress relaxation of about 35% within the first 120 s and a subsequent stress decline of about 2% in the following 120 s. Therefore, we can consider that a time range of 240 s is sufficient to have an almost complete development of viscous phenomena. The stress–relaxation curves show that 90% of stress relaxation takes place in the first minute after the application of the strain.

- Hysteresis: can be defined as the amount of energy lost during a loading–unloading cycle. This concept of the hysteretic behaviour of aponeurotic fascia is illustrated in Figure 3.38. For a specific viscoelastic material, the hysteresis area depends on the rate of loading and unloading. If the loading–unloading cycle is fast, the hysteresis area tends to reduce, resulting in the loading and unloading curves being equal, indicating that energy dissipation is reduced and the mechanical efficiency of the system is increased. In this situation, the behaviour of the aponeurotic fasciae is similar to that of a tendon. Looking at this phenomenon from the point of view of motion analysis, an athlete would desire to have fasciae with a minimum of hysteresis, since that would allow more efficient movement and create more power with less muscular effort. The possible change in the viscosity of the fasciae is important. For example, it was shown that increasing fascial temperature (Matteini et al 2009) decreases fascial viscosity. Decreasing fascial viscosity improves the efficiency of fascial response to stretch and recoil. This reduction of fascial hysteresis explains the importance of warm-up before sports competition.

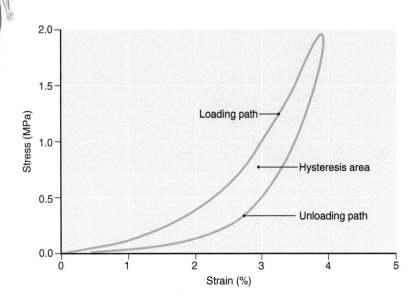

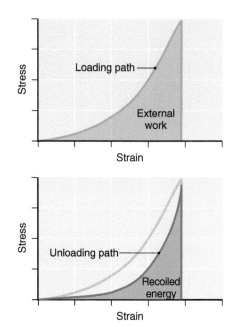

FIGURE 3.38 Typical hysteresis curve of aponeurotic fascia subjected to a loading–unloading cycle. The two curves are not coincident due to the energy dissipated by the tissue through inelastic phenomena. The area under the loading curve is proportional to external mechanical work done; the area under the unloading curve is proportional to the energy stored elastically in loading and returned in unloading; the closed (hysteresis) area is proportional to dissipated energy. If the hysteresis area is small, it indicates that the fascia has a high capability for storing the external mechanical work as strain energy, minimizing energy dissipation.

CLINICAL PEARL 3.7 INVOLVEMENT OF DEEP FASCIAE IN STRETCHING

The aponeurotic fasciae of the limbs work in parallel with respect to the muscles and are, therefore, stiffer than muscles. Consequently, during stretching it is the fascia that is more stressed and therefore plays an important role in determining the limits of stretching. The stress–relaxation curves show that 90% of stress relaxation takes place in the first minute after the application of a strain. From a clinical point of view, this means that it is important to relax the fascia to held a position for at least one minute during static stretching.

MULTILAYERED MECHANICAL RESPONSE

The distinct structural appearance of aponeurotic fasciae that makes it different from other connective tissues is the presence of loose connective tissue between adjacent layers. Histological analysis shows that each layer is reinforced by collagen fibre bundles that run parallel and in a specific direction. This particular arrangement gives each layer the capability of resisting tensile loads along specific fibre directions. This direction differs from layer to layer and is dependent on the particular location in the body. It is probable that this conformation results in:

- the ability to resist loads transmitted to the fasciae through the attachments of the musculoskeletal system

- the adaptability to local effects of muscle contraction.

This multilayered structural characteristic is also related to the mechanical anisotropy of the fasciae discussed in a previous section (p. 84). It is likely that the presence of loose connective tissue interposed between fibre-reinforced layers is the key factor that allows the layers to glide during the contraction of the underlying muscles. As a consequence there is greater fascial adaptability. The annulus fibrosus of the intervertebral disc shows a multilayered conformation, but lacks the gliding phenomena found in aponeurotic fasciae. Deficiencies in gliding adaptability may be a reason for pathological conditions such as compartment syndrome. Gliding capability between fibre-reinforced layers depends on the viscosity of loose tissue and attention should be focused on this aspect.

Epimysial Fascia

The term 'epimysial fascia' refers to all the thin and well-organized fibrous layers that ensheath a muscle and define its form and structure (Figs 3.39 and 3.40). To be classified as fasciae, epimysial fasciae must contain fibrous layers that are able to transmit muscular forces and connect adjacent synergistic muscular fibre bundles. Epimysial fasciae are thinner than aponeurotic fasciae and their range of action is more localized. The epimysial fasciae are specific for each muscle and define its form and volume, while the aponeurotic fasciae envelop several muscles and connect them. The epimysial fasciae transmit forces generated by single muscle bundles, while the aponeurotic

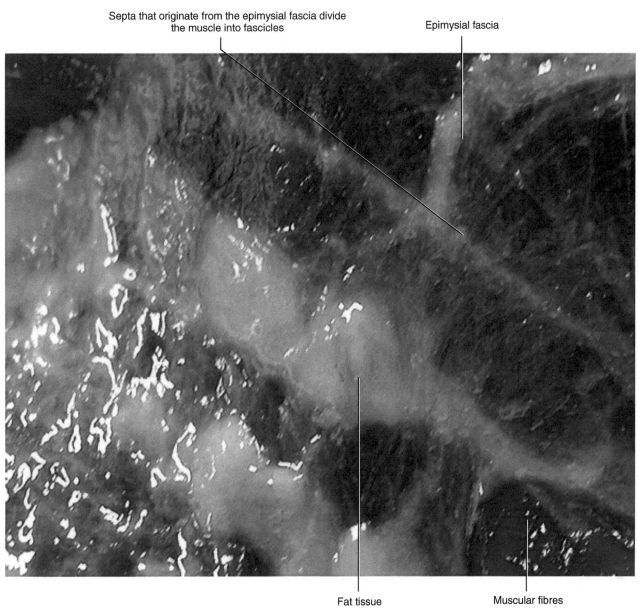

Septa that originate from the epimysial fascia divide the muscle into fascicles

Epimysial fascia

Fat tissue

Muscular fibres

FIGURE 3.39 Macroscopic view of the epimysial fascia of the deltoid muscle. The tissue is a thin, fibrous, white membrane, strongly adherent to the muscle. It forms a gliding surface over the muscle.

fasciae transmit forces generated by whole muscles. The epimysial fasciae provide insertions for muscle fibres.

With the term epimysial fascia we include the deep fascia of some trunk muscles (such as the pectoralis major, latissimus dorsi and deltoid muscles), and the epimysium[4] (see Fig. 3.1) of the muscles of the limbs. Epimysial fasciae are fibrous laminae with a mean thickness of 150–200 μm and are composed of collagen fibre types I and III (Sakamoto 1996), and many elastic fibres (~15%). In fusiform muscles (i.e. biceps brachii), the collagen fibres have an angle of

incidence of 55° with respect to the path of the muscular fibres at rest (Purslow 2010). In pennate muscles (i.e. rectus femoris) the epimysial fasciae mainly reflect the progression of muscular fibres, forming a dense lamina that continues into the tendon of the muscle. One of the most important features of the epimysial fasciae is their tight adherence to underlying muscles via multiple fibrous septa that originate from their inner aspect and penetrate the muscle. For this reason, it is impossible to separate the functions and features of the epimysial fascia and the underlying muscle.

The epimysial fasciae are thinner compared to the aponeurotic fasciae, but Purslow (2010) has demonstrated that they have the same structural organization. He described three superimposed layers of the epimysial fasciae:

---

[4]The terms 'epimysial fascia' and 'epimysium' will be used throughout this text in an interchangeable way.

Deep Fasciae

87

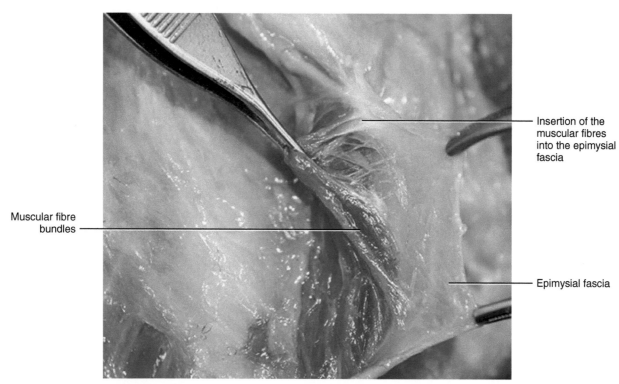

Muscular fibre bundles

Insertion of the muscular fibres into the epimysial fascia

Epimysial fascia

FIGURE 3.40 Epimysial fascia of the pectoralis major muscle: thin, resistant fibrous layer, strongly adherent to the muscle.

- Internal layer: collagen fibres are arranged in a disorganized manner without any precise orientation.
- Middle layer: thin intertwined collagen fibres forming a network.
- External layer: large diameter collagen fibres forming flattened bands that follow a specific direction.

It is important to note that the space between the collagen fibres of the epimysial fasciae is occupied by HA (Fig. 3.41). This allows the collagen fibres to slide with less friction during movement (McCombe et al 2001). HA provides a relative mobility until there is tension at the interfibrillar cross-links. This fundamental substance is a lubricant and simultaneously acts as a binder for the diverse elements of the extracellular matrix (Hukinsa & Aspden 1985). The presence of HA in the epimysial fasciae allows each muscle belly to slide independent of surrounding muscles. Gao et al (2008) demonstrated that the epimysial fasciae from old rats are much stiffer than that of young rats. Age-related increase in the stiffness of the epimysial fasciae could play an important role in the impaired lateral force transmission in the muscles of the elderly and be responsible for alteration of intramuscular motor coordination. This increased stiffness cannot be attributed to variations in the thickness of the epimysial fasciae or in the size of the collagen fibrils. Microscopic analysis does not show any change in the arrangement or size of the collagen fibrils of the epimysial fasciae in older rats (Gao et al 2008). It is probable that the key element explaining this stiffness is the composition of

the extracellular matrix with respect to the presence of HA.

Epimysial fascia also covers the small neurovascular bundles that are present between related muscles and acts to support the vessels and nerves for these muscles. It provides the vessels and nerves with an important autonomy that allows them to adapt to the changes in form of the muscles during movement. Epimysial fascia also prevents two adjoining bellies from separating and facilitates a discrete sliding of muscles in all directions.

Perimysium

The perimysium is a thin fibrous layer that is closely connected with the epimysial fasciae[5] and divides the muscle belly into fascicles (bundles) of different dimensions. From a functional perspective, the perimysium correlates strongly with the epimysial fasciae and this helps to explain the possible role of the epimysial fascia in local motor coordination.

The perimysium comprises collagen fibres, types I, III, VI and XII, and many elastic fibres (Figs 3.42 and 3.43). Compared to the epimysium, the percentage of collagen type I decreases and that of collagen type III increases (Sakamoto 1996). The type I collagen fibres in the perimysium have a diameter of up to 10 times greater than the collagen fibres located in the endomysium (Purslow 1989). This provides the perimysium with a notable resistance to traction as compared to

---

[5]From a functional point of view, the term 'epimysial fasciae' also includes the perimysium.

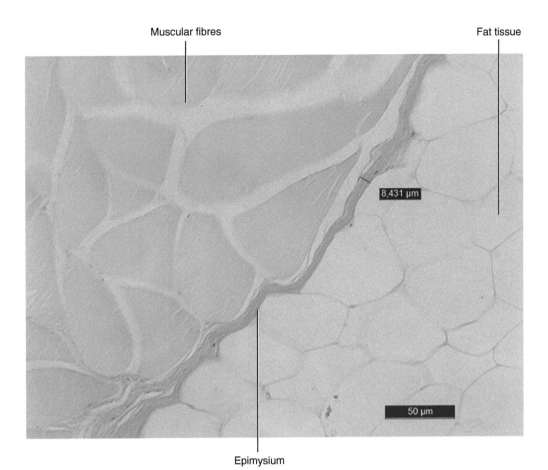

Muscular fibres

Fat tissue

8,431 µm

50 µm

Epimysium

FIGURE 3.41 Epimysium of the muscle of a rat, stained with Alcian blue, that is specific for the glycosaminoglycans. It is evident that the epimysium stains very well demonstrating a high concentration of glycosaminoglycans (HA).

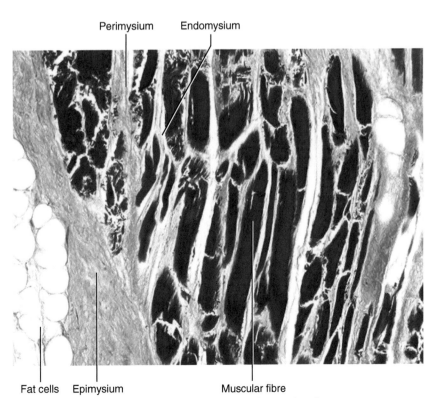

Perimysium   Endomysium

Fat cells   Epimysium

Muscular fibre

FIGURE 3.42 Section of muscle. Azan-Mallory stains the connective tissue blue and the muscle red.

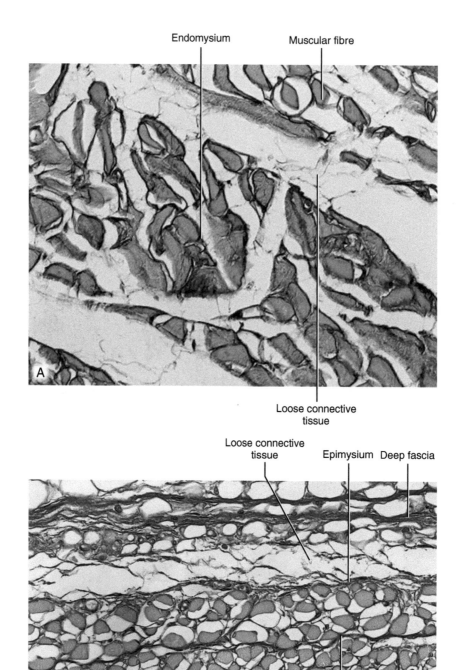

Endomysium   Muscular fibre

A

Loose connective
tissue

Loose connective
tissue   Epimysium Deep fascia

B

Endomysium   Muscular cells   Perimysium

FIGURE 3.43 Stains of endomysium and perimysium. **(A)** The antibody highlights in brown the collagen type III, particularly abundant in the endomysium. **(B)** Immunohistochemical stain: anti-HA binding protein, enlargement 400×, section of a mouse muscle. The HA is stained in brown. It is evident that the epimysium enveloping the muscle stained very well, as did the perimysium and endomysium using this stain. This indicates that the HA is present in high quantities in all these structures, and permits gliding among the single muscular fibres (HA in the endomysium), among fascicles (perimysium) and between muscle and surrounding structures (epimysium).

the endomysium. Rowe (1981) divides the perimysium into three recognizable layers of collagen fibres:

- Superficial: straight fibres with a smaller diameter and spread out without a definite direction. They intersect with each other forming a disorganized network.

- Intermediate: larger diameter fibres, flattened and curved, that intersect in their course with an average angle of 55° with respect to the resting muscular fibres. If the fibres are recruited, the angle increases up to 80° and decreases to 20° when the muscular fibres are stretched.

- Deep: comprises soft lamina that is in direct contact with the endomysium. The space between the collagen fibres is significantly increased giving it a discreet laxity.

It is evident that the perimysium, with its multilayered organization of collagen fibres, is similar to the epimysium. Therefore, both can be classified as dense regular connective tissue with a fundamental role in force transmission generated in the muscle towards the bone levers. The direction of the collagen fibres changes with the state of the muscle, confirming how much the perimysium is related to the activity of the muscle itself. Rowe (1981) postulated that the perimysium connects various muscular fibres and is able to transmit forces between the adjacent synergistic muscular fibre bundles, whether or not they belong to the same motor unit. The presence of a constant basal tone of muscle fibres maintains the perimysium and epimysium in a state of permanent tension more or less elevated. The epimysial fasciae, formed by perimysium and epimysium, could be considered an organized framework that transmits the forces produced in the locomotor system (Passerieux et al 2007, Trotter & Purslow 1992).

The perimysium is rich in HA (McCombe et al 2001) and this helps to assure the autonomy/gliding among the various muscular fibres (Fig. 3.43B). The perimysium also forms the intramuscular neurovascular tracts which are the 'collagen fibre reinforced sheets or bundles of connective tissues that envelop and protect blood vessels, lymph vessels, nerves and their branches' (Huijing & Jaspers 2005). The neurovascular tracts may also be attached to intermuscular septa, interosseal membranes and periostea, creating continuity between epimysial fasciae and aponeurotic fasciae.

Endomysium

The endomysium is the thinner portion of the intramuscular connective tissue and is directly in contact with and surrounds every single muscle fibre, forming its immediate external environment. It extends itself without interruption to the perimysium collagen. According to Trotter and Purslow (1992) and Passerieux et al (2007), it is composed of collagen fibre types III, IV and V, and a few collagen type I. Type IV is associated with the basal lamina that invests each muscle fibre (Standring et al 2008). Järvinen et al

(2002) used a scanning electron microscope to demonstrate three separate networks of collagen fibres in the endomysium of rat skeletal muscles: fibres running longitudinally on the surface of the muscle fibres (the main collagen orientation), fibres running perpendicularly to the long axis of the muscle fibres and having contact with adjacent muscle fibres, and fibres attached to the intramuscular nerves and arteries. With regards to the longitudinal axis of the muscle fibre, the collagen of the endomysium appears wavy and arranged in fascicles that are predominantly oblique. The paucity of collagen type I and the abundance of extracellular matrix rich in HA suggests that the endomysium has a limited role in the transmission of the muscular force. The endomysium is the key element that separates single muscle fibres from one another. It allows their autonomous gliding during muscle contraction. The endomysium is also a highly deformable tissue that adapts itself to the changes of volume that occur during the muscle fibre contraction. Another important function of endomysium is to regulate the metabolic exchange between muscle and blood.

Mechanical Behaviour

The epimysial fasciae are a major contributor to the mechanical strength of muscles. The arrangement and

---

CLINICAL PEARL 3.8 ROLE OF IMMOBILIZATION IN THE INTRAMUSCULAR CONNECTIVE TISSUE

According to the studies of Järvinen et al (2002), immobilization results in a marked increase in the endo- and perimysial connective tissues. The majority of the increased endomysial collagen is deposited directly on the sarcolemma of the muscle cells. Immobilization of the endomysium also results in a substantial increase in the number of perpendicularly orientated collagen fibres that make contact with two adjacent muscle fibres. Further, immobilization clearly disturbs the normal structure of the endomysium making it impossible to distinguish the various networks of fibres from one another.

In the perimysium, immobilization-induced changes were similar. The number of longitudinally orientated collagen fibres increased, the connective tissue became very dense, the number of irregularly orientated collagen fibres markedly increase and, consequently, the different networks of collagen fibres could not be distinguished from each other. Even the crimp angle of the collagen fibres decreased over 10% in all muscles after the immobilization period. It is apparent, from the above mentioned, that quantitative and qualitative changes in the intramuscular connective tissue contribute significantly to the decreased function and deteriorated biomechanical properties of immobilized skeletal muscles.

orientation of the collagen and elastic fibres within the epimysial fasciae helps regulate a muscle's mechanical behaviour. The epimysial fascia provides a definite resistance to tension along the same direction as the muscular fibres, and also takes the role of containment due to its organization into concentric layers of collagen, thereby limiting muscle expansion. The elasticity of epimysial fasciae is essential for allowing volume variations in muscles. Epimysial fascia also participates in the transmission of muscle force by its connection with the perimysium, its direct attachment with fibres from parts of adjoining muscles and the sliding that occurs between muscles and surrounding structures. Every time a muscle is stretched, the epimysial fasciae are stretched and then return to their basal state.

Epimysial fascia, from a physical point of view, could be considered as:

- An isotropic material (of equal physical properties along all axes) that responds to applied pressure, depending on the orthogonally directed forces exerted on its surface by the muscular mass and by the surrounding elements in the three planes of space. All of the above are dependent on the constituents of the extracellular matrix.

- An anisotropic (directionally dependent) material in relation to traction. Its resistance to deformation varies depending on the disposition and orientation of its fibres.

Epimysial fascia, from a functional point of view, relates to:

- Containment, i.e. limiting the expansion of the muscle with its structure of concentric layers of collagen.

- A transmitter of forces received from the muscle. These forces are transmitted directly to the tendons (in series) and to the aponeurotic fascia (in parallel).

- An integral part of the sliding surface for the muscles and surrounding structures.

MUSCULAR FORCE TRANSMISSION

The epimysial fasciae have a highly specific anatomical organization and a strong connection with the underlying muscles. It is evident that the thinness and close relationship between epimysial fasciae and muscles implies that the role of these fasciae in movement cannot be separated from the action of the muscles. The term 'myofascial complex' refers, for example, to both the pectoralis major and the pectoral fascia that transmit the muscular force connecting the upper limb to the trunk. This myofascial complex allows muscles to modulate the transmission of tension between different segments of the body, especially between the upper and lower limbs.

Huijing et al (2005) demonstrated how 30–40% of the force generated by muscles is transmitted not along the tendon, but rather by the connective tissue surrounding the muscle. The presence of a constant basal tone of the muscle fibres maintains the epimysial fasciae in a state of permanent tension: more or less elevated. Many muscle fibres do not necessarily extend from origin to insertion (nonspanning muscles) but have tapered ends in the middle of the muscle belly and end within the muscle belly. These muscles can only transmit force between adjacent muscle fibres via their common perimysium, emphasizing the idea that force transmission can occur by pathways other than myotendinous routes (Huijing & Baan 2001). The force expressed by a muscle depends not only on its anatomical structure but also on the angle at which its fibres are attached to the intramuscular connective tissue and the relation with the epimyseal and aponeurotic fasciae (Turrina et al 2013). According to Van Leeuwen and Spoor (1992), there are several factors responsible for the force of a muscle contraction: the anatomical structure of the muscle, the angle at which its fibres are attached to the epimysium, the tendon components, and the pressure created during the contraction with respect to the internal pressure of the muscle (based on the muscle tissue and blood). Of high importance is the balance of the basal tone of the muscle that counteracts the tension of the epimysial fasciae.

Innervation of the Epimysial Fascia: Role of the Muscle Spindles

The epimysial fasciae have free nerve endings but lack Pacinian and Ruffini corpuscles. Despite this, the epimysial fasciae play a key role in proprioception and peripheral motor coordination due to their close relationship with muscle spindles (Fig. 3.44).

Muscle spindles are small sensory organs inside striated muscles. They are enclosed in a capsule and have both sensory and motor components. The capsule is a specialization of the epimysial fasciae and is in continuity with the perimysium (Cooper and Daniel 1956, Maier et al 1999, Sherrington 1893, 1894). The motor component consists of several small, specialized muscle fibres, known as intrafusal fibres, localized at either end of the muscle spindle. The contraction of these muscular fibres is stimulated by the efferent gamma motor neurons. Another efferent motor neuron, the alpha motor neuron, innervates the extrafusal fibres. The alpha motor neuron and all the extrafusal muscle fibres that it innervates form the motor unit. Gamma motor neurons are 31% of the motor fibres of muscles and this high percentage demonstrates the important role of muscle spindles. The sensory component is localized in the central area of the spindles, where specialized nerve endings termed annulospiral (for their spiral arrangement) and flower spray (because they spread out on the fibre surface like a spray of flowers) are present. The annulospiral endings (Ia) provide information about the length and velocity of muscle contraction, the flower-spray endings (group II afferents) provide information on muscle length, even when the muscle is at rest. For example, they

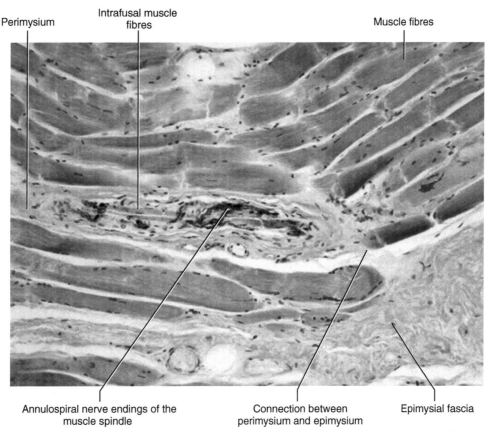

Perimysium | Intrafusal muscle fibres | Muscle fibres

Annulospiral nerve endings of the muscle spindle | Connection between perimysium and epimysium | Epimysial fascia

FIGURE 3.44 Muscle spindle inside the perimysium of a muscle. The perimysium is in continuous contact with the epimysial fascia. Immunohistochemical stain: anti-S100, the nerve elements stain in brown.

indicate the position of an arm after it has stopped moving. When the muscle lengthens and the muscle spindle is stretched, mechanically gated ion channels in the sensory dendrites are opened. This leads to a receptor potential that triggers action potentials in the muscle spindle afferent. Their threshold corresponds to a tension of 3 g. When stretched, the firing of the spindle Ia back to the spinal cord increases, stimulating the alpha motor neurons that cause contraction of the extrafusal fibres. At the same time Ia spindle afferents synapse in the posterior horn of the cord and stimulate inhibitory interneurons. These depress alpha motor activity to the antagonistic muscles. This occurs with the simple myotatic/stretch reflex that acts as a servomechanism to maintain the correct muscle tone. Muscle tone (residual muscle tension or tonus) is the continuous and partial contraction of the muscles, or the muscle's resistance to passive stretch during the resting state. Tone helps maintain posture and it declines during REM sleep (O'Sullivan 2007). Imagine carrying a heavy package for a distance and your biceps become fatigued. Even though the biceps are maximally contracting they will begin to stretch and this will activate the spindle cells, allowing the biceps to increase their contraction. This is an example of how the spindle cells can compensate for muscle fatigue and reflexively create a stronger contraction. If the muscle spindle cannot be activated,

the regulation of muscle tone will be compromised (Leonard 1998).

The role of the gamma motor neurons is generally believed to maintain muscle spindle sensitivity, regardless of muscle length. When the extrafusal fibres have been stimulated to contract by alpha motor neuron activation, the gamma motor neuron is simultaneously excited, stimulating contraction at the two ends of the intrafusal fibre, readjusting the length of the muscle spindle and keeping the central region of the intrafusal fibre taut. This is necessary to keep the muscle spindle afferent responsive and is known as 'alpha–gamma coactivation'.

Ultrasonography shows that movement and tension of the epimysial fascia of a muscle occurs before the contraction of the muscle at its origin and insertion. The muscle belly deforms itself in the three planes of space simultaneously, and the change in volume and form of the belly anticipates its longitudinal shortening. This deformation is due to the contraction of the muscle spindles that work like a probe, discerning the state of the muscle before contraction. If the epimysial fascia is rigid the muscle spindles are unable to change their length, and so the contraction of the extrafusal muscular fibres will be altered, even if the alpha motor neurons stimulate the muscular fibres in the correct way. This results in a diminution of muscular force and limitation of movement.

Considering the relationship between muscle spindles and fascia, the importance of fascia becomes especially evident with regards to its affect on peripheral motor coordination. By analysing the septum of the supinator, Strasmann et al (1990) found that many muscle spindles are inserted directly into the connective tissue of the septum. Von Düring and Andres (1994) studied the evolution of the locomotor system and discovered that muscle spindles are strongly connected to the fascia. Based on this information, it appears that the term 'muscle spindle cell' should be replaced with the term 'fascial spindle cell'. Due to these connections, it is evident that every time a myofascial expansion stretches a portion of deep fascia it also lengthens the muscle spindles connected with it, activating them by passive stretch. This causes the reflex contraction of the extrafusal muscle bundles connected with those spindles. This mechanism can increase the joint stability during movement and could explain the coactivation of different motor units of different segments. If epimysial fascia is overstretched by a myofascial expansion, it is possible that the muscle spindles connected to this portion of the fascia could become chronically stretched and overactivated (Fig. 3.45). This implies that the associated muscular fibres will be constantly stimulated to contract and could explain the increased amount of acetylcholine found in myofascial pain and, in particular, in trigger points (McPartland 2004, Mense 2004). This passive fascial stretch situation could be responsible for muscular imbalances and result in incorrect movement of joints. This may represent a typical case where there is limitation of joint range of motion and associated joint pain. The causation is often found in the proximal muscles that move the joint. Palpation of the proximal muscle belly will often reveal a painful area of localized dense tissue, usually where a significant amount of spindle cells are located.

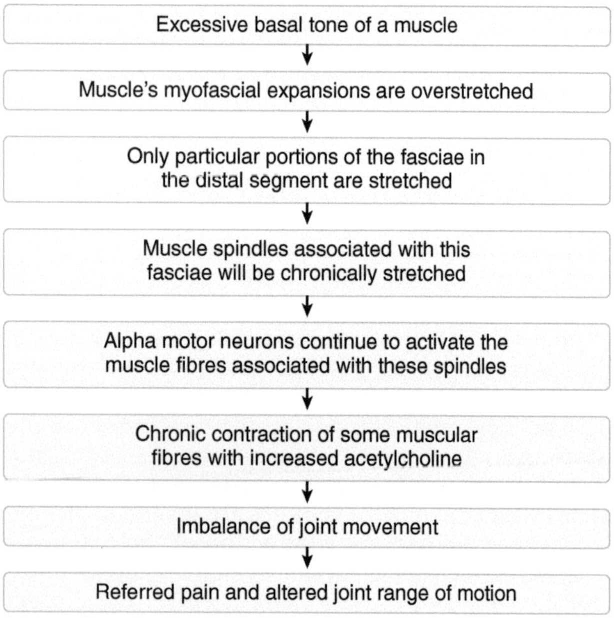

To perceive body position and joint range of motion, it is necessary for muscle spindles to be mapped in a well-defined structure. All the receptors of sensation, such as the vestibular and ocular system and peripheral areas, have neuronal maps emanating from the central nervous system. We suggest that the epimysial fascia could be considered the structure that supports the proprioceptive map peripherally, acting as a coachman: where the horses correspond to the various motor units performing a specific movement. Mense (2011), an expert on muscle pain and neurophysiology, affirms that:

Structural disorders of the fascia can surely distort the information sent by the spindles to the central nervous system and thus can interfere with proper coordinated movement. Particularly, the primary spindle afferents (Ia fibres) are so sensitive that even slight distortions of the perimysium will change their discharge frequency.

For example, if the perimysium is altered after immobilization, as Järvinen et al (2002) have demonstrated, it is probable that the muscle spindles embedded in the perimysium will not function correctly (Fig. 3.46). This emphasizes the fact that normal muscular function is dependent on a normal hydrated functioning fascia. Muscle spindles inform the central nervous system of the continually changing status of muscle tone, movement, loss of normal elasticity, position of body parts, absolute length of the muscle, and rate of change (velocity) of the length of the muscle. For this to occur, muscle spindles must be embedded in an adaptable structure that permits lengthening and shortening. The question arises: what happen to the muscle spindles if the epimysial fascia becomes altered due to trauma, poor posture, surgery or overuse? Fascial densification may inhibit normal spindle cell function (ability to be

---

Excessive basal tone of a muscle
↓
Muscle's myofascial expansions are overstretched
↓
Only particular portions of the fasciae in the distal segment are stretched
↓
Muscle spindles associated with this fasciae will be chronically stretched
↓
Alpha motor neurons continue to activate the muscle fibres associated with these spindles
↓
Chronic contraction of some muscular fibres with increased acetylcholine
↓
Imbalance of joint movement
↓
Referred pain and altered joint range of motion

FIGURE 3.45 Possible effect on motor coordination of chronically overstretched myofascial expansion.

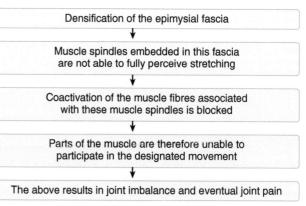

Densification of the epimysial fascia
↓
Muscle spindles embedded in this fascia are not able to fully perceive stretching
↓
Coactivation of the muscle fibres associated with these muscle spindles is blocked
↓
Parts of the muscle are therefore unable to participate in the designated movement
↓
The above results in joint imbalance and eventual joint pain

FIGURE 3.46 Possible consequence of densification of the epimysial fascia. Alteration of the muscle spindle environment prevents stretching of the annulospiral endings of the spindle cell and consequently interrupts the normal function of muscle spindles.

stretched). Inhibition of normal spindle cell stretching could result in abnormal feedback to the central nervous system. If the epimysial fascia becomes dense, then some parts of a muscle will not function normally during movement and will alter the vectors of force acting on a joint. This causes a unbalanced movement of the joint, and results in uncoordinated movement and eventual joint pain. The epimysial fasciae could be considered as a key element in peripheral motor coordination and proprioception.

Imaging of the Deep Fasciae

The aponeurotic fasciae can be successfully evaluated with CT, MRI (particularly in T1-weighted sequences) and ultrasound. Unfortunately, the fascial system is usually not analysed by radiologists and surgeons. To date, very few papers discuss the findings related to the visualization of fascial alterations.

CLINICAL PEARL 3.9 ROLE OF ACIDIFICATION IN FASCIAL GLIDING

The loose connective tissue of the fasciae is an important reservoir for water, salts and other elements. It is also a potential reservoir for the accumulation of degradation products, such as lactate. An accumulation of these products over time could alter the biomechanical properties of the loose connective tissue. Alteration of the loose connective tissue, as we have seen, can adversely affect the sliding motion of fascial layers and can cause myofascial dysfunction. Interactions among HA, lactate and alterations of pH in fascial tissues are of particular interest. Juel et al (2004) documented that when the pH inside muscles reaches 6.6, the athlete is at the stage of exhaustion. At pH 6.6, the viscosity of HA present in the endomysium and perimysium of muscles significantly increases. Gatej et al (2005) documents that at pH 6.6 (normal value is pH 7.4) the complex viscosity of HA approaches 5 Pa•s instead of the typical 3.8 Pa•s. This increase in viscosity can explain the typical stiffness experienced by athletes after prolonged intense activity (marathons, endurance games, etc). This type of stiffness usually disappears with rest and a full restoration of painless range of motion occurs. The acidification of the fascial loose connective tissue is not the only component that creates stiffness. Overuse syndromes or trauma could alter the viscosity of the fascia, promoting stiffness throughout the surrounding areas. One reason for postexercise pain and loss of motion remaining in a percentage of people may be that they have a high-viscosity profile. Overused or post-traumatic areas with increased viscosity may already exist and a high-viscosity profile may be maintained. From a clinical point of view, such areas can be defined as undergoing densification. They constitute potential trigger point
type areas and may be responsible for the myofascial pain syndrome.

In T1-weighted sequences of MRI, the aponeurotic fasciae appear as low-signal intensity lines, sharply delineated in the subcutaneous tissue (Fig. 3.47). They can be better recognized when abundant loose connective tissue is present between the deep fascia and the underlying muscle, while it is difficult to evaluate where strong connections between fascia and the underlying muscles exists. In the axial images the aponeurotic fasciae show a mean thickness of 1 mm (range 0.9–1.2 mm). In general, the axial and coronal T1-weighted spin-echo MR images best depict the anatomic features of the aponeurotic fasciae. This is because of the orientation of these images and the contrast provided by the low-signal intensity of the fasciae and high-signal intensity of the surrounding fat (Numkarunarunrote et al 2007).

With MRI and CT it is possible to appreciate the continuities of retinacula with their respective fasciae. Delineation between retinacula and fasciae is based only on the relative change in thickness of the fascia as it forms the retinacula. Some recent studies have highlighted alterations of the retinacula. Demondion et al (2010) found that with MRI it was possible to analyse differences in thickness between various retinacula. These images showed specific alterations: such as oedema, full or partial interruption of retinacular continuities, thickening or adhesion with the subcutaneous layers and abnormal increased signal on T2-weighted images. All of the above alterations were demonstrated in the ankle retinacula of patients with severe sprains (Stecco et al 2011). In patellofemoral malalignment the medial and lateral retinacula of the knee also demonstrated differences in thickness and/or tension.

With MRI and CT it is possible to appreciate the continuity of the aponeurotic fasciae around the tendons (e.g. the crural fascia forms a basket around the calcaneal tendon) and around the neurovascular bundles. In clinical practice ultrasonoghaphy can be performed less expensively than other noninvasive methods. It allows the practitioner to see the fasciae with high resolution and to measure the thickness of the various sublayers (Figs 3.48 and 3.49). This is the only technique that permits the analysis of sliding between fascia and muscle and between the various fascial sublayers. Langevin et al (2011) used ultrasonoghaphy to demonstrate that TLF shear strain was 20% lower in human subjects with chronic low-back pain. Males seem to have significantly lower shear strain than females in the thoracolumbar fascia. The authors also showed a significant correlation in male subjects among TLF shear strain and echogenicity ($r = -0.28$, $P < 0.05$), trunk flexion range of motion ($r = 0.36$, $P < 0.01$), trunk extension range of motion ($r = 0.41$, $P < 0.01$), repeated forward-bend task duration ($r = -0.54$, $P < 0.0001$) and repeated sit-to-stand task duration ($r = -0.45$, $P < 0.001$). Stecco et al (2014b) recently demonstrated, with ultrasonography, that aponeurotic fascia increases its thickness (mean value 0.4 mm) in pathological conditions. This increase is due more to the increased thickness of the loose connective tissue layers (glycosaminoglycans, hyaluronic acid) than the fibrous

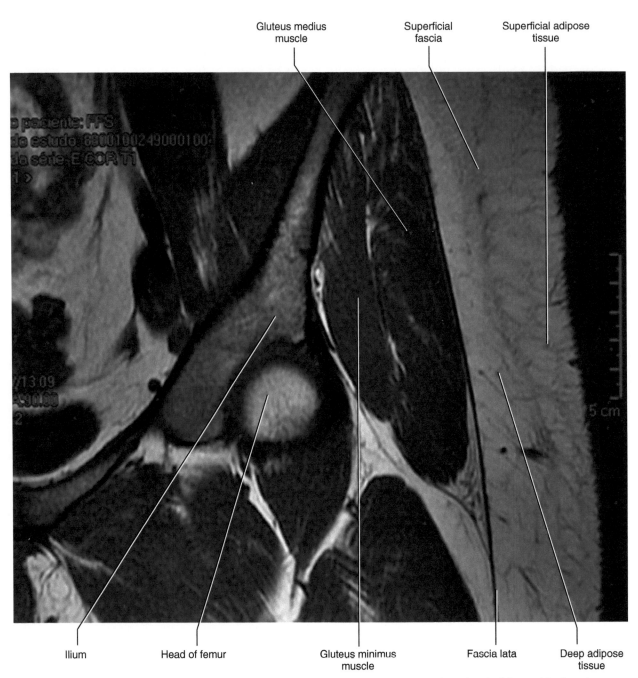

Gluteus medius
muscle

Superficial
fascia

Superficial adipose
tissue

5 cm

Ilium

Head of femur

Gluteus minimus
muscle

Fascia lata

Deep adipose
tissue

FIGURE 3.47 MRI of the hip. The aponeurotic fascia (fascia lata) appear as a low-signal intensity line, sharply delineated in the subcutaneous tissue, thanks to the abundant loose connective tissue present between it and the underlying muscle. The superficial fascia is less defined, but the two different aspects of the DAT and SAT are clearly evident.

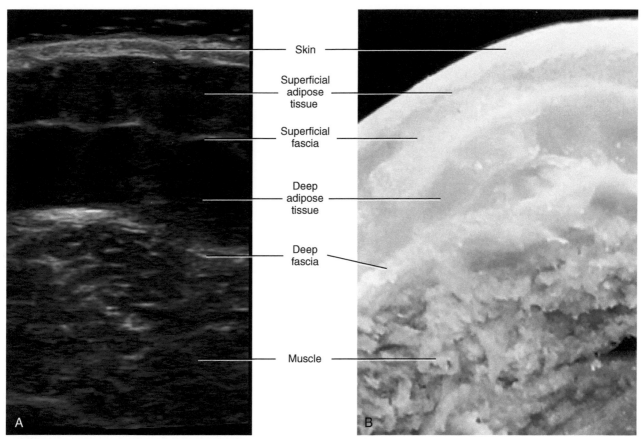

Skin

Superficial
adipose
tissue

Superficial
fascia

Deep
adipose
tissue

Deep
fascia

Muscle

FIGURE 3.48 Comparison of an ultrasound image **(A)** with a cadaver dissection **(B)** at the anterior region of the thigh. The deep fascia is easier to evaluate with dissection **(B)**, appearing as a white fibrous layer distinctly different from the surrounding tissues. Ultrasound **(A)** shows a similar ecogenicity between the deep fascia and the muscle so that the deep fascia can only be evaluated where the loose connective tissue divides the muscle from the deep fascia. Superficial fascia is easier to evaluate with ultrasound since it presents a hyperechogenic layer in the middle of the fatty tissue. In cadavers, only a careful dissection permits us to isolate the superficial fascia from hypodermis. SAT: superficial adipose tissue; DAT: deep adipose tissue.

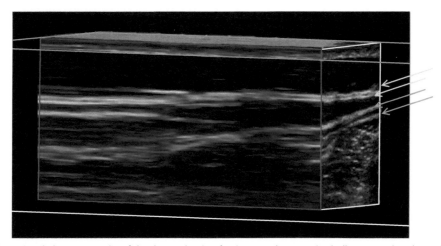

FIGURE 3.49 Three-dimensional ultrasonography of the thoracolumbar fascia. Note the posterior (yellow arrows) and anterior (blue arrows) layers, formed by two fibrous sublayers each. Between the fibrous sublayers, loose connective tissue is present. (Reproduced with permission from Dr Jouko Heiskanen, MD, PT, Senior lecturer in physiotherapy, Helsinki Metropolia University).

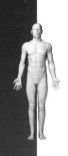

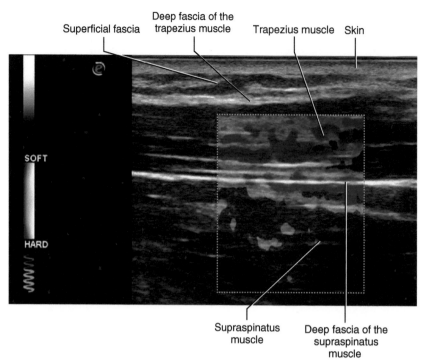

Superficial fascia · Deep fascia of the trapezius muscle · Trapezius muscle · Skin

SOFT

HARD

Supraspinatus muscle · Deep fascia of the supraspinatus muscle

FIGURE 3.50 Elastosonography of the supraspinal region of the shoulder. The machine stains in blue the hard tissues, in red the soft tissues, and in green the in-between tissues. In this patient, the supraspinal fascia is the hardest tissue.

CLINICAL PEARL 3.10 FIBROSIS VERSUS DENSIFICATION

From an anatomical point of view it has not always been easy to distinguish between fascial dysfunction and fascial pathology. Recently, imaging and dissections have helped to clarify these differences. Pathology correlates with a rearrangement of the composition and structure of the dense connective tissue (collagen types I and III). We suggest that fibrosis can, therefore, be defined as an alteration of dense connective tissue. This can be recognized by an increase in quantity of the collagen fibres usually accompanied by a hyperintense signal. This type of fascial pathology is easy to recognize with MRI, CAT scans and ultrasonography.

Fascial densification refers to an alteration of the loose connective tissue (adipose cells, glycosaminoglycans and HA). Densification (dysfunction) can involve an alteration in the quantity or quality of the components of loose connective tissue and an alteration in fascial viscosity. This differs from pathology since there is no macroscopic alteration of the morphology of the fascia that would be seen on dissection or biopsy. We feel that densification of fascia is the underlying reason for what is known as the myofascial pain syndrome.

were unable to diagnose fibromas, as the signals emitted were similar to those for normal fascia. To obtain high-resolution images of fasciae, it is still necessary to use linear probes with operating frequencies of 12–18 MHz.

An evolution of ultrasound is sonoelastography (Fig. 3.50). This is a computational technique that uses cross-correlation methods to quantify tissue motion based on a series of ultrasound images acquired in rapid succession. Wu et al (2011) used sonoelastography to demonstrate that plantar fascia softens with age in subjects with plantar fasciitis.

To conclude, the fasciae can be visualized in vivo both with MRI, CT and ultrasound. Both MRI and CT can provide an objective picture of fasciae and their alterations. It is easier to interpret the location of fascial layers with MRI and CT compared to ultrasound. Ultrasound is less expensive and allows analysis of the gliding and the structure of the sublayers. Sonography and elastography show great promise for the future study of fasciae in medical practices to complement physical examination, support the diagnosis of myofascial pain and evaluate treatment outcomes. It is of course necessary that clinicians using ultrasound to study fasciae have a complete understanding of its anatomy and the concept of fascial layer impairment.

layers (collagen type I), and means that myofascial pain is more likely due to fascial densification than fibrosis.

McNally and Shetty (2010) believe that ultrasound is superior to MRI for the diagnosis of fascial alterations. In evaluating plantar fibromas using MRI they

References

Abu-Hijleh, M.F., Harris, P.F., 2007. Deep fascia on the dorsum of the ankle and foot: extensor retinacula revisited. Clin. Anat. 20 (2), 186–195.

Bednar, D.A., Orr, F.W., Simon, G.T., 1995. Observations on the pathomorphology of the thoracolumbar fascia in chronic mechanical back pain. Spine 20 (10), 1161–1164.

Benetazzo, L., Bizzego, A., De Caro, R., Frigo, G., Guidolin, D., Stecco, C., 2011. 3D reconstruction of the crural and thoracolumbar fasciae. Surg. Radiol. Anat. 33 (10), 855–862.

Benjamin, M., Qin, S., Ralphs, J.R., 1995. Fibrocartilage associated with human tendons and their pulleys. J. Anat. 187 (Pt 3), 625–633.

Benjamin, M., Ralphs, J.R., 1998. Fibrocartilage in tendons and ligaments–an adaptation to compressive load. J. Anat. 193 (Pt 4), 481–494.

Benjamin, M., 2009. The fascia of the limbs and back: A review. J. Anat. 214 (1), 1–18.

Benninghoff, A., Goerttler, K., 1978. Lehrbuch der Anatomie des Menschen, vol. 2. Urban & Schwarzenberg, München-Berlin-Wien, p. 398.

Bhattacharya, V., Barooah, P.S., Nag, T.C., Chaudhuri, G.R., Bhattacharya, S., 2010. Detail microscopic analysis of deep fascia of lower limb and its surgical implication. Indian J Plast Surg 43 (2), 135–140.

Bhattacharya, V., Watts, R.K., Reddy, G.R., 2005. Live demonstration of microcirculation in the deep fascia and its implication. Plast. Reconstr. Surg. 115 (2), 458–463.

Chiarugi, G., 1904. Istituzioni di Anatomia dell'uomo, vol. 1. Società editrice libraria, Milano, p. 146.

Chen, C.S., 2008. Mechanotransduction – a field pulling together? J. Cell Sci. 15 (121), 3285–3292.

Cooper, S., Daniel, P.M., 1956. Human muscle spindles. J. Physiol. 133 (1), 1–3P.

Deising, S., Weinkauf, B., Blunk, J., Obreja, O., Schmelz, M., Rukwied, R., 2012. NGF-evoked sensitization of muscle fascia nociceptors in humans. Pain 153 (8), 1673–1679.

Demondion, X., Canella, C., Moraux, A., Cohen, M., Bry, R., Cotten, A., 2010. Retinacular disorders of the ankle and foot. Semin. Musculoskelet. Radiol. 14 (3), 281–291.

Eames, M.H., Bain, G.I., Fogg, Q.A., van Riet, R.P., 2007. Distal biceps tendon anatomy: a cadaveric study. J. Bone Joint Surg. Am. 89 (5), 1044–1049.

Gao, Y., Kostrominova, T.Y., Faulkner, J.A., Wineman, A.S., 2008. Age-related changes in the mechanical properties of the epimysium in skeletal muscles of rats. J. Biomech. 41 (2), 465–469.

Gatej, I., Popa, M., Rinaudo, M., 2005. Role of the pH on hyaluronan behavior in aqueous solution. Biomacromolecules 6 (1), 61–67.

Geppert, M.J., Sobel, M., Bohne, W.H., 1993. Lateral ankle instability as a cause of superior peroneal retinacular laxity: an anatomic and biomechanical study of cadaveric feet. Foot Ankle 14 (6), 330–334.

Gerlach, U.J., Lierse, W., 1990. Functional construction of the superficial and deep fascia system of the lower limb in man. Acta. Anat. 139 (1), 11–25.

Huijing, P.A., 2009. Epimuscular myofascial force transmission: A historical review and implications for new research. J. Biomech. 42 (1), 9–21.

Huijing, P.A., Baan, G.C., 2001. Myofascial force transmission causes interaction between adjacent muscles and connective tissue: effects of blunt dissection and compartmental fasciotomy on length force characteristics of rat extensor digitorum longus muscle. Arch. Physiol. Biochem. 109 (2), 97–109.

Huijing, P.A., Jaspers, R.T., 2005. Adaptation of muscle size and myofascial force transmission: a review and some new experimental results. Scand. J. Med. Sci. Sports 15 (6), 349–380.

Hukinsa, D.W.L., Aspden, R.M., 1985. Composition and properties of connective tissues. Trends Biochem. Sci. 10 (7), 260–264.

Hurschler, C., Vanderby, R. Jr., Martinez, D.A., Vailas, A.C., Turnipseed, W.D., 1994. Mechanical and biochemical analyses of tibial compartment fascia in chronic compartment syndrome. Ann. Biomed. Eng. 22 (3), 272–279.

Ingber, D.E., 2003. Tensegrity II: How structural networks influence cellular information processing networks. J. cell Science 116 (8), 1397–1408.

Järvinen, T.A., Józsa, L., Kannus, P., Järvinen, T.L., Järvinen, M., 2002. Organization and distribution of intramuscular connective tissue in normal and immobilized skeletal muscles. An immunohistochemical, polarization and scanning electron microscopic study. J. Muscle Res. Cell Motil. 23 (3), 245–254.

Juel, C., Klarskov, C., Nielsen, J.J., Krustrup, P., Mohr, M., Bangsbo, J., 2004. Effect of high-intensity intermittent training on lactate and H+ release from human skeletal muscle. Am. J. Physiol. Endocrinol. Metab. 286 (2), E245–E251.

Klein, D.M., Katzman, B.M., Mesa, J.A., Lipton, F.L., Caligiuri, D.A., 1999. Histology of the extensor retinaculum of the wrist and the ankle. J. Hand Surg. 24 (4), 799–802.

Kumai, T., Benjamin, M., 2002. Heel spur formation and the subcalcaneal enthesis of the plantar fascia. J. Rheumatol. 29 (9), 1957–1964.

Langevin, H.M., Bouffard, N.A., Badger, G.J., Iatridis, J.C., Howe, A.K., 2005. Dynamic fibroblast cytoskeletal response to subcutaneous tissue stretch ex vivo and in vivo. Am. J. Physiol. Cell Physiol. 288 (3), C747–C756.

Langevin, H.M., Bouffard, N.A., Badger, G.J., Churchill, D.L., Howe, A.K., 2006. Subcutaneous tissue fibroblast cytoskeletal remodeling induced by acupuncture: evidence for a mechanotransduction-based mechanism. J. Cell. Physiol. 207 (3), 767–774.

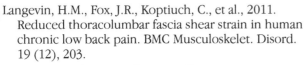

Langevin, H.M., Fox, J.R., Koptiuch, C., et al., 2011. Reduced thoracolumbar fascia shear strain in human chronic low back pain. BMC Musculoskelet. Disord. 19 (12), 203.

Laurent, C., Johnson-Wells, G., Hellström, S., Engström-Laurent, A., Wells, A.F., 1991. Localization of hyaluronan in various muscular tissues. A morphologic study in the rat. Cell Tissue Res. 263 (2), 201–205.

Leardini, A., O'Connor, J.J., 2002. A model for lever-arm length calculation of the flexor and extensor muscles at the ankle. Gait Posture 15 (3), 220–229.

Lee, J.Y., Spicer, A.P., 2000. Hyaluronan: a multifunctional, megaDalton, stealth molecule. Curr. Opin. Cell Biol. 12 (5), 581–586.

Leonard, C.T., 1998. The Neuroscience of Human Movement, Mosby, St Louis, MI, p. 21.

Maier, A., 1999. Proportions of slow myosin heavy chain-positive fibers in muscle spindles and adjoining extrafusal fascicles, and the positioning of spindles relative to these fascicles. J. Morphol. 242 (2), 157–165.

Marshall, R., 2001. Living anatomy: structure as the mirror of function, Melbourne University Press, Melbourne, p. 222.

Matteini, P., Dei, L., Carretti, E., Volpi, N., Goti, A., Pini, R., 2009. Structural behavior of highly concentrated hyaluronan. Biomacromolecules 10 (6), 1516–1522.

McCombe, D., Brown, T., Slavin, J., Morrison, W.A., 2001. The histochemical structure of the deep fascia and its structural response to surgery. J. Hand Surg. 26 (2), 89–97.

McNally, E.G., Shetty, S., 2010. Plantar fascia: imaging diagnosis and guided treatment. Semin. Musculoskelet. Radiol. 14 (3), 334–343.

Mense, S. (2011) Peripheral and central mechanisms of myofascial pain. Presented at Pittsburg Conference on Myofascial Component of Musculoskeletal Pain. University of Pittsburg, May 7–8.

Milz, S., Benjamin, M., Putz, R., 2005. Molecular parameters indicating adaptation to mechanical stress in fibrous connective tissue. Adv. Anat. Embryol. Cell Biol. 178, 1–71.

Milz, S., Rufai, A., Buettner, A., Putz, R., Ralphs, J.R., Benjamin, M., 2002. Three-dimensional reconstructions of the Achilles tendon insertion in man. J. Anat. 200 (Pt 2), 145–152.

Numkarunarunrote, N., Malik, A., Aguiar, R.O., Trudell, D.J., Resnick, D., 2007. Retinacula of the foot and ankle: MRI with anatomic correlation in cadavers. Am. J. Roentgenol. 188 (4), 348–354.

O'Sullivan, S.B., 2007. Examination of motor function: Motor control and motor learning. In: O'Sullivan, S.B., Schmitz, T.J. (Eds.), Physical rehabilitation, fifth ed. FA Davis Company, Philadelphia, pp. 233–234.

Palmieri, G., Panu, R., Asole, A., 1986. Macroscopic organization and sensitive innervation of the tendinous intersection and the lacertus fibrosus of the biceps brachii muscle in the ass end horse. Arch. Anat. Hist. Embr. Norm. Et. Exp. 69, 73–82.

Passerieux, E., Rossignol, R., Letellier, T., Delage, J.P., 2007. Physical continuity of the perimysium from myofibers to tendons: involvement in lateral force transmission in skeletal muscle. J. Struct. Biol. 159 (1), 19–28.

Platzer, W., 1978. Locomotor System. In: Kahle, W., Leonhardt, H., Platzer, W. (Eds.), Color Atlas and Textbook of Human Anatomy, ed. 1. Georg Thieme Publishers, Stuttgart, pp. 148–164.

Piehl-Aulin, K., Laurent, C., Engström-Laurent, A., 1991. Hyaluronan in human skeletal muscle of lower extremity: concentration, distribution, and effect of exercise. J. Appl. Physiol. 71 (6), 2493–2498.

Pisani, G., 2004. Trattato di chirurgia del piede, Minerva Medica, Torino, pp. 25–40.

Purslow, P.P., 1989. Strain-induced reorientation of an intramuscular connective tissue network: implications for passive muscle elasticity. J. Biomech. 22 (1), 21–31.

Purslow, P.P., 2010. Muscle fascia and force transmission. J. Bodywork Mov. Ther. 14 (4), 411–417.

Rowe, R.W., 1981. Morphology of perimysial and endomysial connective tissue in skeletal muscle. Tissue Cell 13 (4), 681–690.

Sakamoto, Y., 1996. Histological features of endomysium, perimysium and epimysium in rat lateral pterygoid muscle. J. Morphol. 227 (1), 113–119.

Sanchis-Alfonso, V., Rosello-Sasrte, E., 2000. Immunohistochemical analysis for neural markers of the lateral retinaculum in patients with isolated symptomatic patellofemoral malalignment. A neuroanatomic basis for anterior knee pain in the active young patient. Me.r J. Sports Med. 28 (5), 725–731.

Schleip, R., Klingler, W., Lehmann-Horn, F., 2005. Active fascial contractility: Fascia may be able to contract in a smooth muscle-like manner and thereby influence musculoskeletal dynamics. Med. Hypotheses 65 (2), 273–277.

Sherrington, C.S., 1894. On the Anatomical Constitution of Nerves of Skeletal Muscles; with Remarks on Recurrent Fibres in the Ventral Spinal Nerve-root. J. Physiol. 17 (3–4), 210.2–258.

Snow, S.W., Bohne, W.H., DiCarlo, E., Chang, V.K., 1995. Anatomy of the Achilles tendon and plantar fascia in relation to the calcaneus in various age groups. Foot Ankle Int. 16 (7), 418–421.

Sobel, M., Geppert, M.J., Warren, R.F., 1993. Chronic ankle instability as a cause of peroneal tendon injury. Clin. Orthop. Relat. Res. 11 (296), 187–191.

Spicer, A.P., Tien, J.Y., 2004. Hyaluronan and morphogenesis. Birth Defects Res. C Embryo Today 72 (1), 89–108.

Standring, S., 2008. Gray's Anatomy, fortieth ed. Elsevier Health Sciences UK, pp. 108–109.

Stecco, A., Gilliar, W., Brad, S., Stecco, C., 2013a. The anatomical and functional relation between gluteus maximus and fascia lata. J. Bodywork Mov. Ther. 17 (4), 512–517.

Stecco, A., Macchi, V., Masiero, S., et al., 2009a. Pectoral and femoral fasciae: common aspects and regional specializations. Surg. Radiol. Anat. 31 (1), 35–42.

Stecco, A., Meneghini, A., Stern, R., Stecco, C., Imamura, M., 2014b. Ultrasonography in myofascial neck pain: randomized clinical trial for diagnosis and follow up. Surg. Radiol. Anat. 36 (3), 243–253.

Stecco, A., Stecco, C., Macchi, V., et al., 2011. RMI study and clinical correlations of ankle retinacula damage and outcomes of ankle sprain. Surg. Radiol. Anat. 33 (10), 881–890.

Stecco, C., Gagey, O., Belloni, A., et al., 2007a. Anatomy of the deep fascia of the upper limb, part 2: study of innervation. Morphologie 91 (292), 38–43.

Stecco, C., Gagey, O., Macchi, V., et al., 2007b. Anatomical study of myofascial continuity in the anterior region of the upper limb. Tendinous muscular insertions onto the deep fascia of the upper limb. First part: anatomical study. Morphologie 91 (292), 29–37.

Stecco, C., Macchi, V., Porzionato, A., et al., 2010a. The ankle retinacula: morphological evidence of the proprioceptive role of the fascial system. Cells Tissues Organs 192 (3), 200–210.

Stecco, C., Macchi, V., Lancerotto, L., Tiengo, C., Porzionato, A., De Caro, R., 2010b. Comparison of transverse carpal ligament and flexor retinaculum terminology for the wrist. J. Hand Surg. [Am] 35 (5), 746–753.

Stecco, C., Pavan, P.G., Porzionato, A., et al., 2009b. Mechanics of crural fascia: from anatomy to constitutive modelling. Surg. Radiol. Anat. 31 (7), 523–529.

Stecco, C., Pavan, P., Pachera, P., De Caro, R., Natali, A., 2014a. Investigation of the mechanical properties of the human crural fascia and their possible clinical implications. Surg. Radiol. Anat. 36 (1), 25–32.

Stecco, C., Porzionato, A., Macchi, V., et al., 2008. The expansions of the pectoral girdle muscles onto the brachial fascia: morphological aspects and spatial disposition. Cells Tissues Organs 188 (3), 320–329.

Stecco, L. (1990) Il dolore e le sequenze neuro-mio-fasciali. IPSA ed, Palermo.

Stilwell, D., 1957. Regional variations in the innervation of deep fasciae and aponeuroses. Anat. Rec. 127 (4), 635–653.

Stedman's Medical Dictionary, ed. 26. 1995. Williams & Wilkins, Baltimore, p. 628.

Strasmann, T., 1990. Functional topography and ultrastructure of periarticular mechanoreceptors in the lateral elbow region of the rat. Acta. Anat. 138 (1), 1–14.

Tanaka, S., Ito, T., 1977. Histochemical demonstration of adrenergic fibers in the fascia periosteum and retinaculum. Clin. Orthop. Relat. Res. Jul-Aug (126), 276–281.

Tesarz, J., Hoheisel, U., Wiedenhöfer, B., Mense, S., 2011. Sensory innervation of the thoracolumbar fascia in rats and humans. Neuroscience. 27 (194), 302–308.

Testut, J.L., Jacob, O., 1905. Précis d'anatomie topographique avec applications medico-chirurgicales, vol. III. Gaston Doin et Cie, Paris, p. 302.

Toumi, H., Higashiyama, I., Suzuki, D., et al., 2006. Regional variations in human patellar trabecular architecture and the structure of the proximal patellar tendon enthesis. J. Anat. 208 (1), 47–57.

Trotter, J.A., Purslow, P.P., 1992. Functional morphology of the endomysium in series fibered muscles. J. Morphol. 212 (2), 109–122.

Turrina, A., Martinez-Gonzalez, M.A., Stecco, C., 2013. The muscular force transmission system: Role of the intramuscular connective tissue. J. Bodywork Mov. Ther. 17 (1), 95–102.

Turvey, M.T., 2007. Action and perception at the level of synergies. Hum. Mov. Sci. 26 (4), 657–697.

Tytherleigh-Strong, G., Baxandall, R., Unwin, A., 2000. Rupture of the ankle extensor retinaculum in a dancer. J. R. Soc. Med. 93 (12), 638–639.

Umidon, M., 1963. Architecture, topography and morphogenesis of the peroneal retinacula and the lateral annular ligament of the tarsus in man. Chir. Organi. Mov. 52, 305–317.

Van Leeuwen, J.L., Spoor, C.W., 1992. Modelling mechanically stable muscle architectures. Philos. Trans. R. Soc. Lond. B. Biol. Sci., Series B-Biological Sciences 336 (1277), 275–292.

Verleisdonk, E.J., Schmitz, R.F., van der Werken, C., 2004. Long-term results of fasciotomy of the anterior compartment in patients with exercise-induced pain in the lower leg. Int. J. Sports Med. 25 (3), 224–229.

Vesalio, A., 1543. De Humani Corporis Fabbrica, Ex officina Joannis Oporini, Basel.

Viladot, A., Lorenzo, J.C., Salazar, J., Rodríguez, A., 1984. The subtalar joint: embryology and morphology. Foot Ankle 5 (2), 54–66.

Von Düring, M., Andres, K.H., 1994. Topography and fine structure of proprioceptors in the hagfish, Myxine glutinosa. Eur. J. of Morph. 32 (2–4), 248–256.

Wavreille, G., Bricout, J., Mouliade, S., et al., 2010. Anatomical bases of the free posterior brachial fascial flap. Surg. Radiol. Anat. 32 (4), 393–399.

101

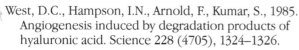

West, D.C., Hampson, I.N., Arnold, F., Kumar, S., 1985. Angiogenesis induced by degradation products of hyaluronic acid. Science 228 (4705), 1324–1326.

Wood, J.F., 1944. Structure and Function as Seen in the Foot, Baillière, Tindall and Cox, London.

Wu, C.H., Chang, K.V., Mio, S., Chen, W.S., Wang, T.G., 2011. Sonoelastography of the plantar fascia. Radiology 259 (2), 502–507.

Yahia, H., Rhalmi, S., Newman, N., 1992. Sensory innervation of human thoracolumbar fascia, an immunohistochemical study. Acta Orthop. Scand. 63 (2), 195–197.

Bibliography

Akhtar, M., Levine, J., 1980. Dislocation of extensor digitorum longus tendons after spontaneous rupture of the inferior retinaculum of the ankle. J. Bone Joint Surg. 62 (7), 1210–1211.

Baldissera, F., 1996. Fisiologia e Biofisica Medica. Poletto ed, Milano, pp. 110–113.

Borg-Stein, J., Simons, D.G., 2002. Myofascial Pain, focused review. Arch. Phys. Med. Rehabil. 83 (Suppl. 1), S40–S47.

Bourne, G.H., 1973. Structure and Function of Muscle, Academic Press, New York and London, pp. 365–384.

Chen, Y., Ding, M., Kelso, J.A.S., 1997. Long memory processes in human coordination. Physics Review Letters 79 (22), 4501–4504.

Engel, A.G., Franzini-Amstrong, C., 2004. Myology, McGraw Hill, New York, pp. 489–509.

Graven-Nielsen, T., Mense, S., Arendt-Nielsen, L., 2004. Painful and non-painful pressure sensations from human skeletal muscle. Exp. Brain Res. 159 (3), 273–283.

Guyton, A.C., 1996. Trattato di fisiologia medica. Piccin-Nuova Libraria, Padova.

Hoheisel, U., Taguchi, T., Treede, R.D., Mense, S., 2011. Nociceptive input from the rat thoracolumbar fascia to lumbar dorsal horn neurones. Eur. J. Pain 15 (8), 810–815.

Huijing, P.A., 1999. Muscular force transmission: A unified, dual or multiple system? A review and some explorative experimental results. Arch. Physiol. Biochem. 107 (4), 292–311.

Huijing, P.A., Bann, G.C., Rebel, G.T., 1998. Non-myotendinous force transmission in rat extensor digitorum longus muscle. J. Exp. Biol. 201 (5), 683–691.

Kjaer, M., 2004. Role of extracellular matrix in adaptation of tendon and skeletal muscle to mechanical loading. Physiol. Rev. 84 (2), 649–698.

Kokkorogiannis, T., 2004. Somatic and intramuscular distribution of muscle spindles and their relation to muscular angiotypes. J. of Theor. Biol. 229 (2), 263–280.

Lee, M.H., Chung, C.B., Cho, J.H., et al., 2006. Tibialis anterior tendon and extensor retinaculum: imaging in cadavers and patients with tendon tear. Am. J. Roentgenol. 187 (2), 161–168.

Mazzocchi, G., Nussdorfer, G., 1996. Anatomia funzionale del sistema nervoso. Ed Cortina Padova, p. 132.

McPartland, J.M., 2004. Travell trigger points: Molecular and osteopathic perspectives. JAOA 104 (6), 244–249.

Mense, S., 2004. Neurobiological basis for the use of botulinum toxin in pain therapy. J. Neurol. 251 (Suppl. 1), I1–I7.

Noble, P.W., 2002. Hyaluronan and its catabolic products in tissue injury and repair. Matrix Biol. 21 (1), 25–29.

Proske, U., Gandevia, S.C., 2009. Kinaesthetic Senses. J. Physiol. 587 (17), 4139–4146.

Purslow, P.P., Trotter, J.A., 1994. The morphology and mechanical properties of endomysium in series-fibred muscles; variations with muscle length. J. Muscle Res. Cell Motil. 15 (3), 299–304.

Sarrafian, S.K., 1983. Anatomy of the Foot and Ankle: Descriptive, Topographic, Functional. JB Lipincott, Philadelphia, pp. 127–129.

Sharafi, B., Blemker, S.S., 2011. A mathematical model of force transmission from intrafascicularly terminating muscle fibers. J. Biomech. 44 (11), 2031–2039.

Sherrington, C.S., 1893. Further experimental note on the correlation of action of antagonistic muscles. Br Med J. 1 (1693), 1218.

Stecco, L., 2004. Fascial Manipulation for Musculoskeletal Pain. Piccin ed, Padova.

Travell, J.G., Simons, D.G., 1998. Dolore Muscolare. Ghedini ed, Milano, pp. 25–38.

Windisch, G., Tesch, N.P., Grechenig, W., Peicha, G., 2006. The triceps brachii muscle and its insertion on the olecranon. Med. Sci. Monit. 12 (8), 290–294.

Zgonis, T., Jolly, G.P., Polyzois, V., Stamatis, E.D., 2005. Peroneal tendon pathology. Clin. Podiatr. Med. Surg. 22 (1), 79–85.

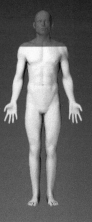

Fasciae of the Head and Neck

4

Introduction

The fasciae of the head and neck serve as an important proprioceptive organ and are often involved in tension-type headaches, temporomandibular joint (TMJ) pain, acute and chronic neck and shoulder pain, pain while chewing or swallowing, tinnitus, sinuses, vertigo and vision, to mention a few. So, knowledge of their anatomy and continuities are crucial for administering fascial treatments. One of the main obstacles to this understanding is that the head is divided into many regions that contain fasciae with different descriptive names (Fig. 4.1) (Davidge et al 2010, Guidera et al 2012). This hinders the description of the fascial continuity between the deep muscles of the head and neck. There are also areas where the superficial and deep fascia fuse at a midline: anteriorly as the cervical linea alba and posteriorly as the nuchal ligament.

Superficial Fasciae

Throughout the head and neck, the superficial fascia forms a continuous fibrofatty layer (Fig. 4.2). This layer has different thicknesses and features in different regions, and these differences are so pronounced that the fascial areas are referred to with different designations. For example, the superficial fascia of the scalp is called the galea capitis, while that of the face is called the superficial musculo-aponeurotic system (SMAS) and that of the neck is referred to as the fibromuscular layer of the platysma muscle. Finally, at the nuchal

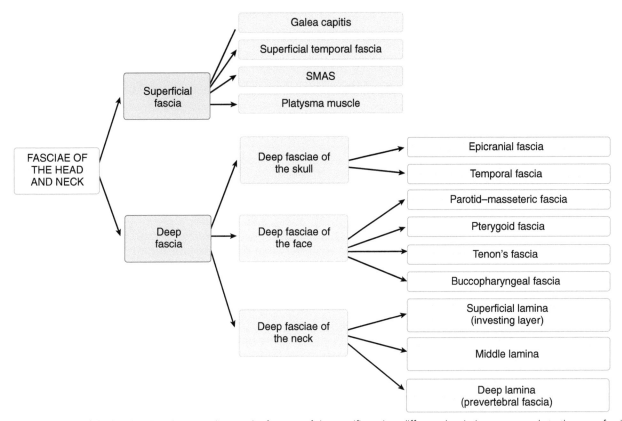

FIGURE 4.1 Fasciae of the head and neck. Depending on the features of the specific region, different descriptive names apply to the same fascia.

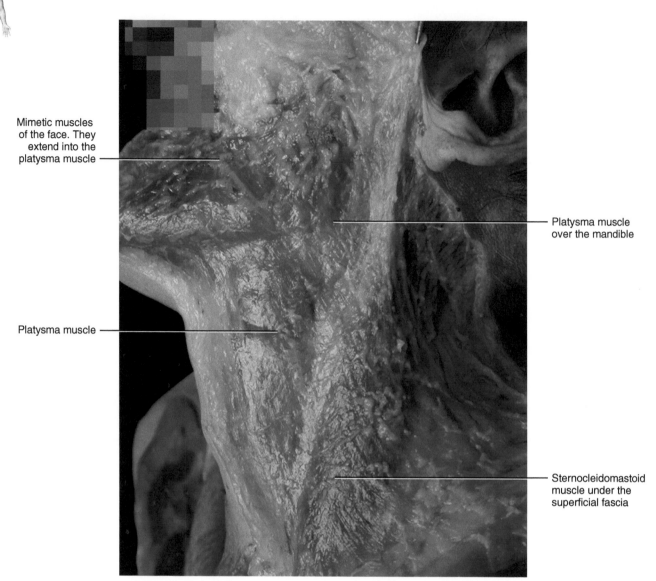

Mimetic muscles of the face. They extend into the platysma muscle

Platysma muscle over the mandible

Platysma muscle

Sternocleidomastoid muscle under the superficial fascia

FIGURE 4.2 Dissection of the lateral region of the neck. Only the skin was removed to show the superficial fascia. It forms a continuous fibrofatty layer throughout the head and neck. It contains striated muscular tissue, such as the mimetic muscles in the face and the platysma muscle in the neck.

(back) region of the neck, the superficial fascia becomes a fibrofatty layer that is harder to identify.

One feature of the superficial fascia of this region is the presence of striated muscular tissue within it. This includes the mimetic muscles and the platysma. In those areas without muscle tissue the superficial fascia becomes thicker and more compact.

A loose areolar tissue plane is just underneath the superficial fascia. Various sources identify this tissue plane by using the terms: 'subgaleal fascia' (Fig. 4.3), 'subaponeurotic plane', 'sub-SMAS plane', 'areolar temporalis fascia', 'innominate fascia', etc. In fact, all loose areolar tissue corresponds to the deep adipose tissue (DAT), which is found throughout the body. This tissue separates, typically, the superficial and deep fasciae and it permits gliding and autonomy between the two fascial systems.

The DAT is well represented in the scalp and is largely responsible for scalp mobility. Near the eyes, it contributes to the formation of the preaponeurotic fat pads of the eye. In the cheek, it forms the Bichat's fat pad between the SMAS and the parotideomasseteric fascia (Fig. 4.4). In the neck it separates the platysma and the underlying muscles. Unlike the superficial fascia in this region, the loose areolar layer (DAT) is discontinuous in three areas: over the zygomatic arch, over the parotid gland and over the anterior border of the masseter muscle. In these areas there are dense attachments between the superficial and the deep fascial systems. In addition, the superficial fascia and deep fascia fuse anteriorly at the linea alba cervicale and posteriorly over the nuchal ligament.

By comparison to the DAT, the superficial adipose tissue (SAT) is scarce in the head and neck (Fig. 4.5)

104

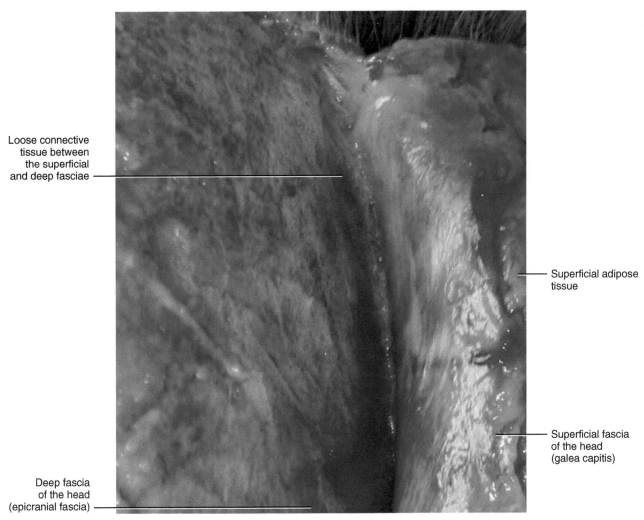

Loose connective tissue between the superficial and deep fasciae

Superficial adipose tissue

Superficial fascia of the head (galea capitis)

Deep fascia of the head (epicranial fascia)

FIGURE 4.3 Dissection of the head. The superficial fascia (together with the skin) was detached from the deep fascia. In the head, the loose connective tissue between superficial and deep fasciae provides an easy plane of separation between the scalp and the epicranial fascia. This layer of loose connective tissue is sometime called "subgaleal fascia". It also provides a plane of access in craniofacial surgery and neurosurgery. In scalping, the scalp (that corresponds to the skin and superficial fascia) is separated through this layer.

and, depending on the region of the face, the relationship between the superficial fascia and skin may vary (Fig. 4.6). For example, the galea capitis (superficial fascia) adheres to the skin via strong and vertical skin ligaments, and, where the mimetic muscles insert into the dermis, the SAT is scant and crossed by muscular fibres.

Superficial Fascia of the Head: Galea Capitis (Galea Aponeurotica)

The superficial fascia of the head (galea capitis) is extremely compact. It resembles aponeurosis and may be confused with the deep fascia (Fig. 4.7). The galea capitis continues to the face with the SMAS and in the neck with the superficial fascia that envelops the platysma muscle (Fig. 4.8).

The galea capitis can be thought of as a large tendon that connects the superficial muscles of the head:

frontalis, occipitalis and superior auricular muscles (Fig. 4.9). These mimetic muscles evolved from the panniculus carnosus of mammals. In monkeys the occipitofrontalis muscles extend almost to the summit of the head so that many muscle fibres weave through the galea capitis. In other mammals, it is evident that the galea capitis is, essentially, the continuation of the superficial fascia of the neck. This blending of the cutaneous musculature with fascial tissue is observed throughout the mammalian body. In humans, however, this musculature has all but disappeared and the galea capitis comprises primarily fibrous tissue.

The galea capitis is highly vascularized and adheres to the skin with many vertical, thick retinacula cutis superficialis (Fig. 4.10). It is separated from the deep fascia by DAT that, in this region, is a thin layer of loose connective tissue with no fat cells. It permits the

Text continued on p. 112

105

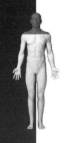

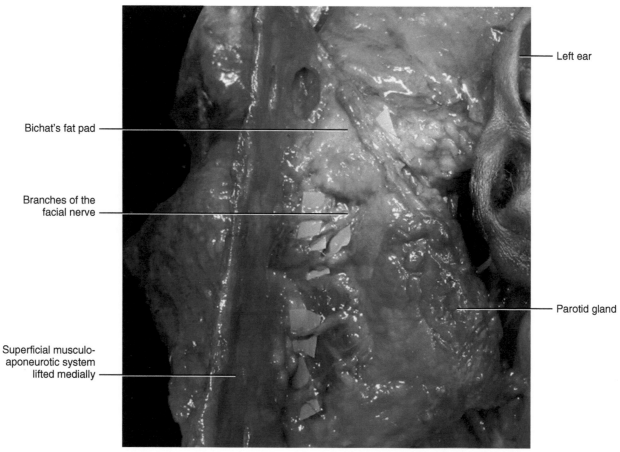

Left ear

Bichat's fat pad

Branches of the
facial nerve

Parotid gland

Superficial musculo-
aponeurotic system
lifted medially

FIGURE 4.4 Dissection of the lateral region of the face, left side. The SMAS was detached from the underlying plane and lifted medially to show the superficial Bichat's fat pad and the branches of the facial nerve. Bichat's fat pad is located between the SMAS and the deep fascia of the face (parotideomasseteric fascia). It augments autonomy between the mimetic muscles and the masticatory muscles and has a filler-type role.

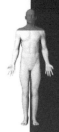
Superficial
adipose
tissue of the
ear region

Superficial
adipose
tissue of
the anterior
region of the
shoulder

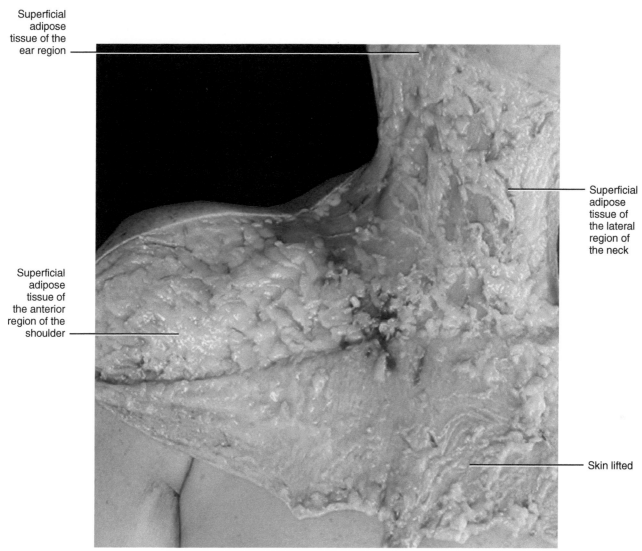

Superficial
adipose
tissue of
the lateral
region of
the neck

Skin lifted

FIGURE 4.5 Anterolateral view of the neck. The skin was lifted to show the SAT. In this region, one typically finds little fat and the retinacula cutis superficialis are also few and thin. This permits great mobility between the skin and the underlying planes.

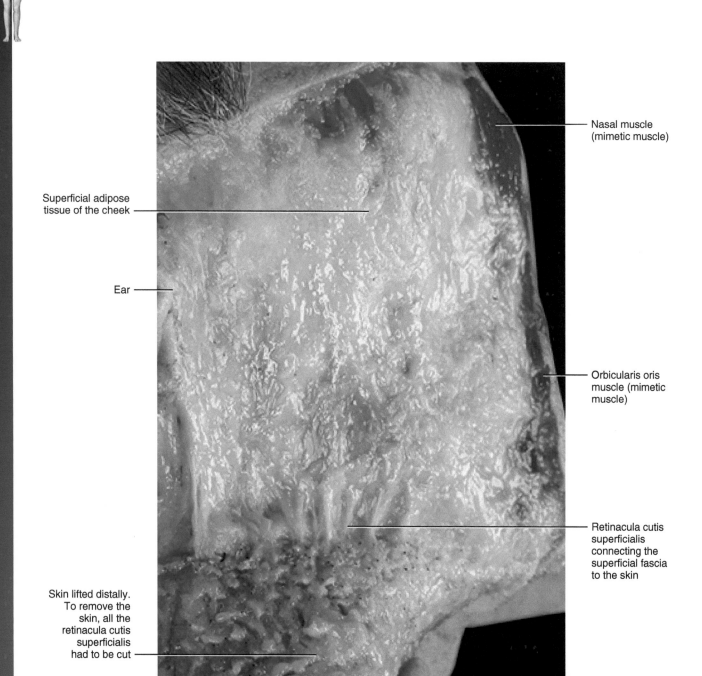

Nasal muscle
(mimetic muscle)

Superficial adipose
tissue of the cheek

Ear

Orbicularis oris
muscle (mimetic
muscle)

Retinacula cutis
superficialis
connecting the
superficial fascia
to the skin

Skin lifted distally.
To remove the
skin, all the
retinacula cutis
superficialis
had to be cut

FIGURE 4.6 Anterolateral view of the right cheek. The skin was removed to show the SAT. Just over the cheek the SAT is abundant, while near the ear the fibrous component increases and near the nose some nasal muscle fibres are evident. The nasal muscle is in the superficial fascia, but its fibres cross the SAT and insert into the dermis.

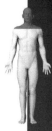

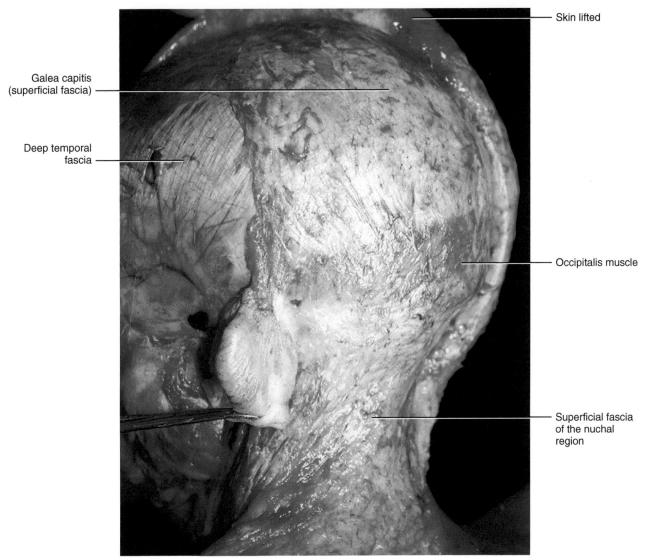

Skin lifted

Galea capitis
(superficial fascia)

Deep temporal
fascia

Occipitalis muscle

Superficial fascia
of the nuchal
region

FIGURE 4.7 Superficial fascia of the head: galea capitis. It is an extremely compact fibrous layer that might be mistaken for the deep fascia. It connects the occipitalis muscle with the frontalis and auricularis muscles.

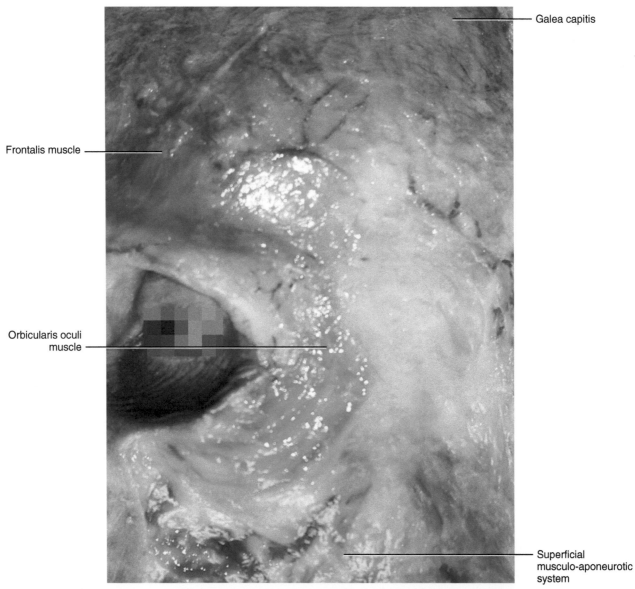

Galea capitis

Frontalis muscle

Orbicularis oculi muscle

Superficial musculo-aponeurotic system

FIGURE 4.8 Continuity between galea capitis and SMAS. Note that the frontalis muscle fibres mingle with the orbicularis oculi fibres.

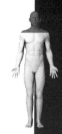

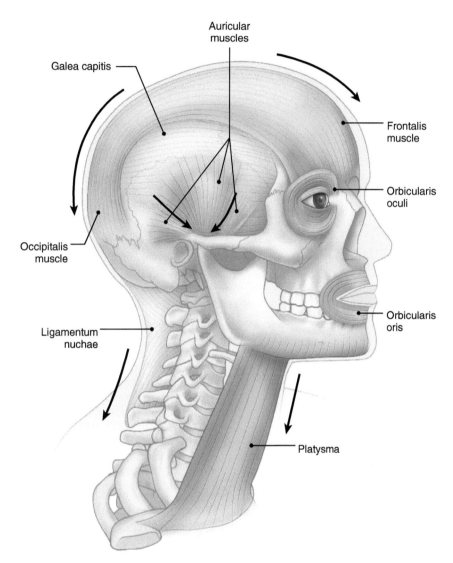

FIGURE 4.9 The galea capitis could be considered a large tendon that connects the superficial muscles of the head: frontalis, occipitalis and auricular. It continues anteriorly with the SMAS and with the platysma muscle, and posteriorly with the superficial fascia of the neck, which adheres to the nuchal ligament. The nuchal ligament is attached to many fibres of the trapezius muscle, as well as the deeper muscles of the neck. Thanks to these connections, the galea capitis is always tensioned in all planes. When a muscle contracts, it also increases the stretch of the galea capitis in a specific direction. If some of these muscles are tight, they could stretch the galea capitis in an altered manner.

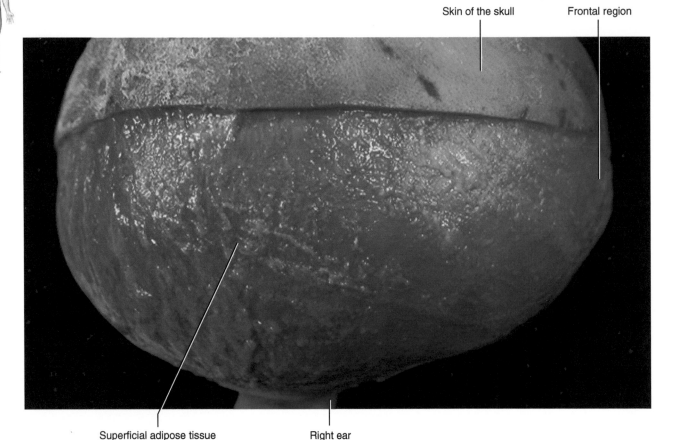

Skin of the skull   Frontal region

Superficial adipose tissue   Right ear

FIGURE 4.10 SAT of the head. The skin was removed cutting all the vertical fibrous septa that usually connect the skin to the galea capitis.

critical gliding between the superficial and deep fascia and contributes to scalp mobility (Fig. 4.11).

Superficial Temporal Fascia (Temporoparietal Fascia)

The superficial temporal fascia (Fig. 4.13) is a single unit of highly vascularized connective tissue. It is thin but can easily be distinguished as a single, distinct layer. Loose connective tissue is found under this layer and separates it from the deep fascia. Superficially, the temporal fascia is joined firmly to subcutaneous tissue and, in fact, a sharp dissection in a plane just deep to the hair follicles is required to separate this fascia from the overlying skin. The attachment to the skin is looser near the zygomatic arch but it becomes progressively firmer as the layers approach the vertex. The anterior portion of the superficial temporal fascia is continuous with the frontalis and orbicularis oculi muscles. Posteriorly, it blends with the occipitalis and posterior auricular muscles. The superior border merges with the galea capitis. Although there may be some disagreement, most studies suggest that the temporoparietal fascia is continuous inferiorly with the SMAS. The continuity of this fascia, the galea and the SMAS has appeared to some as a separate specific tissue in need of additional nomenclature: 'galeal extension', 'extension of epicranial aponeurosis' and 'suprazygomatic/temporal extension of the SMAS'. However, the variety

in terminology only confirms the confusion that may be present in the description of fascial anatomy[1]. The superficial temporal vessels, the auriculotemporal nerve and its branches, and the temporal branches of the facial nerve are found in the superficial temporal fascia, or just under it. The superficial temporal vessels provide most of the vascular supply to the superficial temporal fascia. The zygomatico-orbital, zygomatico-temporal, zygomaticofacial and transverse facial arteries provide only minor contributions.

Superficial Musculo-Aponeurotic System of the Face

In the face, the superficial fascia is quite distinctive due to its relation to the mimetic muscles. In fact, this superficial fascia envelops and connects all the mimetic muscles, creating an organized fibrous, muscular network (Figs 4.14 and 4.15). The mimetic muscles embedded into the superficial fascia of the face are: procerus, nasalis, orbicularis oculi, corrugator supercilii, depressor supercilii, orbicularis oris, depressor anguli oris, risorius, levator labii superioris, depressor labii inferioris, levator anguli oris and mentalis (Figs 4.16 and 4.17). This fibromuscular network is

Text continued on p. 120

---

[1]For an extensive review of the superficial fascia of the temporal region refer to Davidge et al (2010).

CLINICAL PEARL 4.1 GALEA CAPITIS AND THE CERVICAL PROPRIOCEPTIVE SYSTEM

The ligamentum nuchae connects the deep *neck* muscles with the superficial fascia of the neck. The superficial fascia of the neck continues with the galea capitis (Fig. 4.12) that connects the eyes (orbicularis and frontalis muscles) with the ears (auricular muscles) and the occipitalis muscle. The deep muscles of the neck are rich in proprioceptors and muscle spindles that regulate the control of the head position, together with the eyes and the labyrinth. The fasciae link all these proprioceptive elements. In clinical practice, an excessive tension in the deep muscles of the neck is often associated with vertigo.

The cervical proprioceptive system (CPS) consists of mechanoreceptors of cervical intervertebral joints, deep cervical fasciae, ligaments, and muscle spindles located in the deep, short muscles of cervical spine (Grgic 2006). Sensory information from neck proprioceptive receptors is processed in tandem with information from the vestibular system. There are extensive anatomical connections between neck proprioceptive input and vestibular input (Luan et al 2013, Yahia et al 2009). If positional information from the vestibular system or neck proprioceptors is inaccurate or fails to be appropriately integrated in the central nervous system, then errors in head position may occur. Clinical and neurophysiological studies have shown that functional disorders and/ or organic lesions of the CPS cause symptoms similar to vestibular diseases: vertigo, nystagmus and balance disorders. The increased activity of mechanoreceptors due to hypertonus of the neck muscles results in confusion of the vestibular system. Therefore, the impulses from the CPS do not correspond to the impulses from the vestibular organ and other sensory systems that take part in maintaining bodily balance. This disharmony of impulses results in an inadequate vestibulospinal and vestibulo-ocular reaction and manifests as vertigo and nystagmus. Hyperactivity of craniocervical mechanoreceptors also causes disturbances in reflex regulation of postural muscle tonus and manifests as 'general instability'.

Headaches are often due to excessive tension of the galea capitis. The tenderness of pericranial myofascial tissues and the number of myofascial trigger points are considerably increased in patients with tension-type headache (Bendtsen and Peñas 2011, Jensen et al 1998). Sensitization of pain pathways, in the central nervous system, due to prolonged nociceptive stimuli from pericranial myofascial tissues seems to be responsible for the conversion of episodic to chronic tension-type headache. Treatment directed towards muscular factors includes electromyography biofeedback, which has a documented effect in patients with tension-type headaches, as well as physiotherapy and muscle relaxation therapy, which may also be effective.

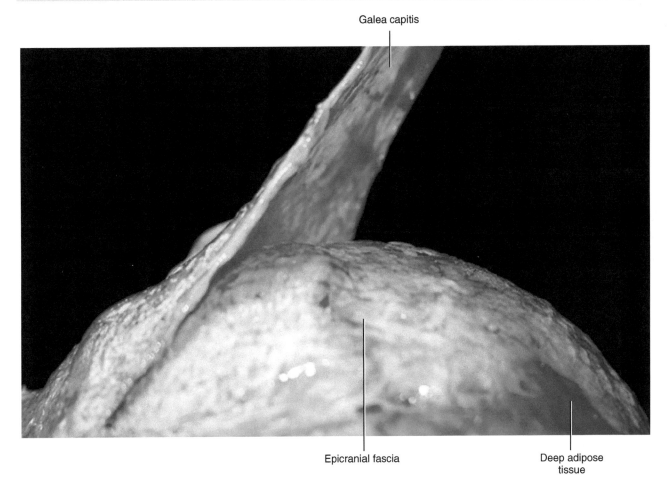

Galea capitis

Epicranial fascia

Deep adipose tissue

FIGURE 4.11 The galea capitis was lifted to show the epicranial fascia. Loose connective tissue separates the two fascial layers. An adherence is present only along the posterior nuchal line.

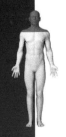

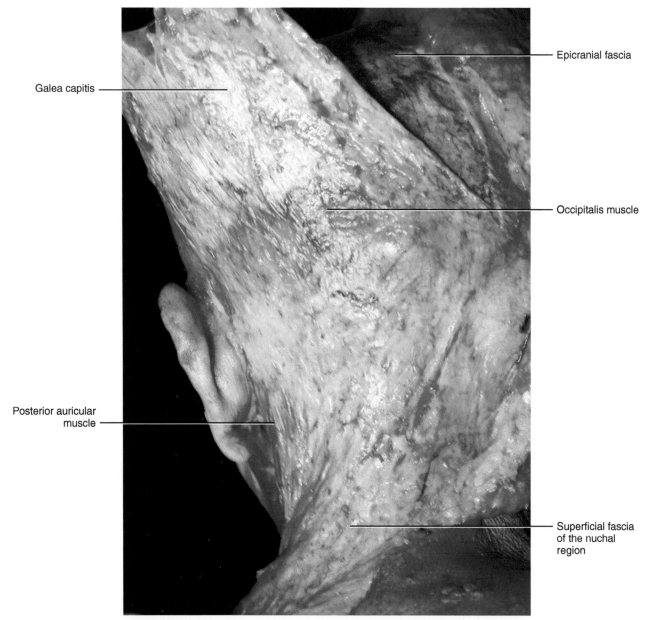

Galea capitis

Posterior auricular muscle

Epicranial fascia

Occipitalis muscle

Superficial fascia of the nuchal region

FIGURE 4.12 Dissection of the posterior region of the head and neck. The skin was removed and the galea capitis detached from the epicranial fascia and stretched cranially to highlight the continuity between the galea capitis and the superficial fascia of the neck. Inside the galea capitis, the occipitalis muscle is seen.

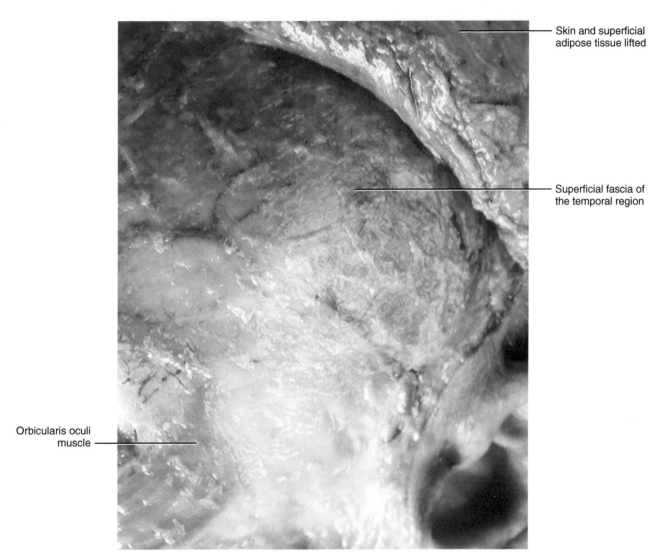

Skin and superficial
adipose tissue lifted

Superficial fascia of
the temporal region

Orbicularis oculi
muscle

FIGURE 4.13 Left temporal region of the head. The superficial temporal fascia is continuous with the galea capitis and the SMAS.

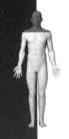

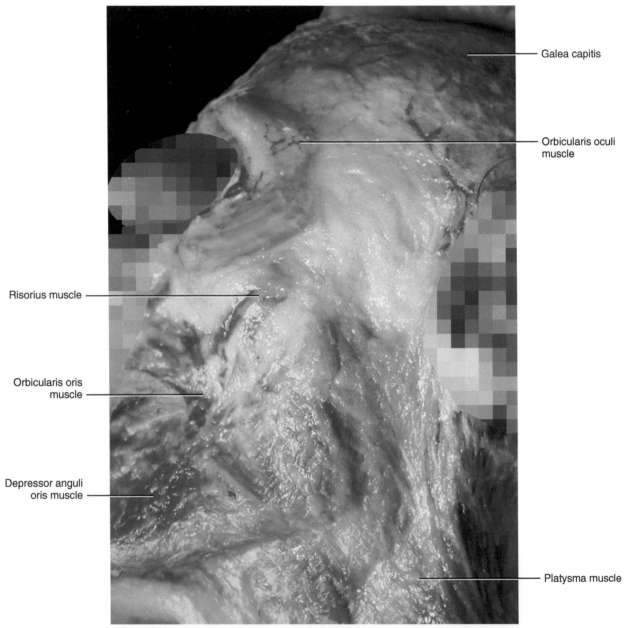

Galea capitis

Orbicularis oculi
muscle

Risorius muscle

Orbicularis oris
muscle

Depressor anguli
oris muscle

Platysma muscle

FIGURE 4.14 Dissection of the lateral region of the face. The skin was removed to expose the superficial fascia of the face with the mimetic muscles embedded inside. These together form a fibromuscular layer, which is called the SMAS of the face. The SMAS here is the centre of an elaborate three-dimensional network that transmits and coordinates mimetic muscle contractions.

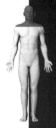

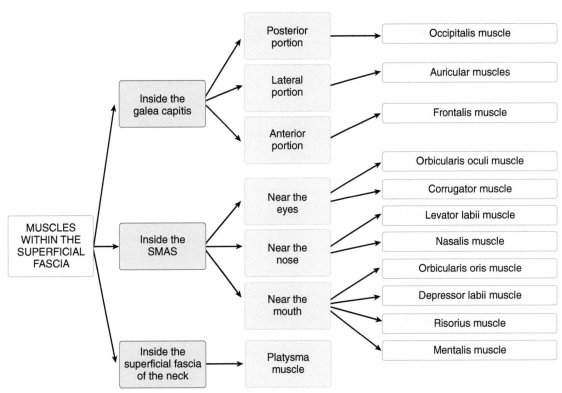

FIGURE 4.15 Muscles within the superficial fasciae of the head and neck.

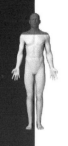

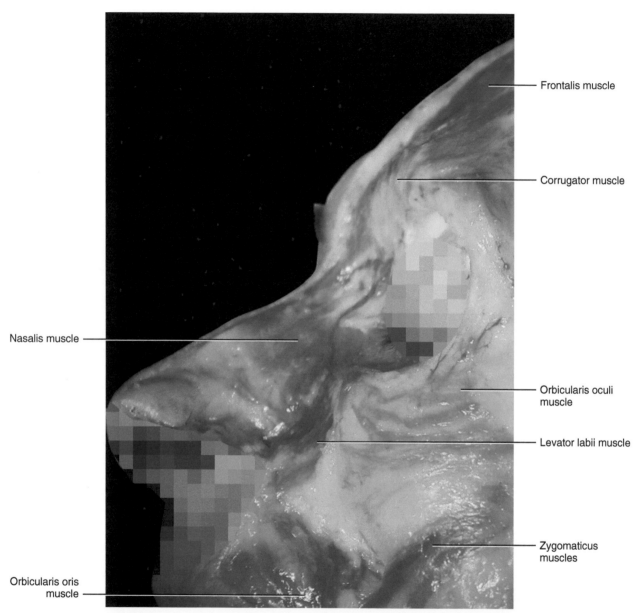

FIGURE 4.16 SMAS of the nasal region. Note that the distal portion of the zygomaticus muscles merge into the superficial fascia.

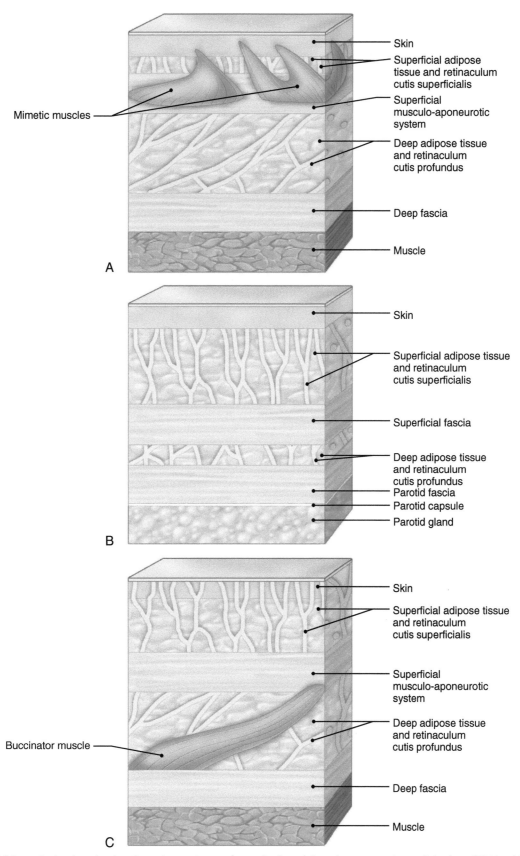

FIGURE 4.17 Schematic drawing showing the various patterns of organization of the subcutaneous tissue of the face. **(A)** Nasolabial fold: the mimetic muscles are inside the superficial fascia and cross the superficial adipose tissue (SAT) to insert into the dermis. **(B)** Parotid region: the deep adipose tissue (DAT) is scarce and the superficial and deep fasciae (parotid fascia) adhere. **(C)** Position of the buccinator muscle with respect to the fasciae of the face. This muscle originates from the buccopharyngeal fascia, crosses the DAT and inserts into the superficial fascia near the corner of the lips.

119

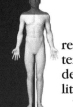
referred to as the superficial musculo-aponeurotic system (SMAS) of the face. Mitz and Peyronie (1976) first described this system that is now accepted in scientific literature and clinical practice.

The SMAS continues caudally with the platysma muscle and cranially with the galea capitis and superficial temporal fascia. Thaller et al (1990) suggest that the SMAS might be considered an evolutionary platysma muscle. During soft tissue facial development, through mesenchymal interaction, the superficial fascia of the face remains the central tendon of the mimetic muscles, with the role of transmitting and modulating the muscular contractions affecting the skin.

From a microscopic point of view, the SMAS is a fibro-elastic tissue with a mean thickness of 600 μm (Macchi et al 2010). The elastic fibres are numerous in the young, and progressively decrease with age. The arrangement of the SMAS shows a centrifugal thinning: becoming thinner almost to the point of invisibility when observed in the proximity of the orbicularis (which is enveloped by two layers of the SMAS). Thanks to the consistency of the SMAS, it is possible to isolate this with the platysma complex in a solid distinct formation. Its surgical dissection, mobilization and traction have become standard techniques in aesthetic facial surgery.

In the face, the SAT is usually thin and laced with the muscular fibres of the mimetic muscles that move from the SMAS to the dermis. Histological analysis of the SAT reveals vertically orientated fibrous septa (superficial retinacula cutis or skin ligaments) that further connect the dermis to the SMAS. Many authors have demonstrated the importance of these ligaments in supporting the normal anatomical position of the facial soft tissues. With ageing, the elasticity of the skin ligaments and the superficial fascia diminishes, and causes ptosis of the skin, prominent separate nasolabial folds and the formation of wrinkles (Stuzin et al 1992).

The DAT is usually easily recognized as it separates the SMAS from the deep fascia. Usually, the fibrous septa of the DAT (retinacula cutis profundis) are thin, rich in elastic fibres, predominantly horizontally orientated, and loosely connect the SMAS to the deep fasciae. Thus, the deep subcutaneous layer could constitute a 'shock absorber' system for muscles as they slide horizontally, separating the actions of the masticatory muscles from those of the mimetic muscles. In the cheek the DAT is particularly evident and rich in adipose tissue, forming the Bichat's fat pad. Only in the parotid region does the DAT disappear and here the SMAS adheres to the deep fascia. At the level of the zygomatic arch and nasolabial fold, the DAT is very thin and the buccinators and zygomatic muscles cross the DAT and connect the deep fascia with the superficial (Fig. 4.17).

Superficial Fascia of the Neck: Platysma Muscle

In the neck, the superficial fascia envelops the platysma muscle (Figs 4.18 and 4.19) and it is impossible to

separate these two elements. The platysma does not insert proximally on the jaw, as some sources allege, but instead it continues beyond the border of the mandible to fuse with the SMAS and, in particular, with the risorius muscle of Santorini (Fig. 4.19). Distally, the platysma is continuous with the superficial fascia of the thorax and the deltoid region. Posteriorly, the superficial fascia of the neck continues cranially with the galea capitis and distally with the thick superficial fascia of the back. Occasionally, there are muscular fibres inside, in a similar manner to the anterior platysma muscle (Fig. 4.20).

The SAT is generally scarce in this region, but between the superficial and deep fascia there is loose

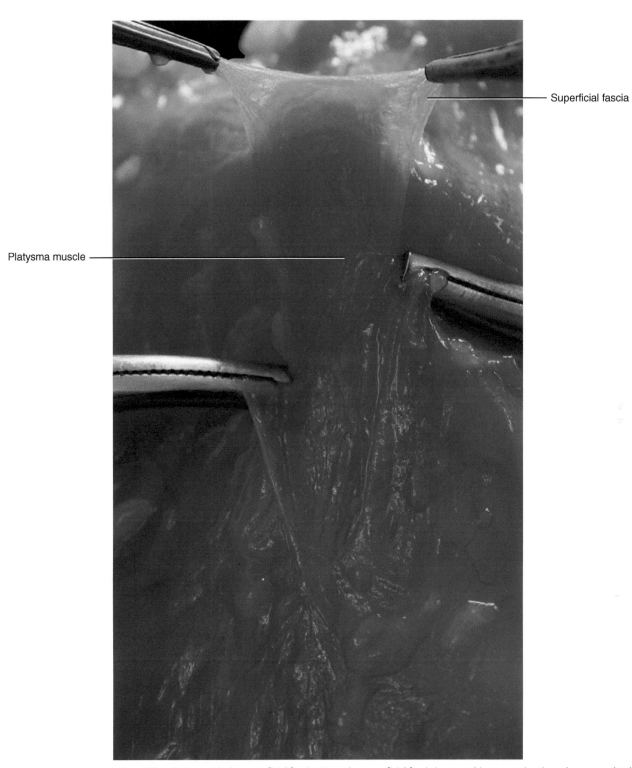

Superficial fascia

Platysma muscle

FIGURE 4.18 Platysma muscle and its relations with the superficial fascia. Here, the superficial fascia is a very thin connective tissue layer completely adherent to the muscle.

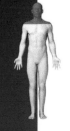

Platysma muscle
embedded in the
superficial fascia

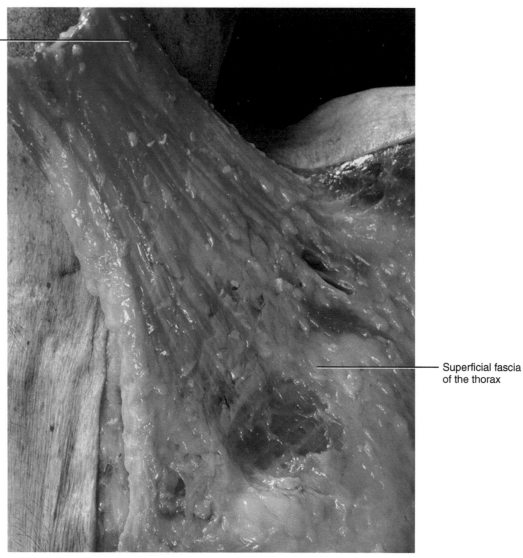

Superficial fascia
of the thorax

FIGURE 4.19 Dissection of the left lateral region of the neck. The superficial fascia of the neck was detached from the deeper structure and stretched cranially. The muscular fibres of the platysma muscle are evident. The superficial fascia of the neck also contains some adipose cells forming little fat lobules. Due to the layer of loose connective tissue under it, the superficial fascia can be easily detached from the underlying planes, which constitute the superficial lamina of the deep fascia of the neck. The superficial fascia of the neck continues down to become the superficial fascia of the thorax. Stretching the superficial fascia in a caudocranial direction shows this fascial connection between the neck and thorax as the stretching is clearly evident across the clavicle and into the superficial fascia of the thorax.

connective tissue that allows the sliding of the two fascial layers. The DAT only disappears at the cervical linea alba and the nuchal ligament. At these two points the superficial and deep fasciae fuse.

Deep Fasciae of the Head

Below the superficial fascia is the deep fascia that is present throughout the head and neck. The deep fascia of the two regions is treated separately because in the head one single layer is present and in the neck the deep fascia has three layers. The deep fascia of the head is usually presented as discrete, isolated areas that envelop the masticatory muscles and the salivary

glands. These are usually referred to with names derived from the embedded tissue (Fig. 4.21); for example, the deep fascia covering the temporalis muscle is called the temporal fascia and the fascia over the masseter muscle is called the masseteric fascia. In fact, the fasciae are not isolated masses but are all part of a continuous sheet that splits to surround muscles and glands and then extends to become the epicranial fascia of the scalp. Although a variety of names are used to designate different areas of the deep fascia, we must emphasize that these divisions are entirely artificial. **It is important to comprehend** the unitary nature of the deep fascia of the head, as it embeds the muscles and glands as part of a single sheath of

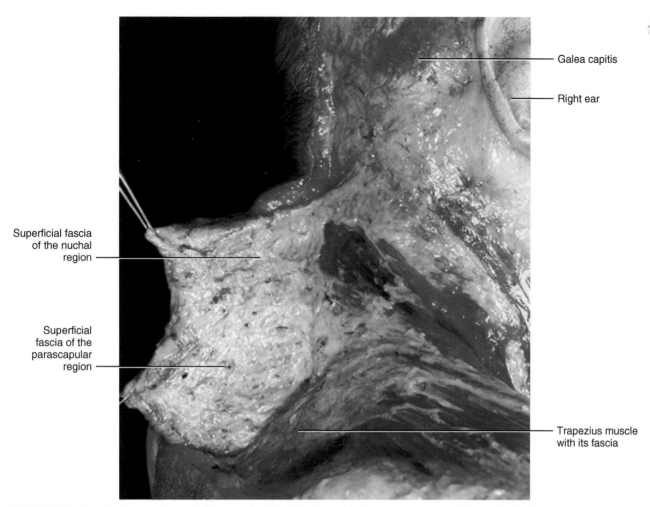

Galea capitis

Right ear

Superficial fascia of the nuchal region

Superficial fascia of the parascapular region

Trapezius muscle with its fascia

FIGURE 4.20 Posterolateral view of the neck. The superficial fascia in the neck is thin and progressively thickens distally. In the parascapular region it is very thick and vascularized. Proximally it continues with the galea capitis. Along the midline it adheres to the ligamentum nuchae.

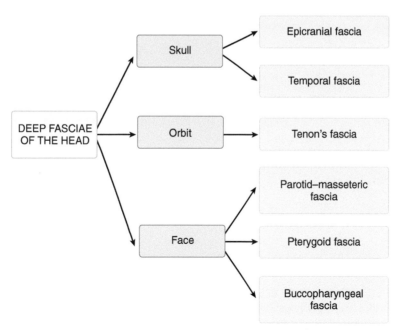

DEEP FASCIAE OF THE HEAD

Skull → Epicranial fascia

Skull → Temporal fascia

Orbit → Tenon's fascia

Face → Parotid–masseteric fascia

Face → Pterygoid fascia

Face → Buccopharyngeal fascia

FIGURE 4.21 Diagram of the terminology used to describe the components of the deep fascia of the head.

123

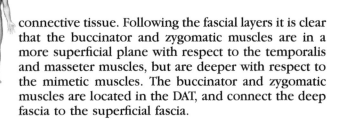

connective tissue. Following the fascial layers it is clear that the buccinator and zygomatic muscles are in a more superficial plane with respect to the temporalis and masseter muscles, but are deeper with respect to the mimetic muscles. The buccinator and zygomatic muscles are located in the DAT, and connect the deep fascia to the superficial fascia.

Deep Fascia of the Skull: Epicranial Fascia

In the areas of the skull lacking deep muscles, the epicranial fascia is referred to as the 'pericranium' (pericranial membrane). In other words, it is the external periosteum that covers the outer surface of the skull (Figs 4.22–4.24). The epicranial fascia continues with the temporal fascia, covering the temporalis muscle, and anteriorly it becomes Tenon's fascia (fascia between the eyeball and the fat of the orbit). The epicranial fascia is separated from the galea capitis by richly vascularized, loose connective tissue.

The epicranial fascia, typical of all deep fasciae, has two sublayers. Habal and Maniscalco (1981) describe the outer layer as loose areolar tissue with fibroblasts, while the inner layer contains osteoblasts. There is a network of vessels, near the inner layer, that permits the pericranial fascia to be used as a flap based on a narrow pedicle.

Deep Fascia of the Orbit: Tenon's Fascia (or Capsule)

Tenon's capsule is the deep fascia of the eyes. It is a fibrous layer surrounding the globe of the eye from the ciliary margin of the cornea backwards to the entrance of the optic nerve. Its anterior third firmly adheres to the back of the ocular conjunctiva and its middle third sends fascial extensions to the muscles of the eye, forming the sheaths of the four recti and the two oblique muscles. Tenon's fascia forms a similar sheath for the elevator muscle of the upper eyelid. Its posterior third is in contact with the orbital fat and then becomes continuous with the sheath of the optic nerve.

The insertions of the ocular muscles are so tightly bound to Tenon's fascia that one may consider these insertions and the fascia as one unit. Sappey (1888) discovered that this fascia attaches to the wall of the lacrimal sac (Fig. 4.25). Along the border of the orbit, the fascia continues to the back of the eyelid and inserts into the periosteum. This fascia varies in thickness and is strengthened by fibrous bands. Its posterior part is thinner but becomes thicker at the equator of the bulb. The fibrous bands that reinforce the fascia are called 'orbital tendons' and they could also be considered accessory insertions for the ocular muscles.

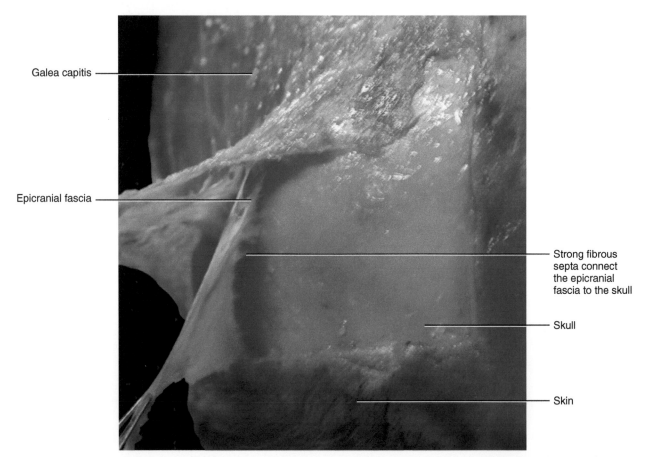

FIGURE 4.22 Dissection of the skull. Two fascial layers are viewed: the superficial fascia (galea capitis) and the deep fascia (epicranial fascia). The deep fascia usually adheres to the skull, and so it could be considered as its periosteum. Loose connective tissue is present between the galea capitis and the epicranial fascia.

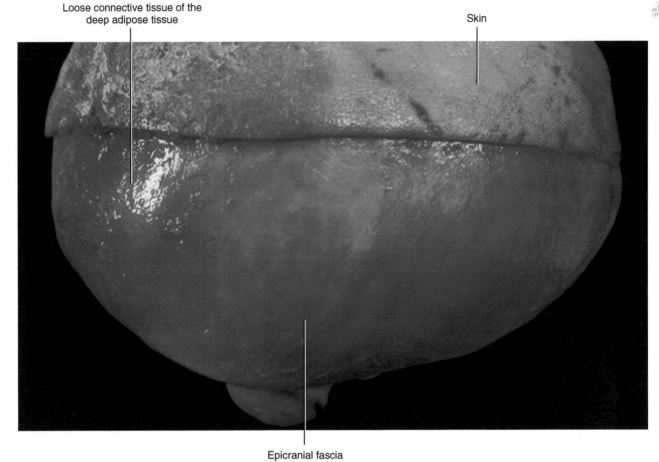

Loose connective tissue of the
deep adipose tissue

Skin

Epicranial fascia

FIGURE 4.23 Deep fascia of the skull: the epicranial fascia. The epicranial fascia is a fibrous layer well vascularized which adheres to the bone by way of many fibrous septa.

CLINICAL PEARL 4.3 ROLE OF TENON'S FASCIA IN EYE MOTILITY

It is impossible to separate the role of the eye muscles from Tenon's fascia. Tenon's fascia modulates and connects the muscles thereby reinforcing the action of single muscles. Each individual muscle needs the tension of its associated orbital tendon and Tenon's fascia. This relationship prevents excessive muscular contraction that might create a damaging force within the limited region of the globe.

The internal surface of Tenon's fascia is in close proximity to the sclera. Loose connective tissue is present between these two structures, except anteriorly where the capsule actually adheres to the sclera. This layer is considered important for lymphatic drainage.

Deep Fascia of the Skull: Temporal Fascia

The temporal fascia is the dense fibrous layer that covers the temporalis muscle (Fig. 4.26) and its broad surface provides attachments to the superficial fibres of this muscle (Fig. 4.27). Superiorly, the temporal fascia continues with the epicranial fascia and is partially attached along the length of the superior temporal line. Inferiorly, it splits into superficial and deep laminae that run down to attach, respectively, to the lateral and medial margins of the zygomatic arch. Between these two layers there is an intrafascial fat pad. This fat pad contains the zygomatico-orbital branch of the superficial temporal artery and a cutaneous nerve, the zygomaticotemporal branch of the zygomatic nerve (itself a branch of the maxillary nerve). Distally, these two layers continue as the parotideomasseteric fascia, which, in turn, is connected to the superficial layer of the deep fascia of the neck.

Another fat pad is found in this region located between the deep leaflet of the temporal fascia and the temporalis muscle. Most researchers call this pad the 'deep temporal fat pad' or 'subfascial fat pad'. This pad begins just superior to the zygomatic arch and extends inferiorly, protecting the masticatory space and allowing the temporalis muscle to glide smoothly under bony prominences. Finally, in this region there is a third fat pad, called 'temporoparietal or suprafascial fat pad', which is between the superficial fascia and the deep temporal fascia (that is the DAT).

125

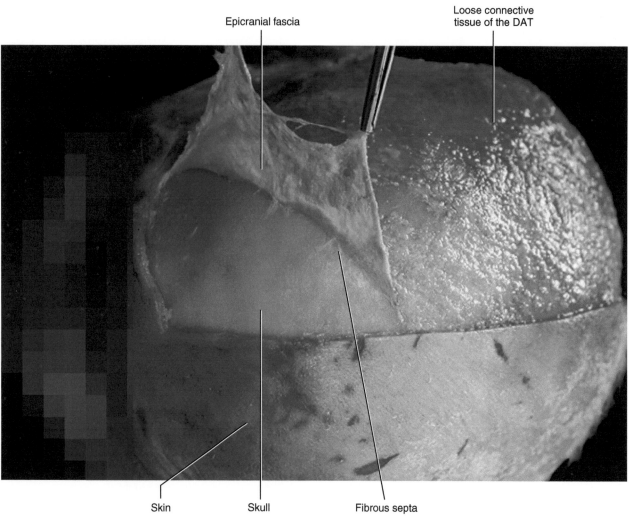

Epicranial fascia

Loose connective
tissue of the DAT

Skin

Skull

Fibrous septa

FIGURE 4.24 The epicranial fascia was lifted to show its relationships with the skull.

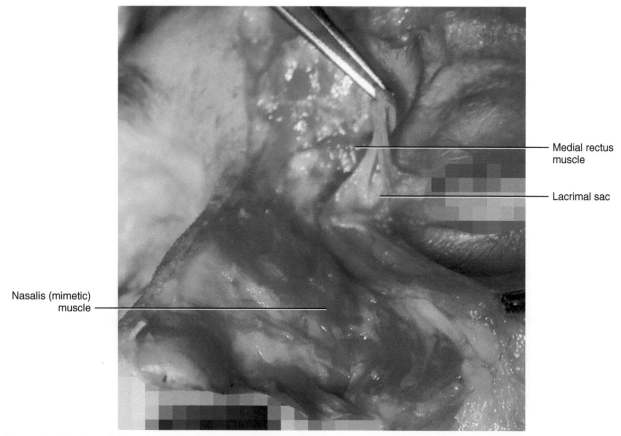

Medial rectus
muscle

Lacrimal sac

Nasalis (mimetic)
muscle

FIGURE 4.25 Dissection of the ocular region. The forceps lift the lacrimal sac.

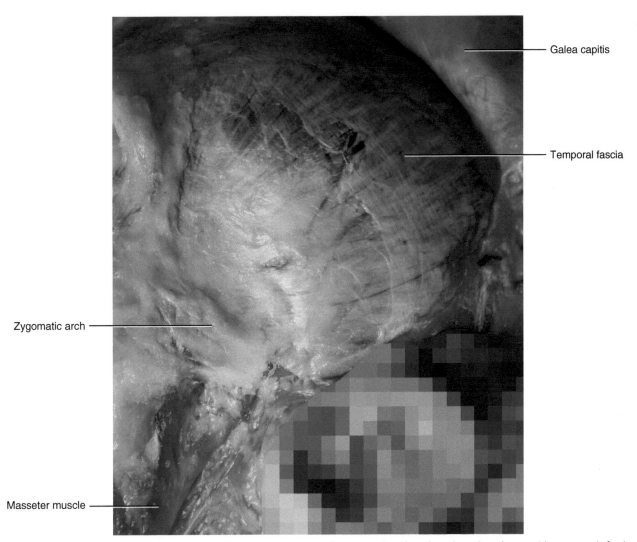

Galea capitis

Temporal fascia

Zygomatic arch

Masseter muscle

FIGURE 4.26 The superficial layer of the temporalis fascia as it passes over the zygomatic arch and continues into the parotideomasseteric fascia. The temporal fascia appears as a white, fibrous layer of connective tissue covering the temporalis muscle.

Deep Fascia of the Face: Parotideomasseteric Fascia

The parotideomasseteric fascia originates from the zygomatic arch and is a continuation of the temporal fascia. It forms the walls of the compartment for the parotid gland and covers the anterior part of the masseter muscle. On the posterior border of the masseter muscle, this fascia connects with the periosteum of the mandible (Fig. 4.28). It also connects with the perichondrium of the external acoustic meatus, the styloid process of the temporal bone, the stylomandibular ligament and the fascia of the posterior belly of the digastric muscle. It then continues with the fascia covering the external carotid artery and the posterior facial vein. The parotid fascia continues in the neck with the superficial layer of the deep cervical fascia. Under the parotid fascia, the capsule of the parotid gland lies. It is a fibrous layer varying in thickness and is thickest on its external surface. Numerous septa radiate out from it and extend between the lobes of the parotid gland.

Deep Fascia of the Face: Pterygoid Fascia

The pterygoid fascia covers the medial and lateral pterygoid muscles. It originates from the lamina lateralis of the pterygoid process and extends to the spina angularis, the petrotympanic fissure and the mandible above the insertion of the pterygoid muscles. It also continues with the capsule of the temporomandibular joint (TMJ). On the entire medial side of the TMJ, the articular disc and its capsular attachments are in close contact with the fascia of the lateral pterygoid muscle. A small portion of the upper head of this muscle inserts directly into the anteromedial part of the articular disc. Thus, the lateral pterygoid muscle and its fascia are likely to influence directly the position of the articular disc during TMJ movement. Schmolke (1994) contends that the masseteric and temporal fasciae are also connected with the ligaments and disc of the TMJ, but, since these attachments are relatively weak, neither the temporalis nor the masseter muscles are considered to act directly on the articular disc. Rather, they may, through afferents from muscle spindles, take part

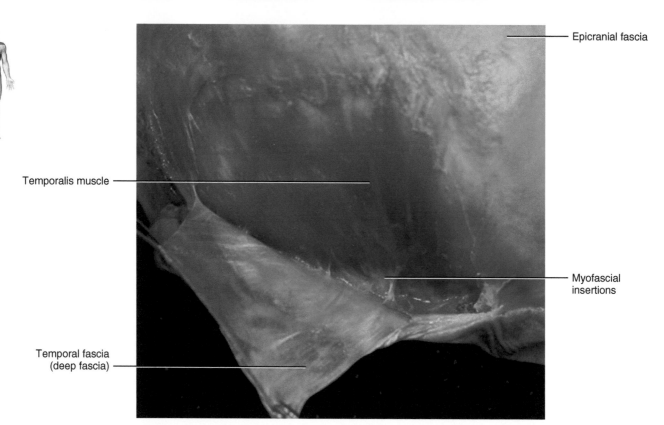

Epicranial fascia

Temporalis muscle

Myofascial insertions

Temporal fascia (deep fascia)

FIGURE 4.27 The temporal fascia was detached from the temporalis muscle and lifted. The temporal fascia is a dense fibrous layer that covers the temporalis muscle. Many fibres of this muscle originate from the inner side of this fascia, making it difficult to detach the fascia from the muscular belly. This means that every time the temporalis muscle contracts, the temporal fascia is stretched.

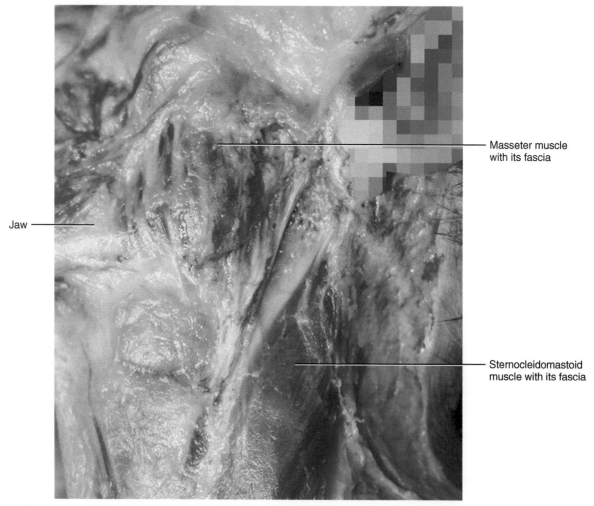

Masseter muscle with its fascia

Jaw

Sternocleidomastoid muscle with its fascia

FIGURE 4.28 Parotideomasseteric fascia covering the masseter muscle. This fascia adheres strongly to the masseter muscle, due to many intramuscular septa that originate from its inner surface. This fascia also connects the periosteum of the mandible.

CLINICAL PEARL 4.4 ROLE OF THE FASCIAE IN CHEWING AND SWALLOWING

All the muscles involved in chewing and swallowing are interconnected by fasciae. The temporal fascia that envelops the temporalis muscle continues into the parotideomasseteric fascia that envelops the masseter muscle. The masseter muscle connects with the pterygoid internus muscle to the degree that the two might be considered a digastric sling-like muscle. The pterygoid fascia joins with the temporomandibular joint capsule and with the buccopharyngeal fascia, which covers the superior pharyngeal constrictor muscles and attaches to the buccinator muscle. The buccinator muscle crosses the DAT to insert into the SMAS near the mouth. A perfect fascial tension in this network assures the coordination necessary for chewing and swallowing. The open-mouth position changes the normal tensional relationship in this fascial network, resulting in abnormal activity of the muscle spindles connected to the swallowing muscles. This explains why swallowing with the mouth open is almost impossible.

CLINICAL PEARL 4.5 MYOFASCIAL PAIN OF THE JAW MUSCLES

Myofascial pain of the jaw muscles is the commonest form of temporomandibular disorder (TMD). Patients with myofascial pain often, from a psychological as well as a social viewpoint, show high rates of chronic pain-related disability and depression/somatization scores. Management of myofascial symptoms is an intriguing challenge for clinicians both at the diagnostic and therapeutic levels, and several treatment approaches have been proposed in the literature. Some techniques that have proved to be helpful are: rhythmic stabilization, postisometric relaxation, hold–relax (Skaggs & Liebenson 2000) and intra-oral massage therapy. Indeed, the lateral and medial pterygoid muscles frequently refer pain to the TMJ and maxillary sinus (Travell & Simons 1983). These muscles are involved in opening the jaw, protrusion of the mandible and lateral deviation of the mandible to the opposite side, by unilateral action of either muscle.

To better understand what conservative approach could be useful for these patients, a randomized controlled trial was performed to compare the short-term effectiveness of botulinum toxin injections and physiatric treatment, provided by means of Fascial Manipulation® technique, in the management of myofascial pain of jaw muscles (Guarda Nardini et al 2012). Thirty patients with a research diagnostic criteria for temporomandibular disorders (RDC/TMD) and diagnosis of myofascial pain were randomized to receive either single-session botulinum toxin injections (group A) or three sessions of Fascial Manipulation (group B). Maximum pain levels (visual analogue scale ratings) and jaw range of motion in millimetres (maximum mouth opening, protrusion, right and left laterotrusion) were assessed at baseline, at the end of treatment, and at a three-month follow-up. Both treatment protocols provided significant improvement over time for pain symptoms and both seem to be almost equally effective. Fascial Manipulation, however, was slightly superior in reducing subjective pain perception, and botulinum toxin injections were slightly superior in increasing jaw range of motion. Differences between the two treatment protocols in changing the outcome parameters at the three-month follow-up were not relevant clinically.

in signalling the position of the TMJ components and the articular disc.

Testut (1905) affirms that the internal pterygoid muscle is distally connected to the masseter muscle via the continuities of their fasciae with the periosteum of the mandible. Thus, the medial pterygoid muscle and masseter muscle form a common tendinous sling that allows these muscles to be powerful elevators of the jaw. Proximally, the internal pterygoid muscle forms the lateral wall of the pharynx and assists in swallowing. As the pterygomandibular ligament and buccopharyngeal fascia originate from the pterygoid process, then this process could be considered a key point, joining the ptyerygoid fascia with the buccopharyngeal fascia.

Deep Fascia of the Face: Buccopharyngeal Fascia

The buccopharyngeal fascia forms a distinct layer just up to the posterior part of the buccinator muscle and envelops the superior pharyngeal constrictor muscle. Many muscular fibres of the buccinator muscle originate from this fascia, and then insert into the buccal fat pad and into the connective tissue of the lips. The buccinator muscle crosses the DAT of the face, connecting the deep fascia (buccopharyngeal fascia) with the superficial fascia of the face (and also with the skin, as the SMAS adheres to the skin near the lip canthus) (Fig. 4.29). From a functional point of view, the buccinator muscle has both a mimetic and masticatory function. Its position permits it to connect and modulate the action of the mouth with that of the pharynx.

The buccopharyngeal fascia fuses with the periosteum on the posterior part of the alveolar process of the maxilla and with the periosteum of the inner plate of the pterygoid process. The fascia extends backwards from this point, over the superior pharyngeal constrictor of the pharynx and then continues into the tunica adventitia of the pharynx and the oesophagus. The buccopharingeal fascia forms the pterygomandibular raphe, between the hamulus of the medial pterygoid

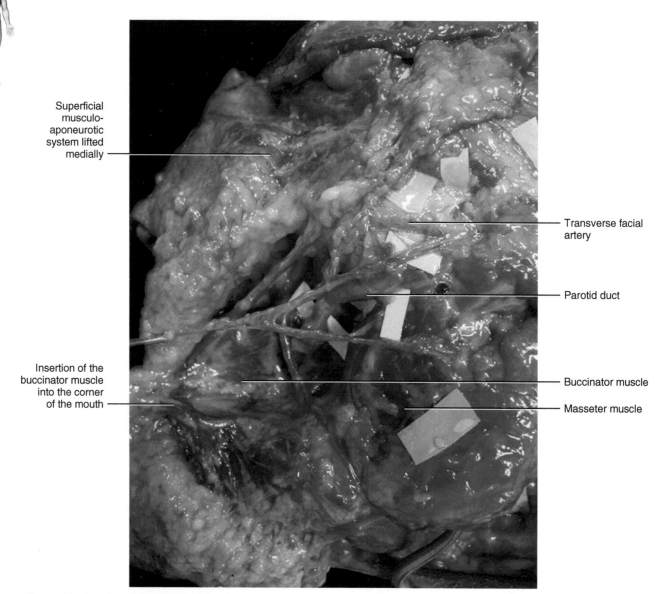

Superficial musculo-aponeurotic system lifted medially

Transverse facial artery

Parotid duct

Insertion of the buccinator muscle into the corner of the mouth

Buccinator muscle

Masseter muscle

FIGURE 4.29 Dissection of the left side of the check. The buccinator muscle originates from the deep fascia near the maxilla and inserts into the superficial fascia near the corner of the mouth.

plate and the posterior end of the mylohyoid line of the mandible, providing attachment for the superior pharyngeal constrictor muscle.

Deep Fasciae of the Neck (Deep Cervical Fascia)

The deep fasciae of the neck have been a controversial subject since their first description by Burns in 1824. Modern anatomical and surgical texts continue the confusion by describing them either too briefly or inaccurately. Poirier (1912) describes these difficulties: 'the cervical fasciae appear in a new form under the pen of each author who attempts to describe them'. The fasciae of the neck are important to clinicians: they have been analysed in relation to chronic neck pain and tension headaches. They have a role in the diffusion of regional anaesthetics and are of importance

in planning neck and head surgery. These altered/thickened fasciae, in addition to their importance in muscular, nervous and vascular function (Melzack et al 1977), may be responsible for nerve compression and nonphysiological tightness of neck muscles.

The deep fasciae of the neck are arranged into three fascial laminae (layers) that envelop the neck muscles: superficial, middle and deep laminae (Fig. 4.30). All three layers of the deep cervical fasciae adhere strongly to their underlying muscles. This is particularly noted in the fascia of the trapezius muscle. This fascia has a series of intramuscular septa that extend out from its internal surface and divide the muscle into many bundles. A number of muscular fibres originate from the inner side of the fascia and directly from the intramuscular septa. The functions of these fasciae cannot be separated from the functions of the underlying muscles themselves. Therefore, during muscular

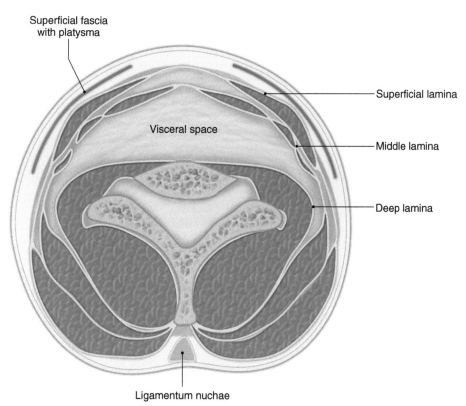

Superficial fascia
with platysma

Superficial lamina

Visceral space

Middle lamina

Deep lamina

Ligamentum nuchae

FIGURE 4.30 Diagram of the three laminae of the deep fasciae of the neck.

contraction, the neck fasciae are always stretched without the necessity of adjoining myofascial expansions.

Deep Fascia of the Neck: Superficial Lamina (Investing Layer or Layer I)

The superficial lamina of the deep fascia surrounds the neck like a collar. The thickness of this lamina varies. Over the belly of the sternocleidomastoid muscle (SCM), it has a mean thickness of 1.1 mm as measured by ultrasound, but it becomes thicker over the upper part of the SCM where it adheres to the superficial fascia and the tendon of the SCM (Stecco et al 2014). It splits around the SCM and trapezius muscles (Fig. 4.31). A fat cushion (corpus adiposum colli) is situated over the gap between the SCM and the trapezius muscle in the supraclavicular fossa. The supraclavicular lymph glands lie under this cushion. In the anterior region of the neck, the fascia extends medially beyond the muscle to join with the contralateral fascia forming the spatium suprasternalis (space of Burns). This fascia fuses along the midline with the superficial fascia and forms the cervical linea alba. Over the hyoid bone, the superficial lamina is firmly anchored to the periosteum. From this point it continues over the anterior belly of the digastric muscle and forms the loggia of the submandibular glands (Fig. 4.32).

Superiorly, this lamina partially attaches to the lower border of the mandible, the mastoid process, the superior nuchal line and the external occipital protuberance. It then partially continues with the parotidomasseteric fascia anteriorly and with the epicranial

fascia posteriorly. Between the angle of the mandible and the tip of the mastoid process it is very compact, forming the angular ligament of the mandible. The superficial lamina of the deep fascia of the neck has another thickening between the styloid process and the angle of the mandible, called the stylomandibular ligament.

Posteriorly, the superficial lamina blends into and covers the (Gray's Anatomy (40th ed, 2008) states that the ligamentum nuchae is not a ligament of the neck since it does not connect adjacent bones nor have the structure of a ligament). At this point the ligament is not separable from superficial fascia. Testut (1905) asserts that the posterior margin of the ligamentum nuchae intermingles with numerous tendinous fibres from the trapezius muscle.

Inferiorly, the superficial lamina partially attaches to the spine and acromion of the scapula and to the clavicle and the sternum, and partially (its superficial part) continues with the fascia of the pectoralis major, deltoid and latissimus dorsi muscles.

Deep Fascia of the Neck: Middle Lamina (Layer II)

Testut (1905) indicates that there are four muscles in the second layer of the neck: splenii, levator scapulae, rhomboids and serratus posterior superior and inferior (Fig. 4.33). All of these muscles are enveloped by the middle lamina of the neck fascia. Standring et al (2008) states that the fascia enveloping the rhomboids

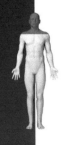

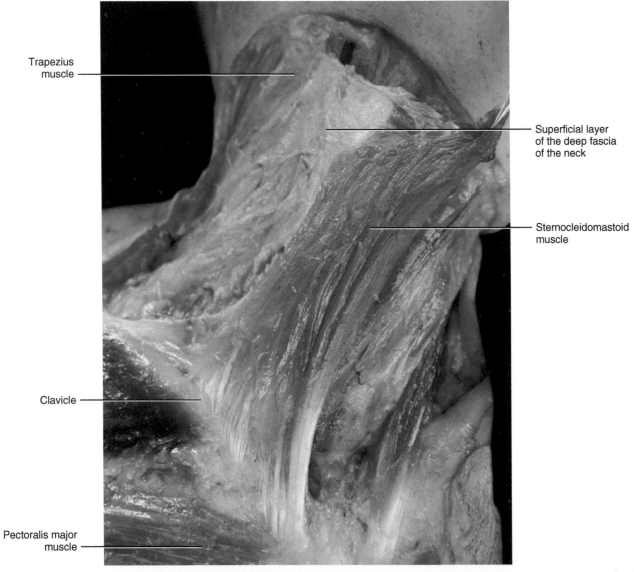

Trapezius muscle

Superficial layer of the deep fascia of the neck

Sternocleidomastoid muscle

Clavicle

Pectoralis major muscle

FIGURE 4.31 Dissection of the lateral region of the neck, right side. The skin and all the subcutaneous tissue were removed to show the superficial lamina of the deep fascia of the neck. The continuity between the SCM and the trapezius muscles is clearly in evidence.

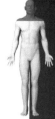

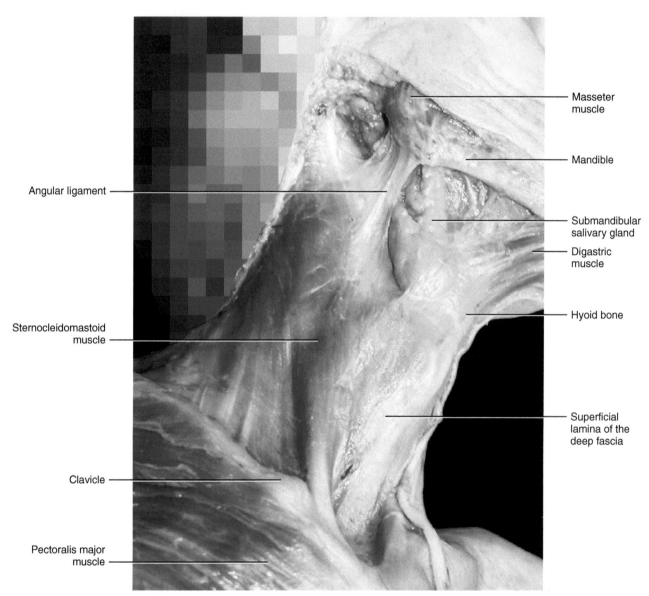

Masseter muscle

Mandible

Submandibular salivary gland

Digastric muscle

Hyoid bone

Superficial lamina of the deep fascia

Angular ligament

Sternocleidomastoid muscle

Clavicle

Pectoralis major muscle

FIGURE 4.32 Dissection of the anterolateral region of the neck. The skin and the superficial fascia were removed to highlight the superficial lamina of the deep fascia of the neck. This lamina envelops the SCM and extends medially to join with the contralateral fascia. Over the hyoid bone, it is firmly anchored in the periosteum. Cranially, it covers the digastric muscles and forms the visceral space for the submandibular **salivary** glands. Between the SCM and the angle of the mandible, the superficial lamina presents a reinforcement forming the angular ligament.

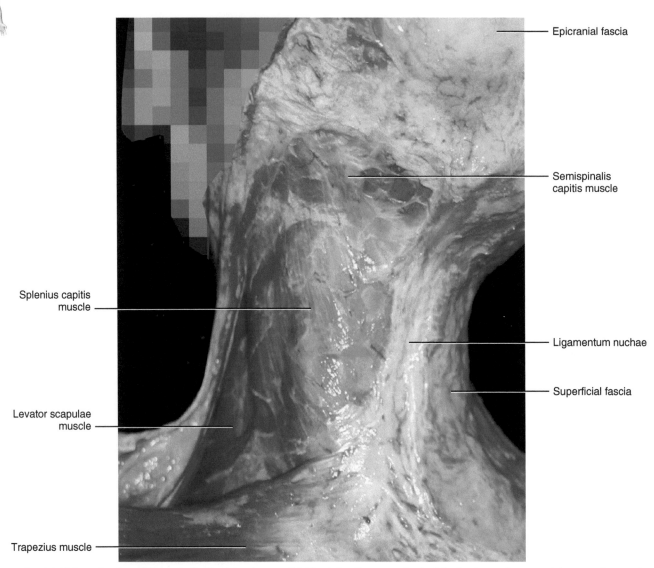

Epicranial fascia

Semispinalis
capitis muscle

Splenius capitis
muscle

Ligamentum nuchae

Superficial fascia

Levator scapulae
muscle

Trapezius muscle

FIGURE 4.33 Posterior view of the neck. On the right, the superficial fascia is still present. On the left, the descending part of the trapezius muscle was removed to show the middle myofascial layer, formed by levator scapulae and splenius muscles. The semispinalis muscle is in a deeper plane.

fuses with the fascia of the serratus anterior muscle. Thus, the middle lamina of the neck fascia forms a continuum with the middle lamina of the thorax, both anteriorly and posteriorly. In addition, the middle lamina of the deep cervical fascia envelops the omohyoid, the sternohyoid and the sternothyroid muscles (Figs 4.34–4.36). This fascia is attached to the posterior surface of the periosteum of the clavicle, where it continues as the internal wall of the sheath of the subclavius muscle. The middle lamina creates the visceral space, where all the viscera of the neck enveloped by the visceral fasciae are located.

The middle lamina must be distinguished from the pretracheal fascia (Fig. 4.37). The middle lamina is considered to be a muscular fascia, while the pretracheal is considered a visceral fascia. The pretracheal fascia envelops the thyroid and distally merges with the connective tissue of the pericardium. Proximally, it attaches to the periosteum of the hyoid bone where it fuses with the middle lamina. Posteriorly, the middle lamina is partially in continuity with another visceral fascia, the alar fascia, which is a connecting band between the sheaths of both common carotid arteries. Finally, the trachea and oesophagus are enveloped by another visceral fascia, which is a continuation of the buccopharyingeal fascia. This visceral fascia inferiorly enters the thorax as parietal pleura and, laterally, forms the ligaments that suspends the cupula pleurae.

Deep Fascia of the Neck: Deep Lamina (Prevertebral Fascia or Layer III)

While the deep lamina of the neck is sometimes referred to as the prevertebral fascia, the prevertebral fascia itself covers mainly the anterior vertebral muscles and extends laterally on the scalenus anterior, medius and posterior (Standring 2008). The deep lamina also has a posterior portion that covers the longissimus and the semispinalis muscles. It also contains the rectus and longus capitis muscles and the sympathetic nerves. A

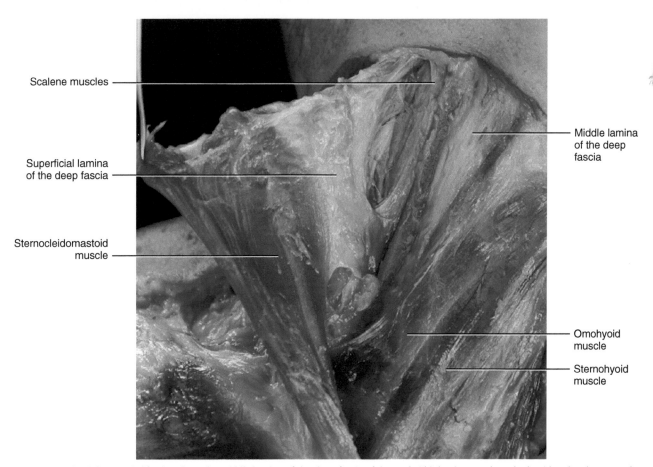

Scalene muscles

Superficial lamina of the deep fascia

Sternocleidomastoid muscle

Middle lamina of the deep fascia

Omohyoid muscle

Sternohyoid muscle

FIGURE 4.34 The right SCM is lifted to show the middle lamina of the deep fascia of the neck. This lamina envelops the hyoid and scalene muscles.

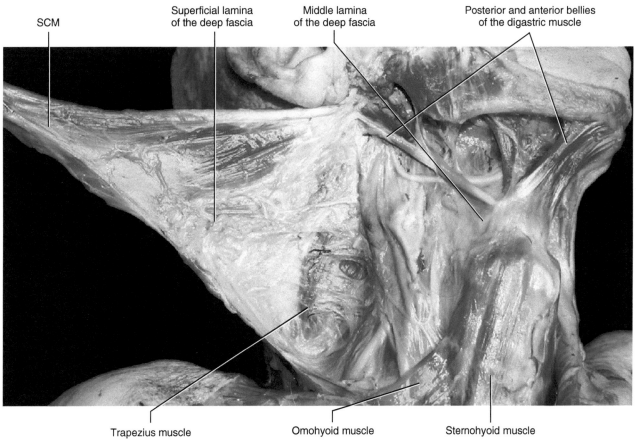

SCM

Superficial lamina of the deep fascia

Middle lamina of the deep fascia

Posterior and anterior bellies of the digastric muscle

Trapezius muscle

Omohyoid muscle

Sternohyoid muscle

FIGURE 4.35 The right SCM is detached from clavicle and lifted to show the middle lamina of the deep fascia of the neck. In this image the fascial continuity between SCM and trapezius muscle (superficial lamina) is clearly evident.

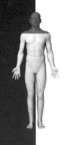

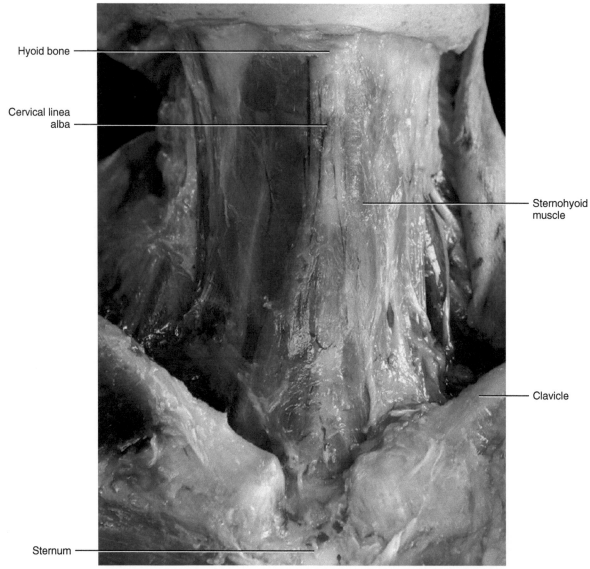

Hyoid bone

Cervical linea alba

Sternohyoid muscle

Clavicle

Sternum

FIGURE 4.36 The superficial lamina was removed together with the SCM to show the middle lamina of the deep fascia of the neck. This lamina envelops the hyoid muscles and covers the thyroid.

CLINICAL PEARL 4.6 ROLES OF THE VISCERAL CERVICAL FASCIAE

According to Allan Burns (1824), the main function of the cervical fasciae is to permit correct breathing:

So long as the superficial and deep fasciae, accompanied by the sternohyoid and thyroid muscles remain normal, breathing is performed with ease; but whenever these fasciae and muscles are removed, then, on every attempt to increase the size of the chest, the atmospheric air pushes back the unresisting skin on the trachea, compressing that tube to such a degree that it will create severe difficulty in breathing. The sternohyoid and thyroid muscles are capable of steadying the hyoid bone and thyroid cartilage, or of depressing these parts, but their great use is to co-operate with fasciae in preventing the gravitation of the air on the windpipe.

According with Richet (1857), the cervical fasciae permit the main vessels to remain open during breathing and neck movements. Indeed there are strong connections between the adventitia of the veins and the fasciae that form their sheaths. Richet also highlighted the role of the omohyoideus muscle as a fascial tensor. Indeed, this muscle could be considered a tensor of the middle layer of the deep cervical fasciae. Thanks to this tension, this fascial layer maintains the patency of the walls of the jugular and thyroid veins.

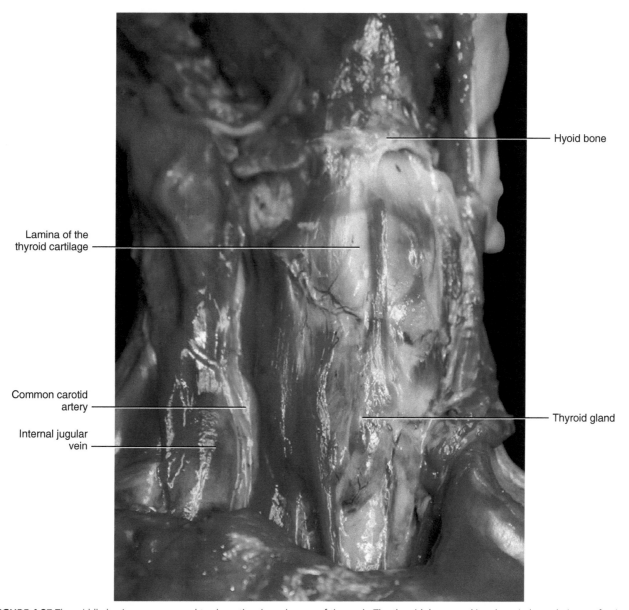

Hyoid bone

Lamina of the thyroid cartilage

Common carotid artery

Internal jugular vein

Thyroid gland

FIGURE 4.37 The middle lamina was removed to show the visceral space of the neck. The thyroid, larynx and jugular vein have their own fasciae, which protects them and guarantees their autonomous function with respect to muscular contraction.

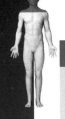

CLINICAL PEARL 4.7 MYOFASCIAL NECK PAIN

Chronic neck pain (CNP) is a very prevalent condition, affecting 10–24% of the population: 30–50% of adults present with neck pain in the course of a year, and 11–14% have loss of work productivity due to neck pain every year. However, a definitive diagnosis of its causes is often not possible in the clinical setting and the terms 'nonspecific neck pain' and 'myofascial pain' are often used, although these diagnoses are made for purposes of exclusion and are based only on clinical determinants (Gerwin 2001). There are, in fact, very few studies which describe objective and clinically applicable methods for identifying and classifying myofascial pain: Shultz et al (2007) quantified the most painful regions with electrodermal instruments, and Arokoski et al (2005) demonstrated increasing superficial soft tissue stiffness. Thermographic studies in areas reported to be painful provide variable results (Giamberardino et al 2011). Stecco et al (2013) demonstrated that there were significant differences in the thickness of the sternocleidomastoid fascia and scalene fascia between healthy subjects and patients with nonspecific CNP. The analysis of the thickness of the sublayers showed a significant increase in the thickness of the loose connective tissue layers rather than the fibrous sublayers.

The authors suggest that the loose connective tissue inside the fasciae plays a significant role in the pathogenesis of CNP. A thickness value of 0.15 cm for the SCM fascia can be considered as a cut-off value allowing clinicians to make a diagnosis of myofascial disease in a subject with CNP. Therefore, the thickness of the deep fascia was due to the increase in quantity of loose connective tissue rather than the overlying dense connective tissue. The probable cause of the increased viscosity is related to hyaluronan (HA) found in loose connective tissue. Piehl-Aulin et al (1991) demonstrated retention of HA after exercise. In overuse syndromes, an increase in the quantity of HA probably occurs in and on the surface of fascia. At high concentrations, HA behaves like a non-Newtonian fluid and becomes more viscous (Knepper et al 1995); this reaction may explain the decrease in gliding action between the fibrous layers. The increased viscosity of the loose connective tissue inside the fascia may cause decreased gliding between the layers of collagen fibres of the deep fasciae, which may be perceived by patients as stiffness. We postulate that increased viscosity alters the dynamic response of the mechanoreceptors within the fascia, causing pain and alteration in proprioception.

study of Miyake et al (2011) indicates that prevertebral lamina develops as an intermediate aponeurosis for the bilateral bellies of the longus colli muscles.

The prevertebral fascia originates from the base of the skull. It attaches to the transverse processes of the vertebrae and extends inferiorly between the oesophagus and the spine to the posterior mediastinum, where it blends with the anterior longitudinal ligament. Loose connective tissue separates it from the buccopharyngeal fascia and from the tunica adventitia of the oesophagus (retropharyngeal space). The deep lamina defines the retrovisceral space. Laterally, it fuses with the superficial and middle laminae forming a boundary between the neck and the nape. In the lower part of the neck, the deep lamina forms a tube that covers the brachial plexus. Thus, the deep lamina continues downwards and laterally, behind the clavicle, as the axillary sheath.

References

Arokoski, J.P., Surakka, J., Ojala, T., Kolari, P., Jurvelin, J.S., 2005. Feasibility of the use of a novel soft tissue stiffness meter. Physiol. Meas. 26 (3), 215–228.

Bendtsen, L., Fernández de-la-Peñas, C., 2011. The role of muscles in tension-type headache. Curr. Pain Headache Rep. 15 (6), 451–458.

Burns, A., Pattison, G.S. 1824. Observations on the Surgical Anatomy of the Head and Neck. Wardlaw & Cunninghame, Glasgow, pp. 31–34.

Davidge, K.M., van Furth, W.R., Agur, A., Cusimano, M., 2010. Naming the soft tissue layers of the temporoparietal region: unifying anatomic terminology across surgical disciplines. Neurosurgery 67 (3 Suppl.), 120–129.

Gerwin, R.D., 2001. Classification, epidemiology, and natural history of myofascial pain syndrome. Curr. Pain Headache Rep. 5 (5), 412–420.

Giamberardino, M.A., Affaitati, G., Fabrizio, A., Costantini, R., 2011. Myofascial pain syndromes and their evaluation. Best Pract. Res. Clin. Rheumatol. 25 (2), 185–198.

Grgić, V., 2006. Cervicogenic proprioceptive vertigo: etiopathogenesis, clinical manifestations, diagnosis and therapy with special emphasis on manual therapy. [Article in Croatian] LijecVjesn 128 (9–10), 288–295.

Guarda-Nardini, L., Stecco, A., Stecco, C., Masiero, S., Manfredini, D., 2012. Myofascial pain of the jaw muscles: comparison of short-term effectiveness of botulinum toxin injections and fascial manipulation technique. Cranio. 30 (2), 95–102.

Guidera, A.K., Dawes, P.J., Stringer, M.D., 2012. Cervical fascia: a terminological pain in the neck. ANZ J. Surg. 82 (11), 786–791.

Habal, M.B., Maniscalco, J.E., 1981. Observations on the ultrastructure of the pericranium. Ann. Plast. Surg. 6 (2), 103–111.

Jensen, R., Bendtsen, L., Olesen, J., 1998. Muscular factors are of importance in tension-type headache. Headache 38 (1), 10–17.

Knepper, P.A., Covici, S., Fadel, J.R., Mayanil, C.S., Ritch, R., 1995. Surface-tension properties of hyaluronic acid. J. Glaucoma 4 (3), 194–199.

Luan, H., Gdowski, M.J., Newlands, S.D., Gdowski, G.T., 2013. Convergence of vestibular and neck proprioceptive sensory signals in the cerebellar interpositus. J. Neurosci. 33 (3), 1198–1210a.

Macchi, V., Tiengo, C., Porzionato, A., et al., 2010. Histotopographic study of the fibroadipose connective cheek system. Cells Tissues Organs 191 (1), 47–56.

Melzack, R., Stillwell, D.M., Fox, E.J., 1977. Trigger points and acupuncture points for pain: correlations and implications. Pain 3 (1), 3–23.

Mitz, V., Peyronie, M., 1976. The superficial muscoloaponeurotic system (SMAS) in the parotid and cheek area. Plast Recontr Surg. 58 (1), 80–88.

Miyake, N., Takeuchi, H., Cho, B.H., Murakami, G., Fujimiya, M., Kitano, H., 2011. Fetal anatomy of the lower cervical and upper thoracic fasciae with special reference to the prevertebral fascial structures including the suprapleural membrane. Clin. Anat. 24 (5), 607–618.

Piehl-Aulin, K., Laurent, C., Engström-Laurent, A., Hellström, S., Henriksson, J., 1991. Hyaluronan in human skeletal muscle of lower extremity: concentration, distribution, and effect of exercise. J. Appl. Physiol. 71 (6), 2493–2498.

Poirier, A., 1912. Les muscles de la to te et du cou. In: Poirier, A., Charpy, A. (Eds.), Traité d'anatomie humaine. Tome 2-1: Myologie, Masson, Paris, France, pp. 216–228.

Richet, L.A., 1857. Traite Practique d'anatomie medico chirurgicale, F. Chamerot, Paris, pp. 161–170.

Sappey, P.H.C., 1888. Traité d'anatomie descriptive, A. Delahaye, E. Lecrosnier, tome II, Myologie, Paris, pp. 94–107.

Schmolke, C., 1994. The relationship between the temporomandibular joint capsule, articular disc and jaw muscles. J. Anat. 184 (2), 335–345.

Shultz, S.P, Driban, J.B., Swanik, C.B., 2007. The evaluation of electrodermal properties in the identification of myofascial trigger points. Arch. Phys. Med. Rehabil. 88 (6), 780–784.

Skaggs, C., Liebenson, C., 2000. Orofacial Pain. Top Clin. Chiropr. 7 (20), 43–50.

Standring, S., 2008. Gray's Anatomy: The Anatomical Basis of Clinical Practice, fortieth ed, Elsevier Health Sciences UK, pp. 524–584.

Stecco, A., Meneghini, A., Stern, R., Stecco, C., Imamura, I., 2014. Ultrasonography in myofascial neck pain: randomized clinical trial for diagnosis and follow up. Surg. Radiol. Anat. 36 (3), 243–253.

Stuzin, J.M., Backer, T.J., Gordon, H.L., 1992. The relationship of the superficial and deep facial fascias: relevance to rhytidectomy and aging. Plast. Reconstr. Surg. 89 (3), 441–449.

Testut, J.L., Jacob, O., 1905. Précis d'anatomie topographique avec applications medico-chirurgicales, Gaston Doin et Cie, Paris.

Thaller, S.R., Kim, S., Patterson, H., et al., 1990. The submuscularaponeurotic system (SMAS): a histologic and comparative anatomy evaluation. Plast. Reconstr. Surg. 86 (4), 690–696.

Travell, J.G., Simons, D.G., 1983. Myofascial Pain and Dysfunction, The Trigger Point Manual, Williams & Wilkins, Baltimore, pp. 260–272.

Tsukahara, K., Tamatsu, Y., Sugawara, Y., Shimada, K., 2012. Relationship between the depth of facial wrinkles and the density of the retinacula cutis. Arch. Dermatol. 148 (1), 39–46.

Yahia, A., Ghroubi, S., Jribi, S., et al., 2009. Chronic neck pain and vertigo: Is a true balance disorder present? Ann. PhysRehabil Med. 52 (7–8), 556–567.

Bibliography

Gardetto, A., Daberning, J., Rainer, C., Piegger, J., Piza-Katzer, H., Fritsch, H., 2002. Does a superficial muscoloaponeurotic system exist in the face and neck? An anatomical study by the tissue plastination technique. Plast. Reconstr. Surg. 111 (2), 664–672.

Kirolles, S., Haikal, F.A., Saadeh, F.A., Abul-Hassan, H., el-Bakaury, A.R., 1992. Fascial layers of the scalp. A study of 48 cadaveric dissections. Surg. Radiol. Anat. 14 (4), 331–333.

Levi, A.C., 1969. Development, configuration and structure of the temporal fascia in humans. Arch. Sci. Med. 126 (9), 567–576.

Lockwood, C.B., 1885. The anatomy of the muscles, ligaments, and fasciae of the orbit, including an account of the capsule of Tenon, the check ligaments of the recti, and the suspensory ligaments of the eye. J. Anat. Physiol. 20 (1), 12–25.

McKinney, P., Gottlieb, J., 1985. The relationship of the great auricular nerve to the superficial musculoaponeurotic system. Ann. Plastic Surgery 14 (4), 310–314.

Tsukahara, K., Osanai, O., Hotta, M., et al., 2011. Relationship between the echogenicity of subcutaneous tissue and the depth of forehead wrinkles. Skin Res. Technol. 17 (3), 353–358.

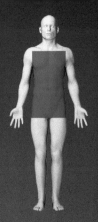

5

Fasciae of the Thorax and Abdomen

Introduction

In the abdomen is the thickest superficial fascia of the body known as 'Scarpa's fascia'. The superficial fascia is present throughout the trunk as a continuous fibro-elastic layer. The deep fascia is arranged into three laminae: superficial, intermediate and deep. Considering that the deep fascia in the thorax is very thin and adherent to the muscles, whilst the superficial fascia is thick and strong, the superficial fascia is often confused with the deep fascia. In this chapter the following will be discussed: the classification and continuation of both the superficial and deep fascia from the thorax into the neck, abdomen and lumbar areas (Fig. 5.1).

Superficial Fascia of the Thorax and Abdomen

In the thorax and abdomen, the superficial fascia is easy to identify. It divides the subcutaneous tissue into two sublayers: the superficial adipose tissue (SAT) and the deep adipose tissue (DAT), and each has its characteristic features. The superficial fascia is a fibroelastic layer mainly composed of collagen and elastic fibres; however, small fat lobules are often observed between the fibres (Fig. 5.2). While macroscopically this fascia appears to be, and can be isolated as, a well-defined membrane (Fig. 5.3), microscopically its structure is better described as lamellar or highly packed and honeycomb like. The superficial fascia can be followed as a dissection plane from the thorax to the inguinal ligament, where it adheres to the deeper planes. It appears to have total continuity with the superficial fascia of the thigh.

The superficial fascia does not have a uniform thickness. It is a well-defined, white layer in the lower abdomen where it is called Scarpa's fascia. It thickens towards the inguinal ligament where a multilayered structure of collagen bundles, extending in different directions, can be perceived both during dissection and in transparency (when a light goes through it). In the lower abdomen of cadavers, the mean resistance to traction of the isolated superficial fascia is 2.8 kg in a transverse direction and 5.5 kg in a craniocaudal direction. This difference demonstrates that the superficial fascia has specific spatial reinforcements rather than being considered a homogeneous tissue. In the upper abdomen, the superficial fascia is much thinner, appearing as a translucid collagen layer through which adipose tissue can be seen. Distally, in males it continues over the penis and spermatic cord to the scrotum, where it helps to form the dartos fascia. The dartos muscle is enveloped by the superficial fascia and in the same manner as the platysma muscle and the fundiform ligament. From the scrotum, it can be traced backwards and is continuous with the superficial fascia of the perineum (fascia of Colles).

According to Sterzi (1910), there are fibrous thickenings inside the superficial fascia of the trunk. These collagen fibrous bundles originate in the back and extend in an oblique direction to the anterior region of the trunk and in a craniocaudal direction. The distribution of these reinforcements of the superficial fascia corresponds to the lines in the dermis described by Langer in 1862.

Occasionally, inside the superficial fascia of the trunk some striated muscle fibres are found. According to Tobler (1902) and Ruge (1905), these muscular fibres inside the superficial fascia are the remains of the panniculus carnosus that is present in all superficial fasciae of mammals. To support this idea, they found well-represented axillary arches in gorillas and monkeys, which also have a large panniculus carnosus. The axillary arch can also be present in human axilla as an anatomical variation, where it can be considered as a possible cause of nerve or vascular compression.

The SAT is typically well represented in both the thorax and the abdomen and shows nearly constant characteristics (Fig. 5.4). The fibrous septa, forming the retinaculum cutis superficialis, generally assume an arrangement perpendicular to the surface. The adipose lobules have an oval shape with their major axis perpendicular to the skin, and they are generally disposed in a single layer. This structure has high-structural stability, mechanical resilience and elastic properties. In particular, if a weight of 1 kg is placed over slices of the flap and then removed, the fat lobules return to their original position and shape. With the augmentation of fat deposition, the fat lobules increase in size and in the lower abdomen they assume a multilayered disposition. This causes a lengthening and thickening of the retinacula cutis, which assume a more oblique orientation forming a second fibrofatty layer parallel to the superficial fascia. This finding could explain why some authors describe an additional fibrofatty fascial

141

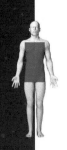

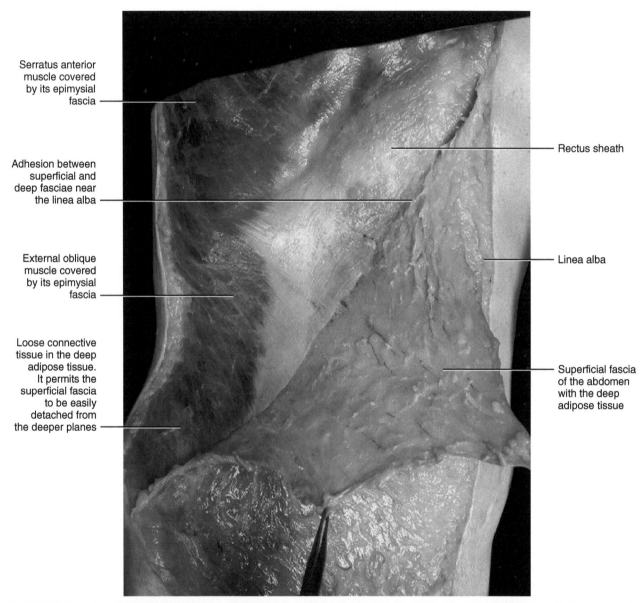

Serratus anterior muscle covered by its epimysial fascia

Adhesion between superficial and deep fasciae near the linea alba

External oblique muscle covered by its epimysial fascia

Loose connective tissue in the deep adipose tissue. It permits the superficial fascia to be easily detached from the deeper planes

Rectus sheath

Linea alba

Superficial fascia of the abdomen with the deep adipose tissue

FIGURE 5.1 Dissection of the abdomen. The superficial fascia was lifted together with the DAT to show its relationships with the deep fascia. Generally, in the abdomen the DAT is scarce and the superficial fascia is free to glide with respect to the underlying planes. Along the linea alba a longitudinal adhesion is present.

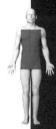

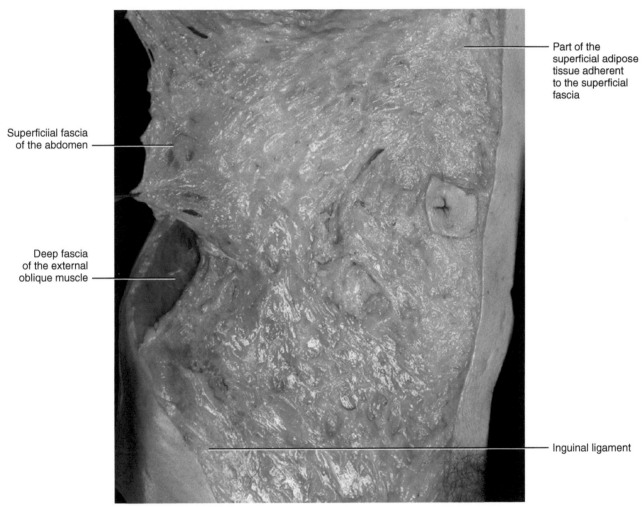

Part of the superficial adipose tissue adherent to the superficial fascia

Superficiial fascia of the abdomen

Deep fascia of the external oblique muscle

Inguinal ligament

FIGURE 5.2 Dissection of the abdominal wall. The skin and the SAT were removed to show the superficial fascia. It appears as a thick fibrofatty layer. Only a careful dissection allows the isolation of its fibrous component (see Fig. 5.3).

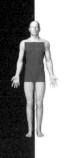

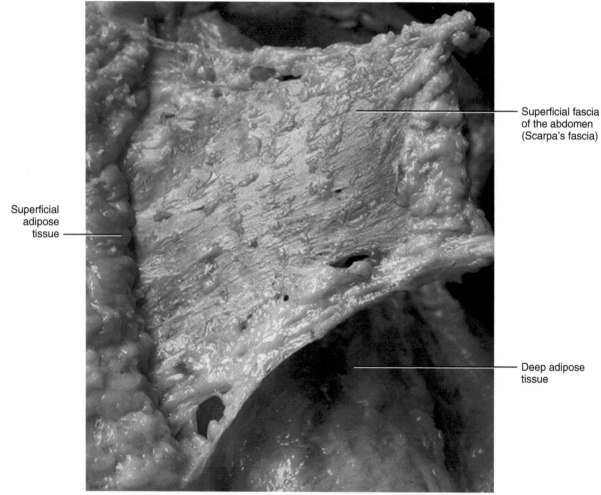

Superficial fascia
of the abdomen
(Scarpa's fascia)

Superficial
adipose
tissue

Deep adipose
tissue

FIGURE 5.3 Dissection of the lower abdomen. The superficial fascia was isolated from DAT and SAT. It appears as a well-defined fibrous layer.

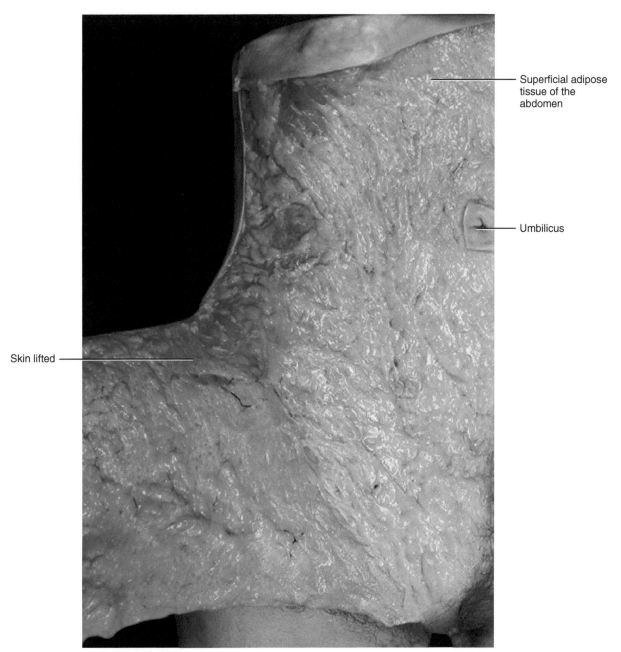

Superficial adipose
tissue of the
abdomen

Umbilicus

Skin lifted

FIGURE 5.4 SAT of the abdomen. The skin was removed after cutting all the retinacula cutis superficialis. In the abdomen SAT is usually abundant.

layer in the subcutis of the abdomen (called 'Camper's fascia'). However, our dissections and imaging studies demonstrate that only one layer of superficial fascia is present; this was also recently confirmed by Chopra et al (2011) in their study of living subjects. These authors, using CT scans of the abdominal region, showed that a membranous layer (corresponding to the superficial fascia based on our findings) is present throughout the anterior abdominal wall. This membranous layer divides the subcutis into three layers: superficial fatty layer (the SAT, based on our findings), intermediate membranous layer (superficial fascia), and deep fatty layer (the DAT, based on our findings). If the membranous layer is not clear on a CT scan, this

could be due to the absence of fat deposited in the deep compartment.

The SAT continues, with a similarly structured layer, over the inguinal ligament into the thigh (Fig. 5.5). No clear border to this layer can be identified either caudally or cranially. This layer is separated from the contralateral layer at the level of the linea alba, where the superficial fascia is adherent to the skin and to the deep fascia.

The deep compartment (DAT) appears to be very different from the SAT. It is usually thinner and formed mostly by loose connective tissue with a few fat cells (Fig. 5.6). The fat lobules are smaller, flatter and less defined, and the fibrous septa are less consistent and

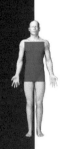

Superficial adipose
tissue of the
abdomen

Rectus sheath
(deep fascia)

Superficial adipose
tissue of the thigh

Superficial adipose
tissue over the
knee

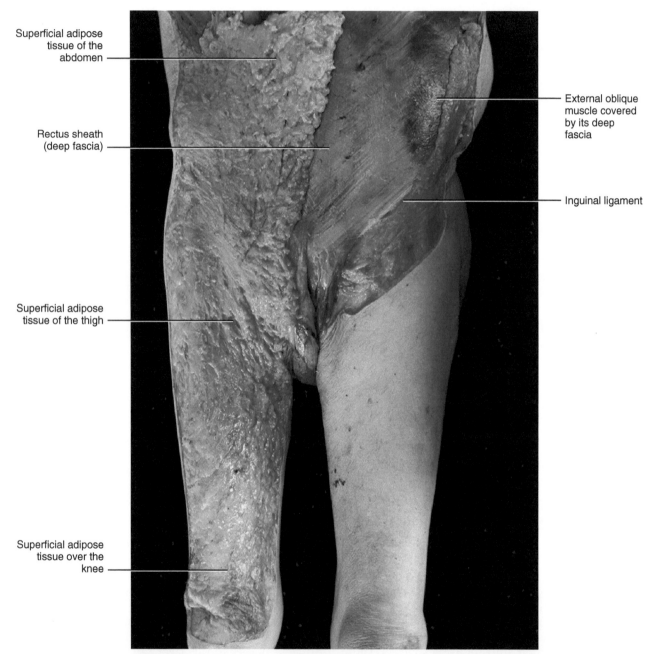

External oblique
muscle covered
by its deep
fascia

Inguinal ligament

FIGURE 5.5 SAT of the abdomen. Note its continuity with the SAT of the thigh. Deeper, along the inguinal ligament, the superficial fascia adheres to the deep fascia, dividing the DAT of the abdomen from the DAT of the thigh (see Fig. 5.10).

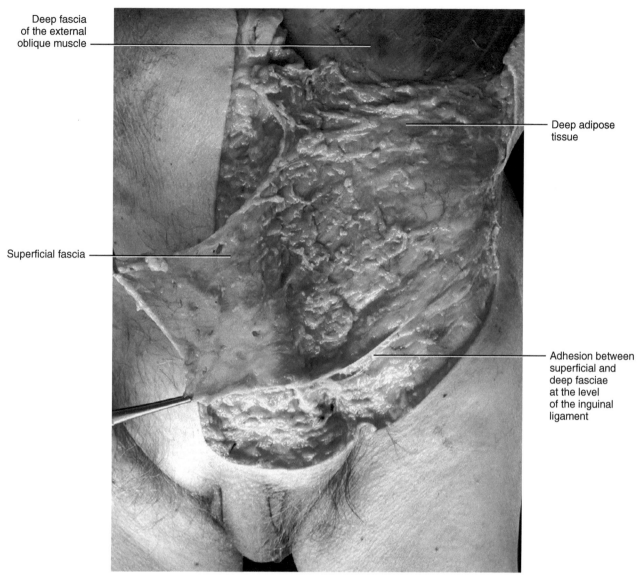

Deep fascia of the external oblique muscle

Deep adipose tissue

Superficial fascia

Adhesion between superficial and deep fasciae at the level of the inguinal ligament

FIGURE 5.6 Dissection of the abdominal region. The superficial fascia is lifted to show the DAT. In the abdomen the DAT is thinner compared to the SAT and has a function of gliding while the SAT is more important for storage.

mostly orientated obliquely. The obliquity of the septa of the DAT, its adequate elastic properties and strength, and its lateral displacement of the fatty lobules creates a perfect plane for sliding of the subcutaneous tissue over the deep fascia. The DAT presents many variations in its structure and in the amount of fat depending on the particular area (Fig. 5.7). Along the sternum and the linea alba the DAT is absent and results in the superficial fascia adhering to the deep fascia (longitudinal adhesion, see Chapter 2). Transverse adhesions are also present between the two fasciae, in particular over the acromion and clavicle, at the level of the sixth rib and over the inguinal ligament (Figs 5.8–5.10). In this way, the DAT of the abdomen is completely divided from the DAT of the thigh, preventing infections or oedema passing from one region to the other. As no fatty tissue is embedded in the DAT of this region the inguinal fold is always easier to see, even in obese people. These adhesions also allow a division of the

CLINICAL PEARL 5.1 ROLE OF THE SUBCUTANEOUS COMPARTMENTS

The cutaneous veins and lymphatic vessels drain in two directions from approximately the level of the umbilicus: upward to the thoraco-epigastric and lateral thoracic veins (thereby providing collateral circulation in caval obstruction) and to the axillary nodes, and downward to the great saphenous vein and superficial inguinal nodes.

subcutis into cervical, thoracic and abdominal compartments. By understanding the various roles of the superficial fascia and subcutis, it may be hypothesized that the compartimentalization of the subcutis play an important role in lymphatic drainage and superficial venous return in this area.

Text continued on p. 152

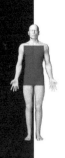

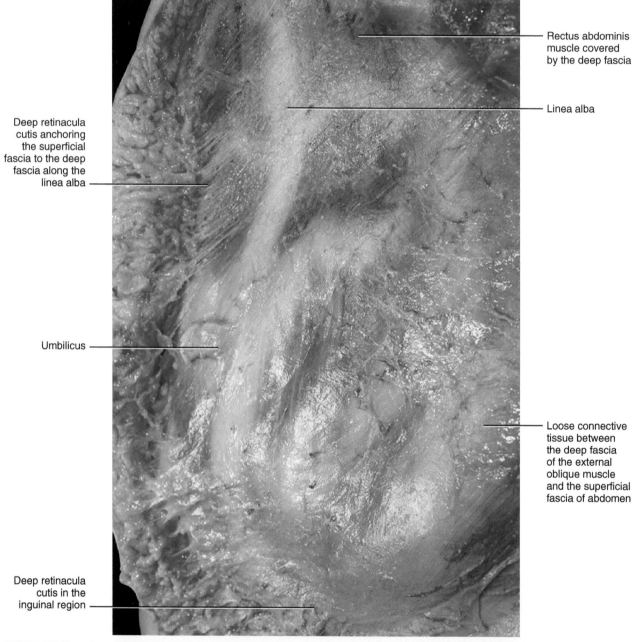

Rectus abdominis muscle covered by the deep fascia

Linea alba

Deep retinacula cutis anchoring the superficial fascia to the deep fascia along the linea alba

Umbilicus

Loose connective tissue between the deep fascia of the external oblique muscle and the superficial fascia of abdomen

Deep retinacula cutis in the inguinal region

FIGURE 5.7 Dissection of the abdomen of an obese subject. The subcutaneous tissue was removed to show the deep fascia. Note the strong retinacula cutis along the midline and in the inguinal region that hinder the dissection of the hypodermis (with respect to the deep fascia).

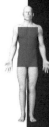

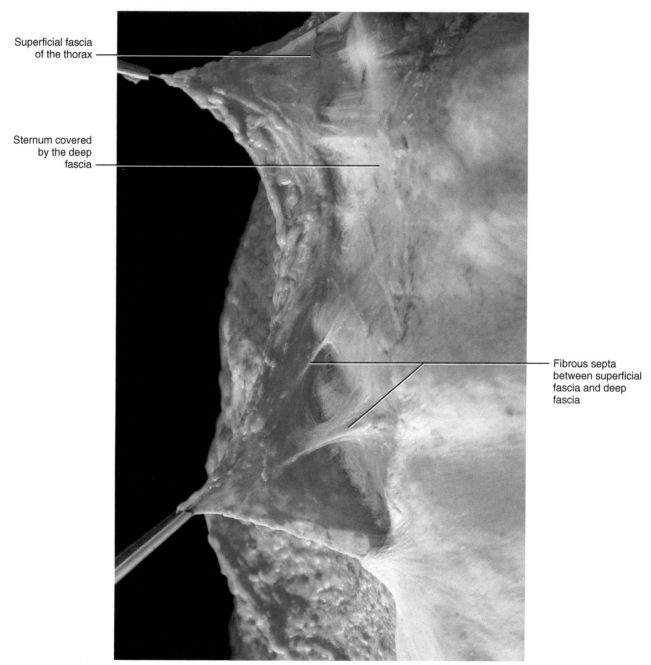

Superficial fascia of the thorax

Sternum covered by the deep fascia

Fibrous septa between superficial fascia and deep fascia

FIGURE 5.8 Dissection of the anterior region of the thorax. The superficial fascia is lifted to show its relationship with the deep fascia. Thick deep retinacula cutis are present over the sternum and form a longitudinal adhesion at the midline.

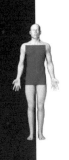

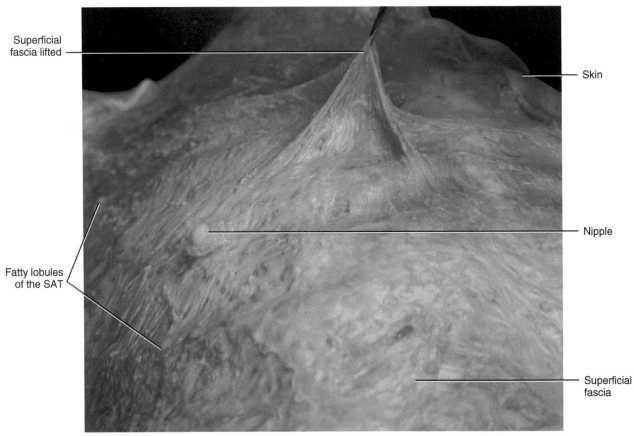

Superficial fascia lifted

Skin

Nipple

Fatty lobules of the SAT

Superficial fascia

FIGURE 5.9 Dissection of the superficial fascia of the thorax of a very thin male subject. The superficial fascia could be easily lifted from the underlying planes thanks to the presence of loose connective tissue in the DAT.

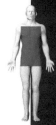

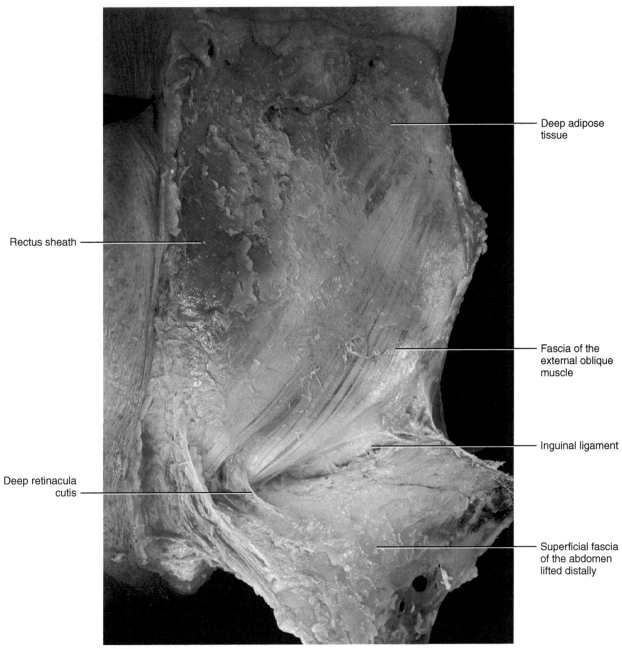

Deep adipose
tissue

Rectus sheath

Fascia of the
external oblique
muscle

Inguinal ligament

Deep retinacula
cutis

Superficial fascia
of the abdomen
lifted distally

FIGURE 5.10 Dissection of the abdomen. The superficial fascia was lifted distally to show the deep adipose tissue and the relationship between the superficial and deep fascia along the inguinal ligament.

HISTORY BOX 5.1 FASCIAE OF CAMPER, SCARPA AND COLLES

The superficial fascia of the abdomen was the first superficial fascia to be described in history. Early in the nineteenth century, Antonio Scarpa described a fascial layer in the abdominal wall and Abraham Colles described one in the perineum. To Petrus Camper is attributed the description of another fibrofatty layer, probably corresponding to the SAT with its retinaculum cutis superficialis.

The description by Colles is more detailed and seems to refer to the continuation in the perineal region of the superficial fascia of the abdomen. Colles, in some points, refers to this as 'superficial' fascia, in contrast to the 'deep' fascia found enveloping the muscles.

The work of Antonio Scarpa deals primarily with the anatomy of the hernia. In the first edition (1809) of his famous text, a short paragraph of the anatomical introduction is dedicated to a description of the layer that he identifies as superficial to the aponeurosis of the external oblique muscle: 'easily and totally dissectable, aponeurotic in character, and strongly connected caudally to the inguinal ligament'. This description corresponds to the superficial fascia that we identified in the abdomen. Scarpa did not use the term 'superficial' in any part of his work. However, the interest that this short paragraph acquired led Professor Scarpa to further investigations which were published in a second edition of *A Treatise on Hernia* (1819). In this book he changed his views, describing the layer as a 'fascia', rich in fat tissue and completely distinct from the fascia lata. This description seems to refer to what we identified as deep adipose tissue of the subcutaneous tissue. The first edition of his work became well known in Italian anatomy schools, the second edition was more popular in France, and both versions, through different channels, found a way into the Anglo-Saxon world. This led to the persisting double definition of Scarpa's fascia as either the membranous layer or the deep adipose layer.

Mammary Region

There is some confusion about the relationship between the superficial fascia and the mammary gland. For some authors the mammary gland is embedded within the superficial fascia, for others the superficial fascia is superficial to it, while others deny the existence of the superficial fascia (Beer et al 2002). Our dissections have revealed superficial fascia in the pectoral region of all subjects. This superficial fascia is a continuation of the superficial fascia of the neck, and the muscular fibres of the platysma muscle extend to the proximal third of the superficial fascia of the thoracic region (Fig. 5.11). The mammary gland at first appears to be enveloped by the superficial fascia.

However, after careful dissection, it is evident that the fascia is always deeper respect to the mammary gland, and that the gland maintains its contact with the skin in the areola region (Figs 5.12 and 5.13). This organization is consistent with the embryologic development of the mammary gland, which is a cutaneous gland that has assumed a specific function. Our findings are confirmed by Sterzi (1910) who studied the superficial fascia of this region in cadavers of different ages. He found that in newborns the superficial fascia is deep with respect to the mammary gland, dividing the abundant SAT from a very thin DAT. In adult females, the superficial fascia adheres intimately to the inner side of the mammary gland. The retinacula cutis of the SAT divides the mammary gland into various lobules (Fig. 5.14). Inside the mammary gland, the fibrous septa of the superficial retinacula cutis are called Cooper's ligaments[1] and they have the role of maintaining the structural integrity of the gland. Without the internal support of these septa, the breast tissue, which is heavier than the surrounding fat, sags under its own weight, and loses its normal shape and contours. Cooper's ligaments play an important role in the changing appearance of the breast that often accompanies development of inflammatory carcinoma, in which blockage of the local lymphatic ducts causes swelling of the breast. As the skin remains tethered by these septa, it takes on a dimpled appearance reminiscent of an orange peel. Carcinomas can also decrease the length of Cooper's ligaments leading to a dimpling.

Between the clavicle and the mammary gland the superficial fascia is thicker, and this thickening forms the suspensory ligament of Giraldes (1851). This ligament is actually a reinforcement of the superficial fascia (rather than a true ligament), and its isolation is an artifact of the dissection. This 'ligament' has the effect of supporting the breast in its normal position and maintaining its normal shape, and it continues medially with the platysma muscle.

Between the superficial and deep fasciae of the thorax there is loose connective tissue that permits the movement of the mammary gland with respect to the underlying muscular plane. So, in the breast region the same organization of the subcutis can be identified as is present throughout the human body. These particular elements are: the presence of the mammary glands in the SAT and the major thickness of the superficial fascia with respect to the deep fascia.

Text continued on p. 157

---

[1]Astley Cooper remarks: 'The margins of the breast do not form a regular disc, but the secreting structure often projects into the surrounding fibrous and adipose tissues so as to produce radii from the nipple of very unequal lengths, hence, a circular sweep of the knife cuts off many of its projections, spoils the breast for dissection, and, in surgical operations, leaves much of the disease unremoved.'

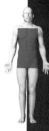

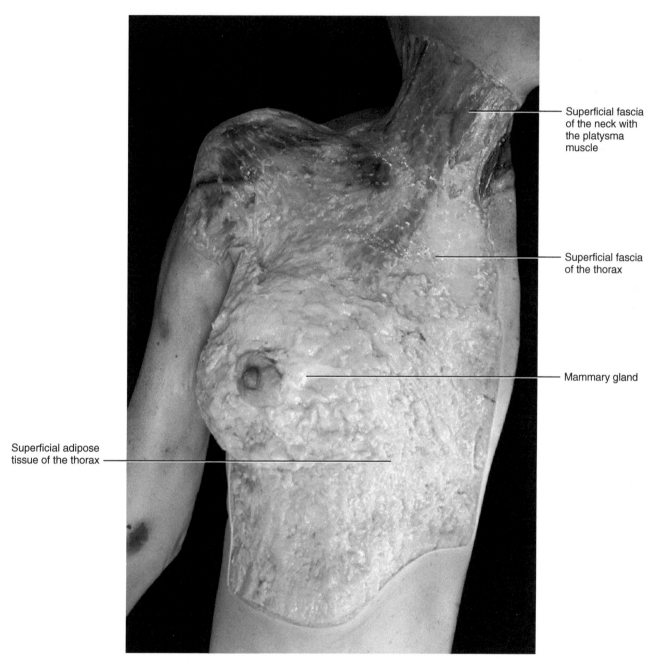

FIGURE 5.11 Dissection of the anterior region of the thorax. The skin was removed to show SAT. In the neck, the SAT is very thin so that the superficial fascia embedded with the platysma muscle is clearly visible.

Superficial fascia of the neck with the platysma muscle

Superficial fascia of the thorax

Mammary gland

Superficial adipose tissue of the thorax

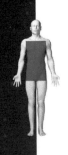

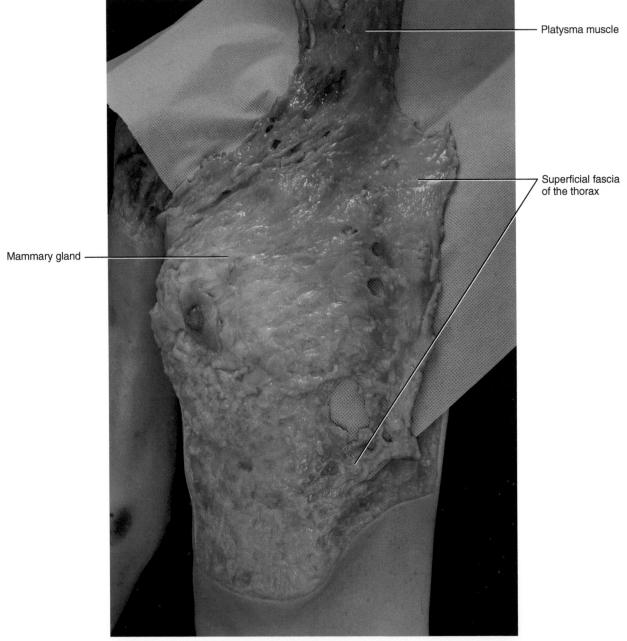

Platysma muscle

Superficial fascia
of the thorax

Mammary gland

FIGURE 5.12 The superficial fascia was detached from the underlying planes and a paper was put in the DAT. The platysma muscle is continuous with the superficial fascia of the thorax and with Cooper's ligaments of the mamary gland.

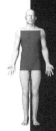

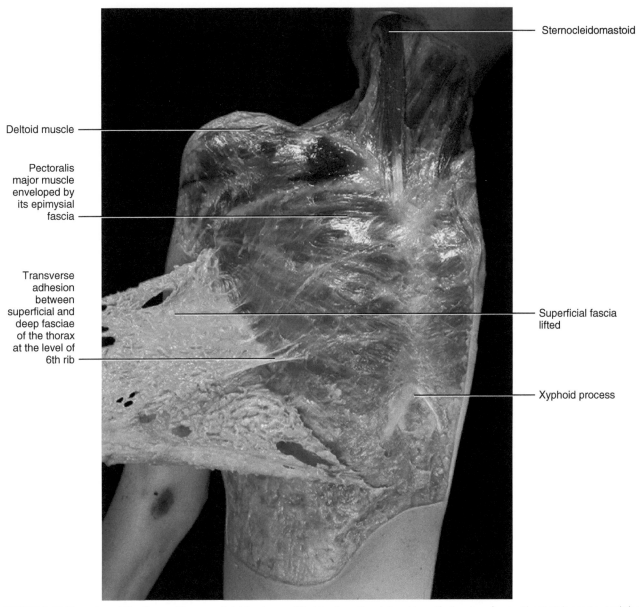

Sternocleidomastoid

Deltoid muscle

Pectoralis major muscle enveloped by its epimysial fascia

Transverse adhesion between superficial and deep fasciae of the thorax at the level of 6th rib

Superficial fascia lifted

Xyphoid process

FIGURE 5.13 Dissection of the thorax. The superficial fascia was lifted to show its relationship with the deep fascia. The DAT is scarce, and the deep fascia is thin and adheres to the muscles.

Adipose tissue of the mammary gland   Dermis

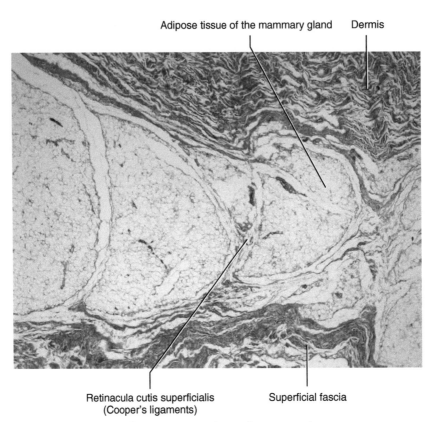

Retinacula cutis superficialis   Superficial fascia
(Cooper's ligaments)

FIGURE 5.14 Histology of the subcutaneous tissue of the mammary region, Mallory–Azan stain.

CLINICAL PEARL 5.2 AXILLARY WEB SYNDROME AND FASCIAL CONNECTIONS WITH THE BREAST

The strong connections between the mammary gland and the superficial fascia of the thorax, and the continuity between this fascia and the axilla, could explain the pathogenesis of the axillary web syndrome and why patients suffering with this syndrome, as a sequela of breast cancer, could be treated successfully using soft tissue techniques (Fourie & Robb 2009). Moskovitz et al (2001) hypothesized that interrupted axillary lymphatics appear to play an important role in the development of this syndrome, proposing a 'lymphovenous injury with stasis' as aetiology. During cancer surgery, the superficial fasciae of the pectoral region and axilla are always removed or damaged, and a scar forms in the subcutaneous tissue. As all the superficial lymphatic vessels are inside the superficial fascia, its damage surely alters lymphatic drainage. The soft tissue techniques could restore the gliding between skin, superficial fascia and deep fascia, restoring the orientation of the collagen and elastic fibres inside the superficial fascia and consequently assisting correct lymphatic drainage.

CLINICAL PEARL 5.3 BREAST PTOSIS

It is known that cigarette smoking, body mass index, number of pregnancies, size of breasts before pregnancy, and age are factors that influence breast sagging. From an anatomical perspective, these factors modify the structure of Cooper's and Giraldes' ligaments; for example, during pregnancy the woman's breasts grow in size and, consequently, Cooper's ligaments are stretched and gradually lose strength. The breast tissues and suspensory ligaments may also be stretched if a woman is overweight, or loses and gains weight in rapid succession.

It has been suggested that reinforcement of the platysma muscle might prevent ptosis of the mammary gland. From an anatomical point of view, this idea could be correct since the platysma muscle is inside the superficial fascia and acts with the Giraldes' ligament to support the mammary gland.

There are different surgical approaches for the emplacement of a breast implant based upon localization of the implant pocket:

- Subglandular: the breast implant is placed in the retromammary space between the mammary gland and the superficial fascia. For a woman with thin pectoral soft tissue: a subglandular position is more likey to show ripples and wrinkles of the underlying implant.
- Subfascial: the breast implant is placed beneath the superficial and deep fascia. This implantation uses the natural pocket given by the adhesion between the superficial and deep fascia, that is always present at the level of the sixth rib. The superficial fascia also provides greater implant coverage and is better at sustaining its position. Plastic surgeons usually refer to this fascial layer as the 'pectoral fascia', but it is the superficial fascia and not the fascia of the pectoralis major muscle. Indeed, the fascia of the pectoralis major adheres to the muscle and so it is impossibile to consider it as a distinct anatomical plane. Therefore, the term 'subfascial' refers to the superficial fascia of the thorax.
- Submuscular: the breast implant is placed beneath the pectoralis major muscle. In breast reconstruction surgery, the submuscular implantation approach results in maximum coverage of the breast implants.

Deep Fascia

The fascial anatomy of the trunk is more complex than that of the limbs. In the limbs, only one aponeurotic fascia connects the ipsodirectional motor units, while in the trunk there are three muscular planes with three fascial layers. Between these fasciae, loose connective tissue is present and permits the sliding between the various muscle bellies (Fig. 5.15). In some places these fasciae fuse, creating specific lines where all the muscular forces converge. The more important of these lines of fusion is the linea alba, but there are also fusions at the borders of the rectus sheath and over the sternum.

Each one of the three muscular layers (laminae) of the trunk have specific fascia with epimysial features. In particular, these fasciae are thin and adhere to the underlying muscles and to the flat tendons of these muscles. Thus, the anatomy and the function of these fascial layers cannot be separated from their respective muscles. Only two aponeurotic fasciae were identified in the trunk: the rectus sheath and the thoracolumbar fascia.

To understand the fascial anatomy of the trunk, it is useful to study their development. According to Skandalakis et al (2006), the deep, intermediate and superficial layers of deep fascia are produced in the embryo as muscular primordial, and originate from somites invading the somatopleura that penetrate the somatic wall connective tissue. This produces epimysial fascia on either side, from which arise the layers of investing fascia. Sato and Hashimoto (1984) report that the pectoralis major, latissimus dorsi and trapezius muscles form an additional myofascial layer with respect to the underlying muscular planes. Indeed, these muscles originate as muscles of the limbs, but then they grow inside the superficial lamina of the deep fasciae of the trunk just up to the connection with the midline (the interspinous processes of the spine in the back and with the sternum in the thorax). Thus an additional muscular plane in the trunk is formed. The development of these muscles in the trunk is probably determined by the necessity to connect firmly the upper and lower limbs to the trunk. The superficial lamina of the deep fascia, enveloping all these muscles, serves to reinforce these connections. The connections are spatially organized and very specific; for example, the expansions of the pectoralis major muscles into the rectus abdominis sheaths connect the muscles of the thorax and abdomen on both sides. The superficial layer of the pectoral fascia passes over the sternum to connect the two pectoralis major muscles.

We can identify three myofascial laminae in the trunk (superficial, middle and deep) (Fig. 5.16). The superficial lamina is formed by a fibrous layer, which is thicker at the level of the neck but becomes thinner as it descends into the abdomen. This fascia envelops all the large muscles of the trunk that work in spiral/rotational movements and connect the trunk with the limbs. At the cervical level it surrounds the sternocleidomastoid and trapezii muscles. At the level of the thorax it surrounds the pectoralis major and the latissimus dorsi muscles. At the level of the abdomen it surrounds the external oblique muscles and covers the rectus sheath on the anterior part. The middle lamina is formed by the infrahyoid, subclavius, pectoralis minor, serratus anterior and internal oblique muscles. These muscles primarily move in the frontal and horizontal planes. This middle layer of the fasciae of the trunk connects and coordinates all of them. The deep lamina is formed by the scalenes, intercostal, rectus abdominis, pyramidalis and transversus abdominis muscles. Most of the muscles in this plane have a longitudinal disposition of their muscular fibres and move primarily in the longitudinal plane. The transversus abdominis muscle and its fascia connect the rectus sheath with the iliopsoas, quadratus lumborum muscles and anterior layer of the thoracolumbar fascia. So, the transversus abdominis muscle becomes the joining element between the anterior and posterior muscular–fascial elements.

Pectoral Fascia

The fascia of the pectoralis major muscle is a thin fibroelastic layer (mean thickness 151 µm±37) firmly connected to the underlying muscle by many intramuscular septa. They originate from its inner surface and penetrate between the muscular fibres, dividing the muscle itself into many bundles (Fig. 5.17). Many

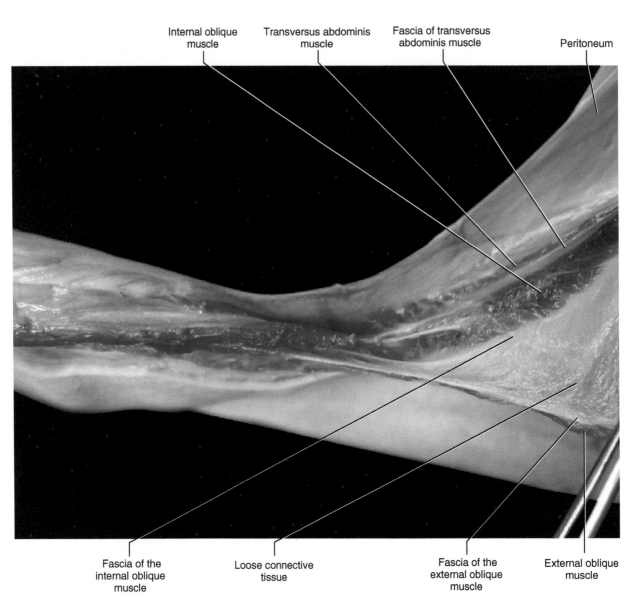

Internal oblique muscle

Transversus abdominis muscle

Fascia of transversus abdominis muscle

Peritoneum

Fascia of the internal oblique muscle

Loose connective tissue

Fascia of the external oblique muscle

External oblique muscle

FIGURE 5.15 Layers of the abdominal wall. The transversus abdominis, internal oblique and external oblique muscles are enveloped by epimysial fascia. Between the various fasciae loose connective tissue is present, assuring autonomy between the various myofascial layers.

	THORAX	ABDOMEN
SUPERFICIAL LAMINA OF THE DEEP FASCIA	Pectoral fascia	Fascia of the external oblique muscles
MIDDLE LAMINA OF THE DEEP FASCIA	Clavipectoral fascia	Fascia of the internal oblique muscle
DEEP LAMINA OF THE DEEP FASCIA	Fascia of the intercostalis muscles	Rectus sheath and fascia of the transversus abdominis muscle

FIGURE 5.16 The three laminae of the deep fascia of the trunk.

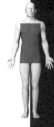

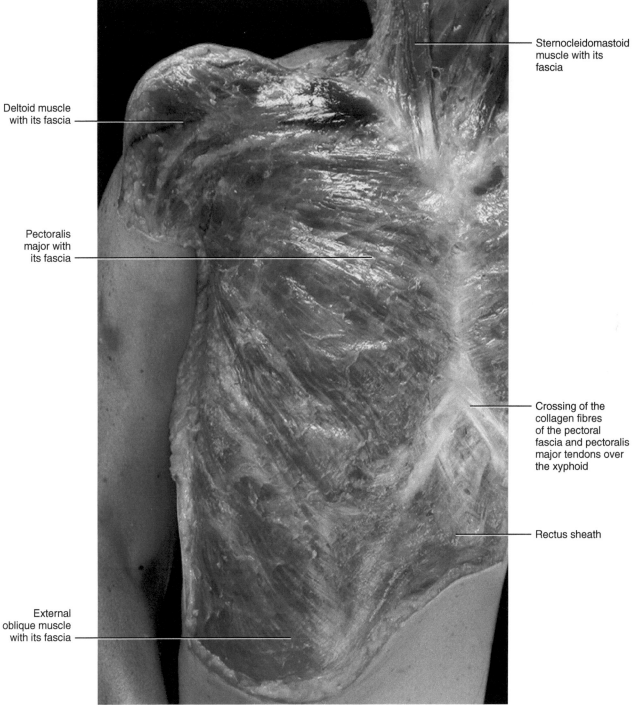

Sternocleidomastoid muscle with its fascia

Deltoid muscle with its fascia

Pectoralis major with its fascia

Crossing of the collagen fibres of the pectoral fascia and pectoralis major tendons over the xyphoid

Rectus sheath

External oblique muscle with its fascia

FIGURE 5.17 The pectoralis major muscle is enveloped by the superficial lamina of the deep fasciae of the trunk. This fascia is thin and adheres to the underlying muscle, showing the typical features of the epimysial fasciae. Over the sternum, the deep layer of this fascia adheres to the periosteum, while the superficial layer glides to connect the two sides. Distally, the fascia continues with the fascia of the external oblique muscle.

muscular fibres insert directly onto the pectoral fascia itself. The pectoral fascia originates from the clavicle and then divides into two layers to envelop the pectoralis major muscle. Proximally, only the deep layer of the pectoral fascia adheres to the clavicular periosteum. Its superficial layer continues with the superficial lamina of the deep cervical fascia, which surrounds the sternocleidomastoid muscle. Laterally, the pectoral fascia continues with the deltoid fascia and with the axillary fascia, extending as a fibrous expansion into the brachial fascia. The deltoid fascia envelops the deltoid muscle, just like the pectoral fascia does with the pectoralis major muscle. Over the serratus anterior, the two layers of the pectoral fascia adhere to form a single fascial lamina (Fig. 5.18) that some authors call the anterolateral thoracic fascia (Sebastien at al 1993). Posteriorly, this single layer divides itself again to enclose the latissimus dorsi muscle in the same manner as the pectoral fascia encloses the pectoralis major muscle. Medially, the deep layer of the pectoral fascia inserts into the periosteum of the sternum, while the superficial layer extends beyond the sternum to continue with the pectoral fascia on the other side (Figs 5.19 and 5.20). Distally, the pectoral fascia continues with some fibrous expansions into the rectus abdominis sheath and into the fascia of the controlateral external oblique muscle. Over the xyphoid process a criss-cross interweaving of fibres is clearly visible (Fig. 5.21).

Histologically, the pectoral fascia appears to be formed by undulated collagen and elastic fibres in an irregular mesh. A true epimysium of the pectoralis major is not identifiable and the deep fascia itself acts as a surrogate.

Clavipectoral Fascia

Detaching the pectoralis major muscle exposes the clavipectoral fascia (Figs 5.22 and 5.23). There is an ample plane of cleavage between the pectoralis major muscle and this fascia due to the presence of loose connective tissue. This loose connective tissue allows the deep layer of the pectoral fascia to glide autonomously with respect to the clavipectoral fascia. The clavipectoral fascia is a strong connective tissue layer arising from the clavicle and extending distally to

enclose the subclavius and pectoralis minor muscles. Under the subclavius muscle, the clavipectoral fascia continues with the middle lamina of the deep fascia of the neck. Laterally, the clavipectoral fascia forms the suspensory ligament of the axilla that drags the axillary fascia upwards when the arm is raised. This forms the 'pit' of the armpit. Singer (1935) divides the clavipectoral fascia into two parts: one covering the pectoralis minor muscle and one that forms a triangular-shaped layer between the upper border of this muscle and the clavicle, called the 'coracoclavicular fascia'. The thicker lateral border of the coracoclavicular fascia extends from the coracoid process of the scapula to the cartilage of the first rib and is known as the costocoracoid ligament. It separates the cavity of the axilla from the anterior chest wall. The anterior thoracic artery and nerve and the cephalic vein pierce the coracoclavicular fascia. In the arm, the coracoclavicular fascia continues with the fascia of the coracobrachialis muscle.

The continuation of the clavipectoral fascia envelops the serratus anterior muscle and then continues posteriorly with the fascia of the rhomboids (forming the 'serratorhomboid complex'). This complex continues proximally with the intermediate layer of the deep

Text continued on p. 167

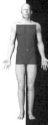

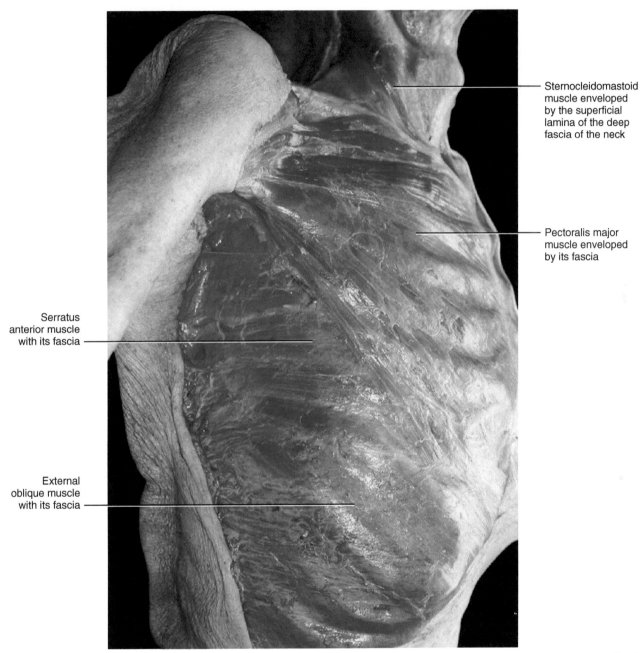

Sternocleidomastoid
muscle enveloped
by the superficial
lamina of the deep
fascia of the neck

Pectoralis major
muscle enveloped
by its fascia

Serratus
anterior muscle
with its fascia

External
oblique muscle
with its fascia

FIGURE 5.18 Anterolateral view of the trunk. The serratus anterior muscle is deeper with respect to the pectoralis major muscle. The pectoral fascia passes over the serratus anterior to envelop the latissimus dorsi muscle.

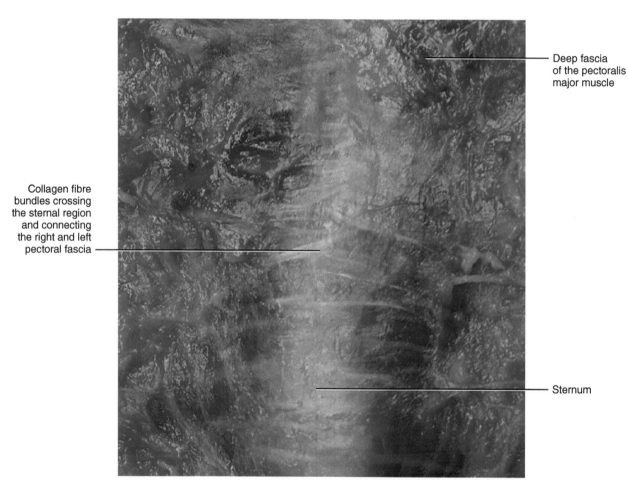

Deep fascia
of the pectoralis
major muscle

Collagen fibre
bundles crossing
the sternal region
and connecting
the right and left
pectoral fascia

Sternum

FIGURE 5.19 Crossing of the fibres of the deep fascia of the pectoralis major muscle over the sternum. In this way the deep fasciae of the two sides are connected, helping the peripheral motor coordination of the two pectoralis major muscles.

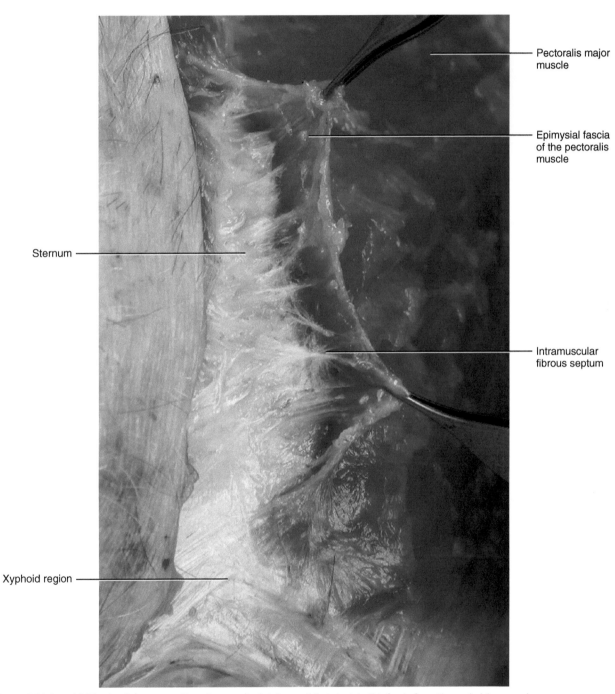

Pectoralis major
muscle

Epimysial fascia
of the pectoralis
muscle

Sternum

Intramuscular
fibrous septum

Xyphoid region

FIGURE 5.20 Epymisial fascia of the pectoralis major muscle. It is impossible to isolate this fascia from the underlying muscle.

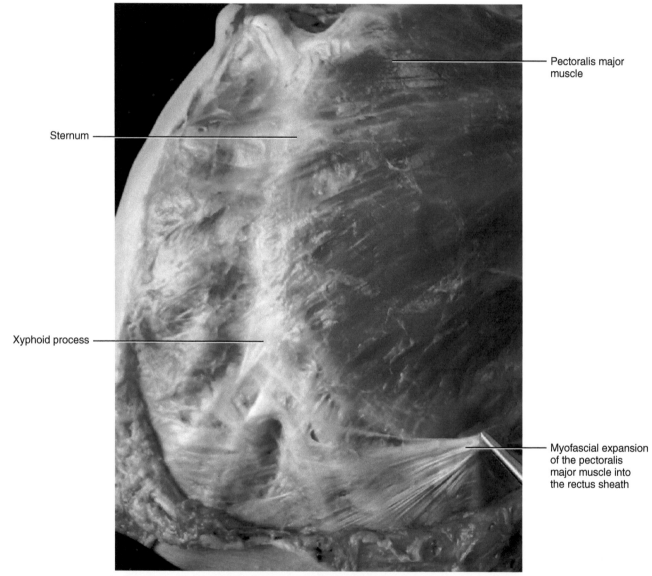

Pectoralis major
muscle

Sternum

Xyphoid process

Myofascial expansion
of the pectoralis
major muscle into
the rectus sheath

FIGURE 5.21 Some of the muscular fibres of the pectoralis major muscle are always inserted into the rectus sheath. Therefore, everytime these fibres contract they stretch the rectus sheath in a craniolateral direction. To show this phenomenon we have stretched the muscular fibres of the pectoralis major in a cranial direction, causing the formation of 'lines of force' in the rectus sheath.

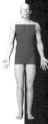

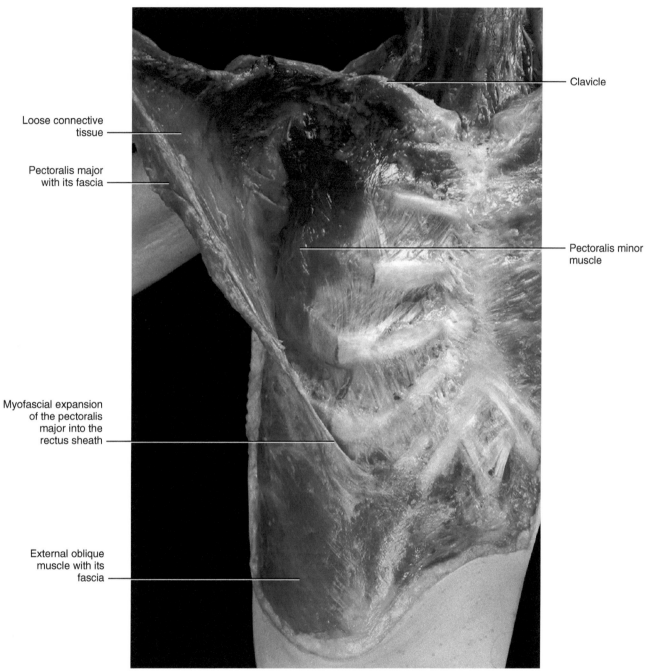

Clavicle

Loose connective tissue

Pectoralis major with its fascia

Pectoralis minor muscle

Myofascial expansion of the pectoralis major into the rectus sheath

External oblique muscle with its fascia

FIGURE 5.22 Dissection of the thorax. The pectoralis major muscle is detached from its sternal and clavicular insertions and lifted laterally. Both the pectoralis major and minor are enveloped by an epimysial fascia. Between the two fasciae, loose connective tissue is present. It permits the easy separation of the two muscles, and the autonomous gliding of the two muscles in a living subject.

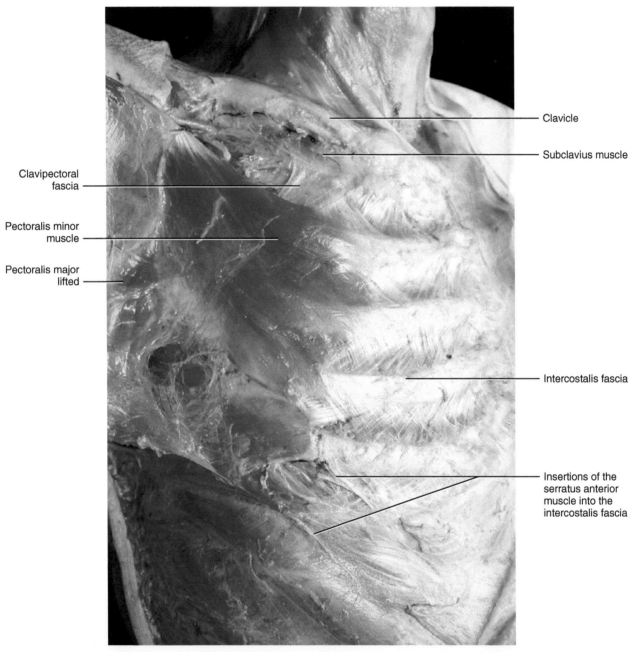

Clavicle

Subclavius muscle

Clavipectoral fascia

Pectoralis minor muscle

Pectoralis major lifted

Intercostalis fascia

Insertions of the serratus anterior muscle into the intercostalis fascia

FIGURE 5.23 Dissection of the thorax. The pectoralis major muscle was lifted laterally to show the clavipectoral fascia enveloping the pectoralis minor and serratus anterior muscles.

fasciae of the neck. 'Serratorhomboid complex' was a term used by Nguyen in 1987 to emphasize the anatomical and functional continuity between the serratus anterior, rhomboid and levator scapulae muscles. Distally, the clavipectoral fascia continues with the fasciae of the internal oblique muscle.

Intercostal and Endothoracic Fasciae

The intercostal muscles are enveloped by a specific fascia that continues over the ribs as periosteum (Fig. 5.24). This fascia forms local fascial compartments between the various ribs, where the internal and external intercostal muscles are present. The intercostal nerves run along this fascia, as described by Kumaki et al (1979). The intercostal fascia continues with the fascia of the transversus abdominis muscle and with the rectus sheath. According to Chiarugi (1975), the lower internal intercostal muscles are in direct contact also with the internal abdominal oblique muscle. At the level of the sternum the intercostal fascia fuses with the periosteum. Internally, this fascia adheres to the parietal pleura to form the endothoracic fascia. Hence, an anatomical connection between visceral fasciae (parietal pleura) and muscular fasciae (intercostal fasciae) is created. This contrasts with the fascial anatomy of the abdomen, where there is a separation between the parietal peritoneum and the muscular fasciae. This difference is functionally significant as the lung needs the muscles to expand and in this way the parietal pleura follows all the movements of the thoracic wall.

Endothoracic fascia is a fascial layer deep to the intercostal spaces and ribs and represents the outermost membrane of the thoracic cavity. Testut (1905) described the endothoracic fascia as formed by three parts: a thin layer of loose connective tissue (probably corresponding to the epimysial fascia of the intercostal muscle), a fibroelastic layer (the true endothoracic fascia), and another layer of loose connective tissue (the parietal pleura). Stopar-Pintaric et al (2012) have studied the endothoracic fascia in rats using electronmicroscopy imaging. These authors located the endothoracic fascia between the parietal pleura and the innermost intercostal muscles or ribs. Its thickness ranges from 15 to 27 μm (mean, 20±3 μm) and it

appears as a condensed, fibroelastic lamina with its fibres primarily orientated transversely and obliquely.

The endothoracic fascia continues distally into the diaphragmatic fascia and, at the level of the oesophageal hiatus, it forms the phrenico-oesophageal ligament. The phrenico-oesophageal ligament is a strong structure firmly attached to the oesophageal wall. It surrounds the upper part of the distal oesophagus like a skirt. Thus, it is reasonable to assume that it plays an important role in the gastro-oesophageal sphincteric mechanism. Apaydin et al (2008) demonstrated that its collagen and elastic fibres decrease with age, which could mean a decrease in the resistance and the elasticity of the ligament. This situation may explain the predisposition towards developing hiatal hernias that is associated with increasing age.

Proximally, the endothoracic fascia forms the suprapleural membrane, which is attached in front to the internal border of the first rib and behind to the anterior border of the transverse process of the seventh cervical vertebra. It contains some muscular fibres which spread from the scalene muscles. Posteriorly, it is attached to the periosteum of the vertebral bodies, where it becomes continuous with the prevertebral fascia that covers the vertebrae and the intervertebral disks. Medially, it becomes part of the phrenopericardial membrane.

The endothoracic fascia has not been well defined as to its make-up, boundries or relationship to the spinal nerves. For example, Karmakar and Chung (2000) place the spinal nerves dorsal to the endothoracic fascia in the paravertebral space, while Naja et al (2004) claim that they are ventral.

Deep Fasciae of the Abdomen

The large muscles of the abdomen have a thin epimysial fascia with proprioceptive function and an aponeurotic fascia with a force transmission function formed by the fusion of their flat tendon and epimysial fascia. Loose connective tissue is present between the epimysial fasciae, permitting the gliding of the various muscular layers. The aponeurotic fasciae fuse with each other to form the rectus sheath. We can, therefore, identify a line of fusion between the three deep fasciae in the lateral border of the rectus muscle (lateral adhesion), and a larger line of fusion comprising the subcutis and skin, along the linea alba.

FASCIA OF THE EXTERNAL OBLIQUE MUSCLE

The fascia of the external oblique muscle is a thin but strong membranous structure, adherent to the underlying muscle and to the rectus sheath (Fig. 5.25). This fascia envelops the muscular belly and then continues to cover the tendinous insertions of the muscle. The oblique external component of the rectus sheath consists of two layers: a superficial layer formed by the true epimysial fascia of the muscle, and a deep layer, which is thicker and formed by the tendon of the oblique external muscle. This description agrees with Rizk (1980), who wrote:

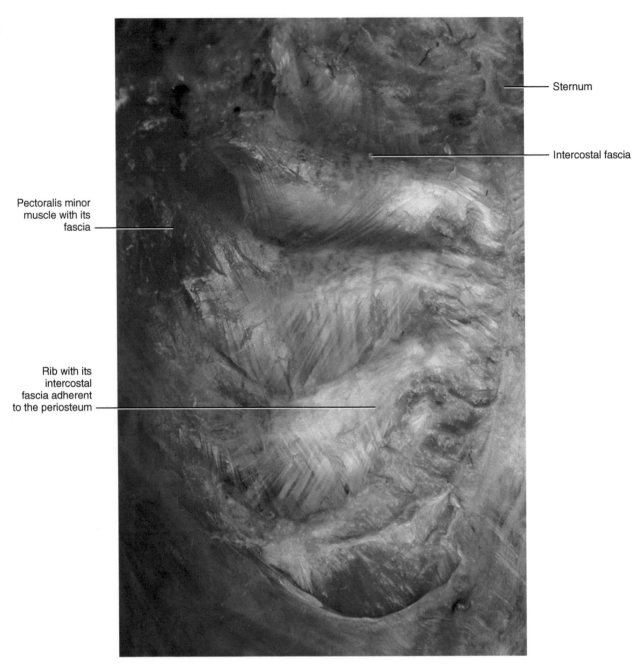

Sternum

Intercostal fascia

Pectoralis minor muscle with its fascia

Rib with its intercostal fascia adherent to the periosteum

FIGURE 5.24 Intercostal fascia at the level of the seventh and eighth ribs on the right side.

The aponeurosis of the external oblique was formed of two layers: superficial and deep. The fibres of each layer were perpendicular to those of the other layer. The fibres of the deep layer were the direct continuation of the fleshy bundles of the external oblique muscle and extended downwards and medially. At the midline they crossed to the opposite side. Some fibres extended superficially to form the superficial layer of the opposite external oblique aponeurosis, while others passed deep to become directly continuous with the fibres of the anterior lamina of the internal oblique of the opposite side.

Rizk (1980) also described the myofascial expansion of the external oblique muscle into the fasciae of the controlateral external oblique and internal oblique muscles. This organization suggests that the muscles of the anterior abdominal wall are to be considered digastric-like muscles and the rectus sheath has the role of harmonizing the action of all these muscles. This prevents the action of an individual muscle or the muscles of one side from working independently. The external oblique muscle is free to glide with respect to the internal oblique muscle because of loose connective tissue between the two (Fig. 5.26). At the level of the rectus sheath, the various layers adhere and then completely merge at the linea alba.

Distally, the fascia of the external oblique muscle is thicker and joins to form the inguinal ligament. The

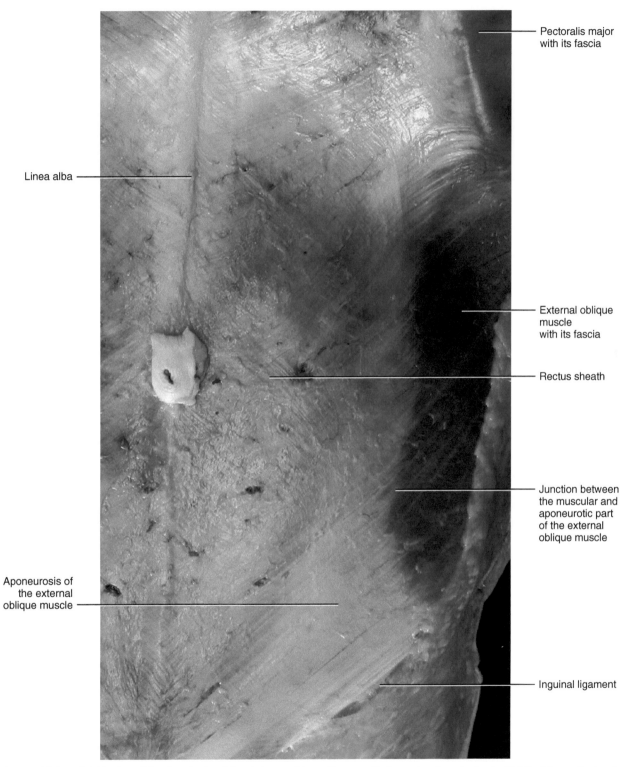

Pectoralis major
with its fascia

Linea alba

External oblique
muscle
with its fascia

Rectus sheath

Junction between
the muscular and
aponeurotic part
of the external
oblique muscle

Aponeurosis of
the external
oblique muscle

Inguinal ligament

FIGURE 5.25 Superficial lamina of the deep fascia of the abdomen. It is continuous with the pectoralis major fascia. Distally, it forms the inguinal ligament. Note the connection between the muscular and aponeurotic part of the external oblique muscle and how the deep fascia covers both the elements. Aponeurosis (flat tendon) differs from aponeurotic fascia (see Chaper 3, p. 13).

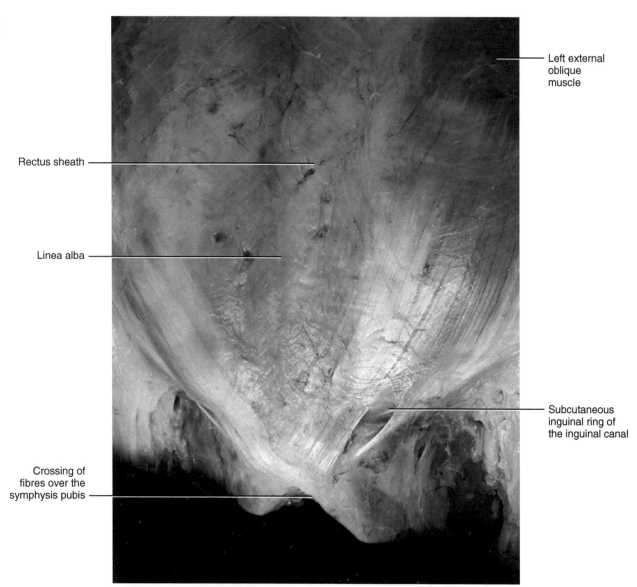

Rectus sheath

Linea alba

Crossing of
fibres over the
symphysis pubis

Left external
oblique
muscle

Subcutaneous
inguinal ring of
the inguinal canal

FIGURE 5.26 Myofascial expansions of the external oblique muscles into the fascia lata of the contralateral side. Note the crossing of the collagen fibres over the symphysis pubis.

superficial fibres of this fascia continue distally to merge with the fascia lata, while the deeper fibres are attached to the anterior superior iliac spine and to the pubic tubercle. The inguinal ligament could thus be considered the lower border of the aponeurosis of the external oblique muscle, and it is also the point of conjunction between the fasciae of the abdomen and the fasciae of the thigh.

An expansion of the inguinal ligament connects the pubic tubercle with the pectineal line and forms the medial boundary of the femoral ring. Due to its expansion, the external oblique fascia is also continuous with the pectineal fascia, which originates from the pectineal line. The external oblique fascia, immediately above the crest of the pubis, has a triangular opening which forms the subcutaneous inguinal ring of the inguinal canal (Fig. 5.27).

FASCIA OF THE INTERNAL OBLIQUE MUSCLE

The fascia of the internal oblique muscle is a very thin fibrous layer that envelops the muscle from both sides. It is connected stongly to the muscle by many intermuscular septa and is separated from the fasciae of the external oblique and transversus abdominis muscles by a thin layer of loose connective tissue (Figs 5.28 and 5.29). This layer disappears over the rectus abdominis muscle where the various fasciae attach to one another to form the rectus sheath. The internal oblique fascia of one side joins with that of the opposite muscle along the midline, to form the rectus sheath and the linea alba. As for the external oblique, the fascia of this muscle, which is located over the rectus sheath, is also formed by two layers: the superficial (corresponding to the epimysial fascia), and the deep (which corresponds to the flat tendon of the muscle). The fascia

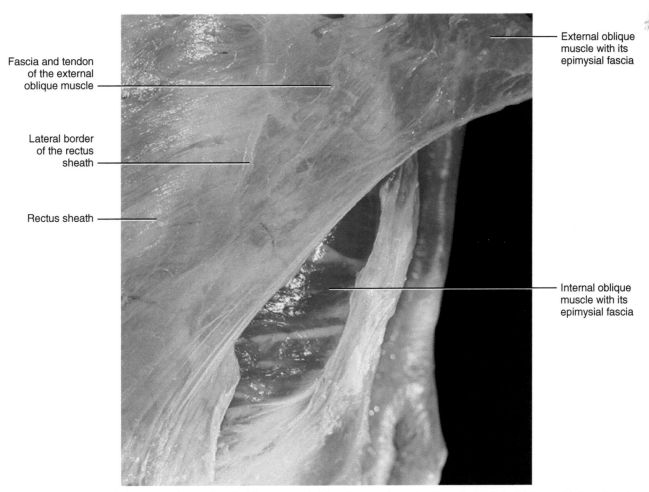

Fascia and tendon of the external oblique muscle

Lateral border of the rectus sheath

Rectus sheath

External oblique muscle with its epimysial fascia

Internal oblique muscle with its epimysial fascia

FIGURE 5.27 The external oblique muscle was detached from the underlying planes and stretched laterally. Medially, it is impossible to isolate due to the adhesions among the various fascial layers that form the rectus sheath.

of the internal oblique muscle arises together with the transversus abdominis muscle from the inguinal ligament, from the iliac crest and from the anterior layer of the thoracolumbar fascia. Some bundles of the internal oblique fascia arise from the inguinal ligament and arch downward and medially across the spermatic cord in the male and to the round ligament of the uterus in the female. They insert, joined together with those of the transversus abdominis fascia, into the crest of the pubis and the pectineal line. These form the inguinal aponeurotic falx.

FASCIA OF THE TRANSVERSUS ABDOMINIS MUSCLE

The transversus abdominis is the most internal of the flat muscles of the abdomen. It is enveloped by an epymisial fascia and usually separated from the internal oblique muscle by a layer of loose connective tissue (Figs 5.30 and 5.31). Distally, the two muscles sometime adhere. The transversus abdominis arises from the inguinal ligament, iliac crest, anterior layer of the thoracolumbar fascia, and inner surfaces of the cartilage of the lower six ribs to interdigitate with the diaphragm. This muscle ends in front in a broad aponeurosis, the lower fibres of which curve downwards and medially;

they are inserted with those of the internal oblique into the crest of the pubis and pectineal line to form the inguinal aponeurotic falx. The rest of its aponeurosis passes horizontally to the midline crossing to the opposite side, and forming a digastric-like muscle linking the two sides together. This aponeurosis is commonly described as having its upper three-fourths lying behind the rectus abdominis and blending with the posterior layer of the aponeurosis of the internal oblique,

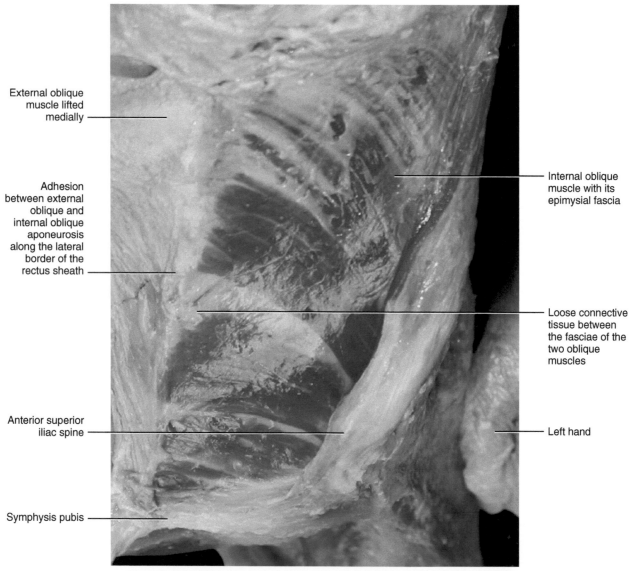

External oblique
muscle lifted
medially

Adhesion
between external
oblique and
internal oblique
aponeurosis
along the lateral
border of the
rectus sheath

Anterior superior
iliac spine

Symphysis pubis

Internal oblique
muscle with its
epimysial fascia

Loose connective
tissue between
the fasciae of the
two oblique
muscles

Left hand

FIGURE 5.28 Internal oblique muscle with its fascia. The external oblique muscle was lifted medially. Note the loose connective tissue that permits gliding between the deep fasciae of these two muscles.

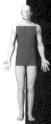

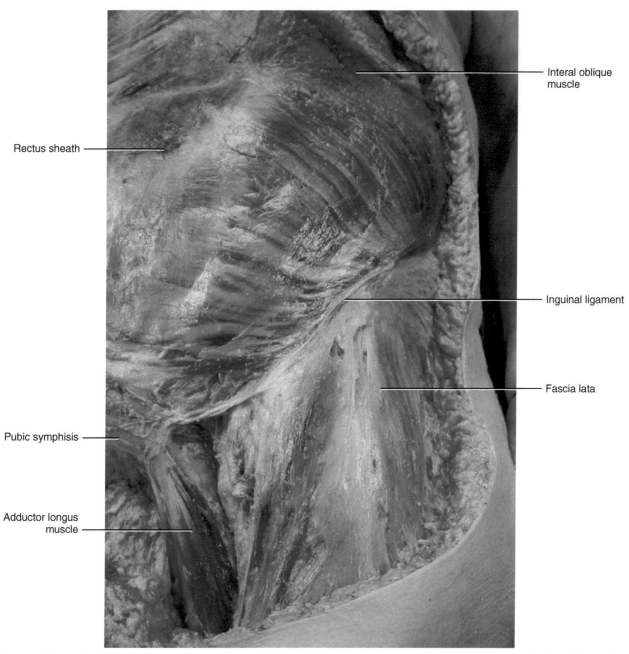

Interal oblique muscle

Rectus sheath

Inguinal ligament

Fascia lata

Pubic symphisis

Adductor longus muscle

FIGURE 5.29 Internal oblique muscle covered by its epimysial fascia. Note it is continuous with the deep fascia of the lower limb at the level of the inguinal ligament. A thin layer of loose connective tissue with some fat is present over the fascia of the internal oblique muscle.

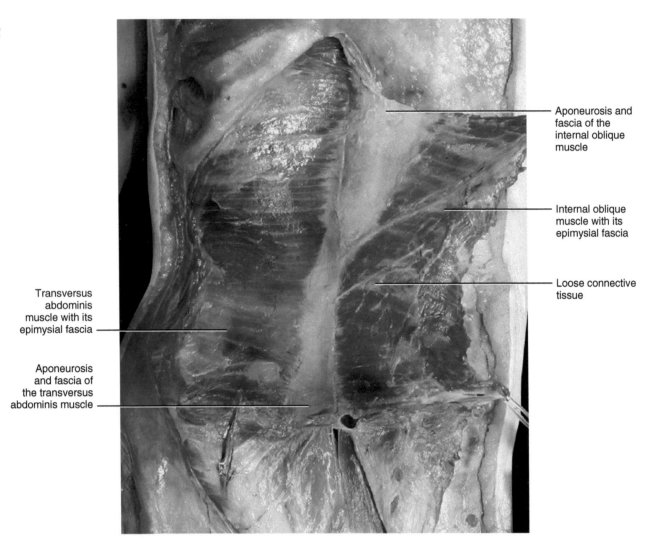

Aponeurosis and
fascia of the
internal oblique
muscle

Internal oblique
muscle with its
epimysial fascia

Loose connective
tissue

Transversus
abdominis
muscle with its
epimysial fascia

Aponeurosis
and fascia of
the transversus
abdominis muscle

FIGURE 5.30 Dissection of the abdominal wall. The internal oblique muscle is detached from the underlying layers up to the rectus sheath, where an adhesion is present. The internal oblique muscle and the transversus abdominis muscle are enveloped by their epimysial fascia. Between the two muscles loose connective tissue is present, allowing autonomy of contraction for these two muscles.

and its lower fourth in front of the rectus. According to Askar (1977) and Rizk (1991), the rate of shifting of the fibres from the posterior to the anterior rectus sheath varies, and so the arcuate line (which demarcates the lower limit of the posterior layer of the rectus sheath) is often a dissector artifact.

RECTUS SHEATH

The rectus abdominis muscle is contained in a sheath made up of the aponeuroses of the three anterolateral abdominal muscles (external oblique, internal oblique and transversus abdominis). These aponeuroses fuse laterally to the rectus abdominis muscle and then pass, in part, over and under the rectus abdominis muscle to form its sheath (Fig. 5.32). Each large abdominal muscle contributes to the formation of the rectus sheath with two layers: the flat tendon and the epymisial fascia. This allows the rectus sheath to have both perceptive and force trasmission components. The layers of the external oblique muscle pass over the rectus abdominis muscle. The internal oblique muscle

passes distally over the rectus abdominis, while proximally it divides into two laminae: a superficial layer that passes over the rectus abdominis muscle, and a deep layer that passes under the muscle. The transversus abdominis muscle passes proximally under the rectus abdominis muscle and distally over the rectus abdominis muscle. The lower border of the posterior layer is called the arcuate line or linea semicircularis of Douglas (Figs 5.33–5.35). It is a horizontal line that occurs about one-third of the distance from the umbilicus to the pubic crest, but this varies from person to person. Rizk (1991) affirms that the arcuate line is not an absolute point of termination of the posterior rectus sheath. It is also where the inferior epigastric vessels perforate the rectus abdominis.

The current understanding of the composition of the rectus sheath is largely the result of the work by Askar (1977) and Rizk (1991), who independently reported their anatomical observations of the anterior abdominal wall and changed the traditional view of the rectus sheath. They described a bilaminar

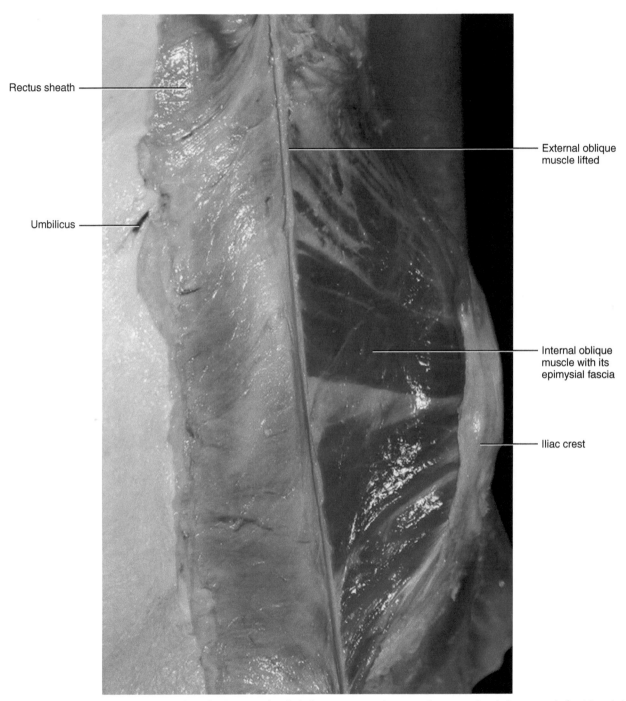

Rectus sheath

External oblique muscle lifted

Umbilicus

Internal oblique muscle with its epimysial fascia

Iliac crest

FIGURE 5.31 Internal oblique muscle with its fascia. Note the dissimilar appearance between the rectus sheath (aponeurotic fascia) and the epimysial fascia of the internal oblique muscle.

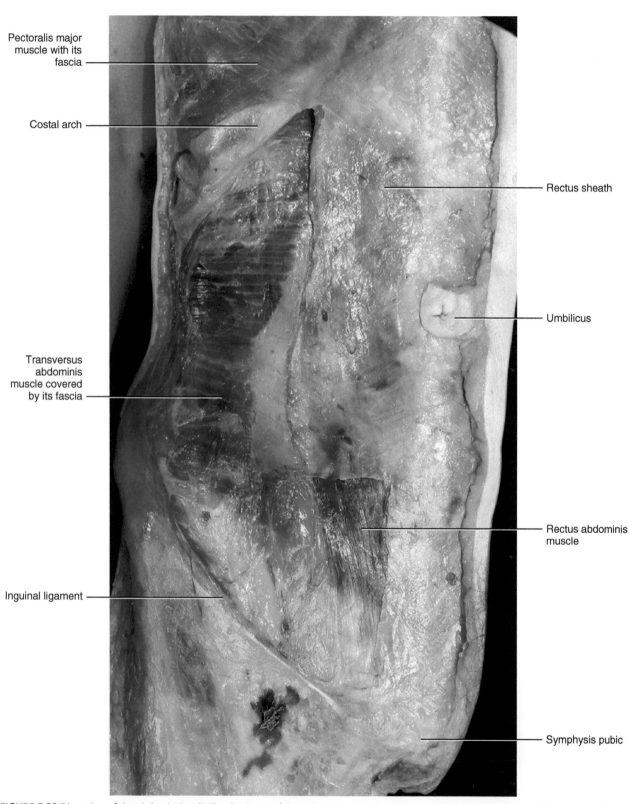

Pectoralis major
muscle with its
fascia

Costal arch

Rectus sheath

Umbilicus

Transversus
abdominis
muscle covered
by its fascia

Inguinal ligament

Rectus abdominis
muscle

Symphysis pubic

FIGURE 5.32 Dissection of the abdominal wall. The distal part of the right rectus sheath was removed to show the rectus abdominis muscle.

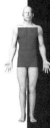

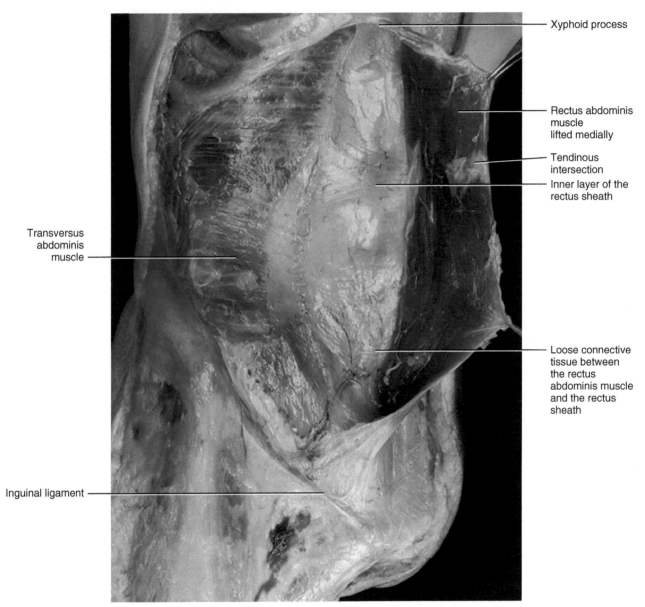

— Xyphoid process

— Rectus abdominis
muscle
lifted medially

— Tendinous
intersection

— Inner layer of the
rectus sheath

Transversus
abdominis
muscle —

— Loose connective
tissue between
the rectus
abdominis muscle
and the rectus
sheath

Inguinal ligament —

FIGURE 5.33 Posterior view of the rectus abdominis muscle. The rectus sheath was cut along the right border and opened. The rectus abdominis muscle was lifted medially. This muscle is formed by two identical lateral sides divided by the linea alba. It is also divided by some tendinous intersections, usually attributable to the original segmentation of the myotomes. The more distal insertion is usually at the level of the umbilicus. These tendinous intersections are less evident posteriorly. At the level of these tendinous intersections, the muscle fuses with the rectus sheath. Thus, the muscle becomes a fascial tensor. Rizk (1991) demonstrated in rats that the tendinous intersections of the rectus abdominis muscle are not seen except postnatally, suggesting that they represent some sort of intermediate tendon of a multigastric, longitudinal muscle.

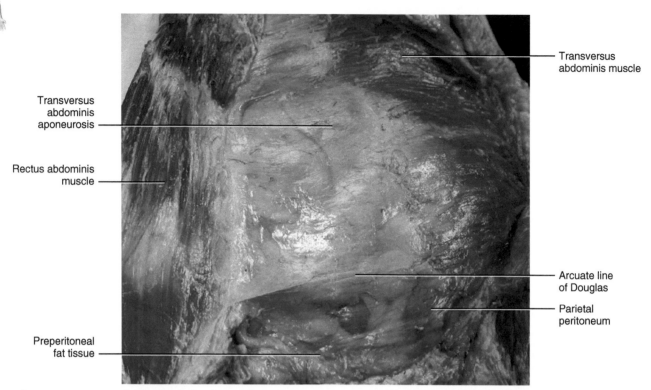

Transversus
abdominis muscle

Transversus
abdominis
aponeurosis

Rectus abdominis
muscle

Arcuate line
of Douglas

Parietal
peritoneum

Preperitoneal
fat tissue

FIGURE 5.34 Dissection of the abdominal wall. The left rectus abdominis was removed to show the arcuate line of Douglas. This is a horizontal line that demarcates the lower limit of the posterior layer of the rectus sheath. The arcuate line occurs about one-third of the distance from the umbilicus to the pubic crest, but this varies from person to person. Inferior to the arcuate line, the internal oblique and transversus aponeuroses merge and pass superficially (i.e. anteriorly) to the rectus abdominis. Under this line, between the peritoneum and the rectus abdominis, only the preperitoneal fat tissue is present.

composition of the flat muscles of the abdominal wall, with each layer contributing fibres to the contralateral side. According to Askar (1977), the linea alba should be considered less as the insertion of the abdominal muscles and more as the common area of decussation of the intermediate aponeurosis. Consequently, the rectus sheath was discovered to be a trilaminar structure of variable thickness with decussating components from the external oblique, internal oblique and transversus abdominis muscles. They described a 'plywood-like' arrangement of the rectus sheath (similar to what we have described for the other aponeurotic fasciae), where there is a close collaboration of the layers without an actual fusion that would interfere with the free mobility of the abdominal wall (Fig. 5.36). In addition, histological analysis reveals a thin layer of loose connective tissue between the various sublayers of the rectus sheath, with complete adhesion only occurring at the level of the linea alba. Along the linea alba, also the superficial fascia connects with the deep fascia. This organization permits the free mobility of each layer, which allows an appreciable capacity for deformation in the resultant fabric of the rectus sheath. The oblique direction in which the collagen fibrous bundles are placed permits the adaptability of the rectus sheath to movements of the trunk. Due to this fascial organization, flexion of the trunk, for example, will produce folds in the skin and subcutis but not in the rectus sheath. This function may be lost as a result of rigid scarring following a midline incision.

The rectus sheath is constantly stretched by the various muscular insertions. Obviously, the abdominal muscles stretch this sheath in a lateral direction, but it is also stretched in a longitudinal direction by the myofascial expansions of the pectoralis major and pyramidalis muscle. The anterior layer of the rectus sheath is reinforced proximally by the myofascial expansions of the pectoralis major muscles that form a cross in front of the xiphoid. Distally, the rectus sheath and particularly the linea alba are tensioned by the pyramidalis muscle, which may also be considered a fascial tensor (Fig. 5.37). This muscle is inside the rectus sheath (Rizk 1980) and is inserted into the pubis and anterior pubic ligament, and proximally it has just a fascial insertion into the linea alba.

There has been confusion over the position of the rectus abdominis with respect to the other muscular layers. Some authors hold that this is a superficial muscle. However, if we consider the embryological origin and the fascial anatomy, then the rectus abdominis is clearly a deep muscle corresponding to the erector spinae. The rectus abdominis originates from the hypaxial muscles and is the antagonist of the erector spinae that originates from the epaxial mass. The transversus abdominis muscle (a hypaxial muscle) with its fascia creates continuity between the epaxial muscles that moved around the visceral cavity during evolution.

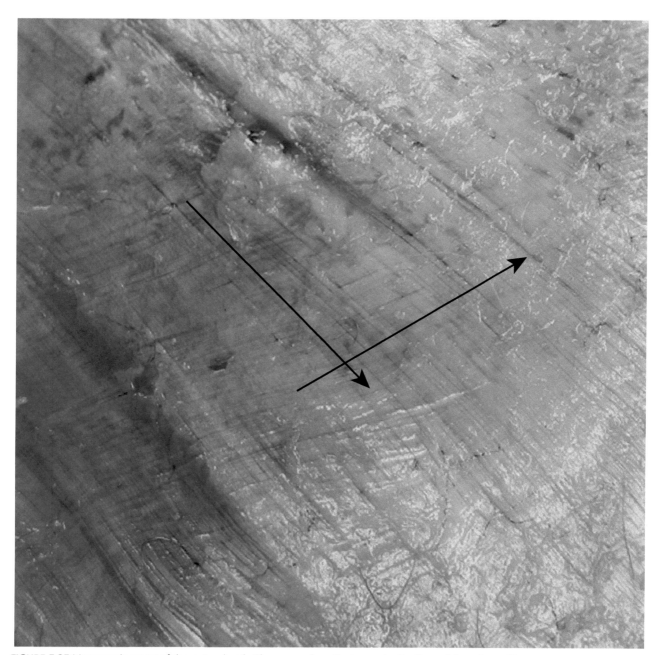

FIGURE 5.35 Macroscopic aspect of the rectus sheath. The arrows show the two main directions of the collagen fibres.

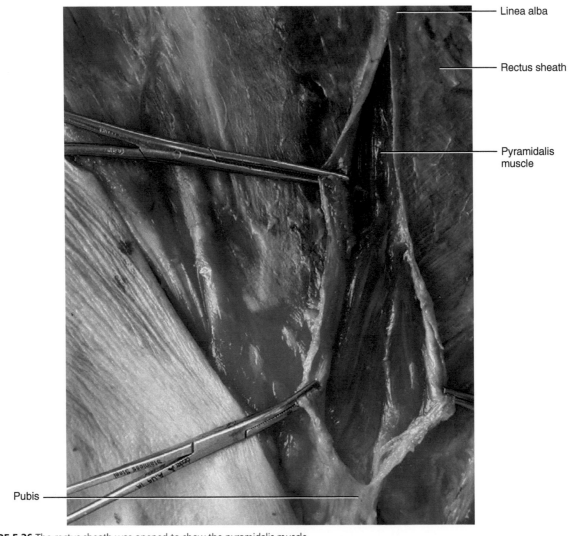

Linea alba

Rectus sheath

Pyramidalis muscle

Pubis

FIGURE 5.36 The rectus sheath was opened to show the pyramidalis muscle.

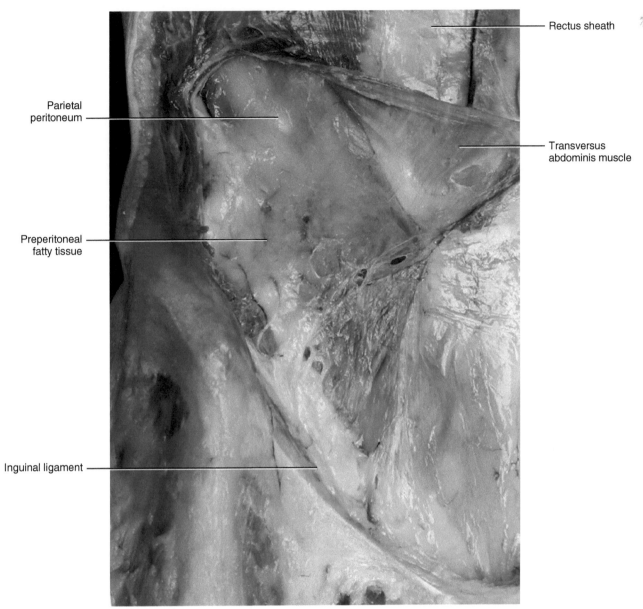

Parietal peritoneum

Preperitoneal fatty tissue

Inguinal ligament

Rectus sheath

Transversus abdominis muscle

FIGURE 5.37 Dissection of the abdominal wall, right side. The transversus abdominis muscle was lifted to show the peritoneum.

In addition, the fascia of the external oblique muscle is inserted posteriorly into the posterior (or 'more superficial') layer of the thoracolumbar fascia, and anteriorly forms the anterior (or 'more superficial') layer of the rectus sheath. The fasciae of the internal oblique and transversus abdominis muscles are inserted posteriorly to the anterior layer of the thoracolumbar fascia, and contribute anteriorly to form the rectus sheath. Thus, myofascial continuity between the thoracolumbar fascia and the rectus sheath is formed. This assures synchronization between the erector spinae and rectus abdominis muscles. Therefore, every time the oblique muscles contract, they stretch both the rectus sheath and the thoracolumbar fascia that envelops the erector spinae. This causes these fasciae to become more rigid, contributing to the increased force of the muscular contraction (see Clinical Pearl 6.4).

TRANSVERSALIS (OR PREPERITONEAL FASCIA)

The transversalis fascia has been an object of discussion. According to Skandalakis et al (2006), the transversalis fascia is the epimysium of the transversus abdominis muscle. Tobin et al (1946) holds that the transversalis fascia is a fascial layer between the peritoneum and the abdominal wall. It forms a continuous lining for the abdomen, pelvis and spermatic cord (Fig. 5.39). He describes three strata: an inner stratum (peritoneum) associated with the digestive system; an intermediate stratum (transversalis fascia) embedding the adrenals, urogenital system, aorta and vena cava; and an outer stratum (muscular fascia) which is the intrinsic fascia of the transversus abdominis muscle. Our dissections reveal a distinct fascial layer between the internal surface of the transversus abdominis muscle and the peritoneum. This is especially evident in

CLINICAL PEARL 5.9 IMPORTANCE OF THE RECTUS SHEATH

The rectus sheath is a region where various muscular forces converge (Fig. 5.38). Chronically increased tonus of the various muscles that insert into the rectus sheath can cause excessive tension of the sheath, and this might prevent the rectus sheath from adapting normally to variations in the rectus muscle volume. Therefore, pain in the abdominal wall could be due to an alteration in one of the various muscles that stretches this sheath. In addition, excessive training of abdominal muscles reduces the rectus sheath's capacity to adapt to multidirectional muscular contractions. Inefficiency of the transversus abdominis muscle could cause a loss of coordination between the anterior hypaxial and posterior epaxial muscles.

the distal part of the abdomen. This fascia is separated from the peritoneum by loose connective tissue that is typically scarce, but in some places may contain a great amount of fat, especially posteriorly and in the pelvis. Inferiorly, it is continuous with the pelvic androvesical fasciae. According to Bendavid (2001), the transversalis fascia corresponds to the investing layer of the bladder or the spermatic cord (Fig. 5.39). This fascia continues in the inguinal canal and in the scrotum. From an embryological point of view, we can affirm that the transversalis fascia comes from the septum transversum[2], and is the element that guides the descent of the testis/ovaries into the pelvis.

---

[2]The septum transversum arises as the most cranial part of the mesenchyme on day 22 of embryo development. It gives rise to parts of the thoracic diaphragm and the ventral mesentery of the foregut.

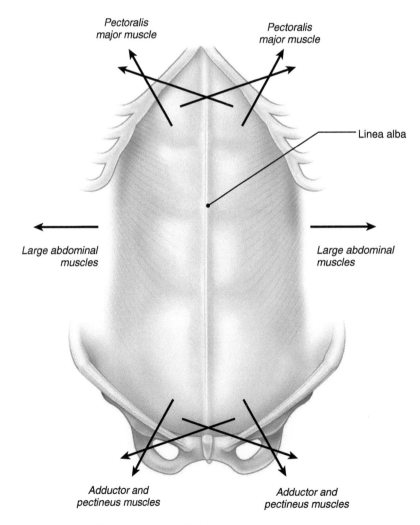

FIGURE 5.38 Scheme of the various myofascial expansions that affect the rectus sheath.

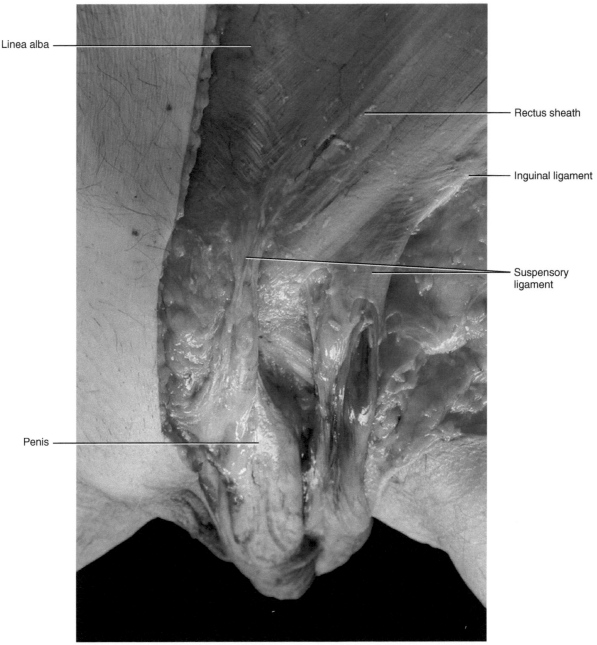

Linea alba

Rectus sheath

Inguinal ligament

Suspensory ligament

Penis

FIGURE 5.39 In the scrotum we found many fascial layers. The testis, during its descent, drags all the fasciae of the abdomen. In the scrotom the following can be found: superficial fascia (dartos fascia), the external spermatic fascia (a continuation of the aponeurosis of the external oblique muscle), the internal spermatic fascia (a continuation of the fasciae of the internal oblique and transversus abdominis), the tunica vaginalis testis (the serous covering of the testicle that is continuous with the peritoneum), and finally, the testicular tissue that is surrounded by the tunica albuginea. A consequence of the strong connection between the testis and the abdom is that often pain in the testicular region is caused by an alteration of the abdominal wall.

References

Apaydin, N., Uz, A., Evirgen, O., Loukas, M., Tubbs, R.S., Elhan, A., 2008. The phrenico-esophageal ligament: an anatomical study. Surg. Radiol. Anat. 30 (1), 29–36.

Askar, O.M., 1977. Surgical anatomy of the aponeurotic expansions of the anterior abdominal wall. Ann. R. Coll. Surg. Engl. 59 (4), 313–321.

Beer, G.M., Varga, Z., Budi, S., Seifert, B., Meyer, V.E., 2002. Incidence of the superficial fascia and its relevance in skin-sparing mastectomy. Cancer 94 (6), 1619–1625.

Bendavid, R., 2001. Abdominal Wall Hernias: Principles and Management, Springer Verlag, New York, pp. 12–19.

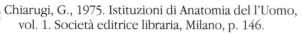

Chiarugi, G., 1975. Istituzioni di Anatomia del l'Uomo, vol. 1. Società editrice libraria, Milano, p. 146.

Chopra, J., Rani, A., Rani, A., Srivastava, A.K., Sharma, P.K., 2011. Re-evaluation of superficial fascia of anterior abdominal wall: a computed tomographic study. Surg. Radiol. Anat. 33 (10), 843–849.

Fourie, J.W., Robb, K.A., 2009. Physiotherapy management of axillary web syndrome following breastcancer treatment: Discussing the use of soft tissue techniques. Physiotherapy 95 (4), 314–320.

Giraldès, Mons, 1851. Anatomie chirurgicale de la region mammaire, Bull, de la Soc. de chir, Paris.

Karmakar, M.K., Chung, D.C., 2000. Variability of a thoracic paravertebral block. Are we ignoring the endothoracic fascia? Reg. Anesth. Pain Med. 25 (3), 325–327.

Kumaki, K., Yamada, M., Kumaki, S., Miaki, K., Kodama, K., Kawai, K., 1979. The extramural nerves on the thoracic region. Acta Anat. Nippon 54, 226–227.

Langer, K., 1862. Zur Anatomie und Physiologie der Haut, vol. II. Uber die Spaltbarkeit der Cutis. Die Spannung der Cutis. Sitzungsberichte der Mathematisch-naturwissenschaftlicher Classe der Kaiserlichen Akademie der Wissenschaften. Wien. 45: 133.

Moskovitz, A.H., Anderson, B.O., Yeung, R.S., Byrd, D.R., Lawton, T.J., Moe, R.E., 2001. Axillary web syndrome after axillary dissection. Am. J. Surg. 181 (5), 434–439.

Naja, M.Z., Ziade, M.F., El Rajab, M., El Tayara, K., Lönnqvist, P.A., 2004. Varying anatomical injection points within the thoracic paravertebral space: effect on spread of solution and nerve blockade. Anaesthesia 59 (5), 459–463.

Nguyen, H.V., Nguyen, H., 1987. Anatomical basis of modern thoracotomies: the latissimus dorsi and the "serratus anterior-rhomboid" complex. Surg. Radiol. Anat. 9 (2), 85–93.

Rizk, N.N., 1980. A new description of the anterior abdominal wall in man and mammals. J. Anat. 131 (3), 373–385.

Rizk, N.N., 1991. The arcuate line of the rectus sheath – does it exist? J. Anat. Apr, 175, 1–6.

Ruge, G., 1905. Der Hautrumpfmuskel der Saugetiere: der M. sternalis und der Achselbogen des Menschen. Morph. Jahrb. 33, 379–531.

Sato, T., Hashimoto, M., 1984. Morphological analysis of the fascial lamination of the trunk. Bull. Tokyo Med. Dent. Univ. 31 (1), 21–32.

Scarpa, A., 1809. Sull'ernie memorie anatomo-chirurgiche, first ed. Reale Stamperia, Milano.

Scarpa, A., 1819. Sull'ernie memorie anatomo-chirurgiche, second ed. Stamperia Fusi e Compagno, Pavia.

Sebastien, C., Regnier, M., Lantieri, L., Pétoin, S., Guérin-Surville, H., 1993. Anterolateral thoracic fascia: an anatomic and surgical entity. Surg. Radiol. Anat. 15 (2), 79–83.

Skandalakis, P.N., Zoras, O., Skandalakis, J.E., Mirilas, P., 2006. Transversalis, endoabdominal, endothoracic fascia: Who's who? Am. Surg. 72 (1), 16–18.

Singer, E., 1935. Fasciae of the human body and their relations to the organs they envelop, Williams & Wilkinns Company, Baltimore.

Sterzi, G., 1910. Il tessuto sottocutaneo (tela subcutanea), Luigi Niccolai, Firenze, pp. 1–50.

Stopar Pintaric, T., Veranic, P., Hadzic, A., Karmakar, M., Cvetko, E., 2012. Electron-microscopic imaging of endothoracic fascia in the thoracic paravertebral space in rats. Reg. Anesth. Pain Med. 37 (2), 215–218.

Testut, J.L., Jacob, O., 1905. Précis d'anatomie topographique avec applications medico-chirurgicales, vol. II. Gaston Doin et Cie, Paris, p. 184.

Tobler, L., 1902. Der Achselbogen des Menschen, ein Rudiment des Panniculus carnosus der Mammalier. Morph. Jahrb. 30 (3), 453–507.

Tobin, C.F., Benjamin, J.A., Wells, J.C., 1946. Continuity of the fascia lining the abdomen, pelvis and spermatic cord. Surg. Gynecol. Obstet. 83 (5), 575–596.

Bibliography

Deschenes, D., Couture, P., Dupont, P., Tchernof, A., 2003. Subdivision of the subcutaneous adipose tissue compartment and lipid–lipoprotein levels in women. Obes. Res. 11 (3), 469–476.

Dugan, D.J., Samson, P.C., 1975. Surgical significance of the endothoracic fascia: The anatomic basis for empyemectomy and other extrapleural technics. Am. J. Surg. 130 (2), 151–158.

Gaughran, G.R., 1964. Suprapleural membrane and suprapleural bands. Anat. Rec. Apr; 148, 553–559.

Kent, G.C., 1978. Comparative Anatomy of the Vertebrates, Mosby Co, Saint Louis, pp. 333–334.

Markman, B., Barton, F.E., 1987. Anatomy of the subcutaneous tissue of the trunk and lower extremity. Plast. Reconstr. Surg. 80 (2), 248–254.

Saito, T., Den, S., Tanuma, K., Tanuma, Y., Carney, E., Carlsson, C., 1999. Anatomical bases for paravertebral anesthetic block: fluid communication between the thoracic and lumbar paravertebral regions. Surg. Radiol. Anat. 21 (6), 359–363.

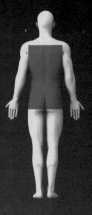

Fasciae of the Back

6

Introduction

This chapter examines the relationships between the superficial and deep fasciae of the back, with particular attention to the thoracolumbar fascia. The fasciae of the back extend from the superior nuchal line of the occipital bone to the lumbopelvic region. Together with the muscles, they form a multilayered myofascial structure whose characteristics vary by location. Three myofascial layers could be identified similar to that in the anterior part of the trunk. In this chapter the connections among the ventral and dorsal fasciae will be analysed. In the back, both epimysial and aponeurotic fasciae can be found. The thoracolumbar fascia (TLF) is a significant aponeurotic fascia that plays an essential role in the transfer of loads between the trunk and the extremities and helps maintain stability of the lumbosacral area.

Superficial Fascia

Dissection of the back exposes the superficial fascia as a fibrous, adipose layer in the middle of the subcutaneous adipose tissue (Fig. 6.1). It is very thick, especially in the proximal portion of the back, while the deep fascia over the trapezius muscle is thin and adheres to the muscle. The superficial fascia is often mistaken for deep fascia in this area. It is important to have an overall view of the fascial layers to understand these differences and to classify fasciae of the trunk properly. Indeed, the superficial fascia is a fibroelastic covering that surrounds the whole trunk, and it is possible to isolate this layer in the middle of the subcutis, from the neck to the lumbar region. This layer continues into the superficial fascia of the thorax and abdomen.

Abu-Hijleh et al (2006) showed that the thickness of the superficial fascia of the back varies significantly among humans, but generally is thicker in females. The superficial fascia of the back is rich in adipose tissue in most areas. The fat cells are usually distributed within the fibrous tissue of the superficial fascia, which gives the appearance that the superficial fascia consists of multiple sublayers. Abu-Hijleh et al (2006) demonstrated that the collagen fibres in two adjacent sublayers run at right angles to one another. Sterzi (1910) identified fibrous thickenings inside the superficial fascia of the trunk. These collagen fibrous bundles originate in the back and run in an oblique direction to the anterior region of the trunk, in a cranial–caudal direction. The distribution of these fibrous reinforcements in the superficial fascia corresponds to the lines in the dermis described by Langer in 1862. In addition, some striated muscular fibres are embedded in the superficial fascia of the trunk. In particular, they are always present and well organized around the anus, forming the external anal sphincter.

The superficial adipose tissue (SAT) of the back is generally thick, homogeneously distributed and with few regional variations. The deep adipose tissue (DAT) may range from a substantial thickness (especially in the lateral lumbar region), to very thin and almost absent over the sacrum (Figs 6.2 and 6.3). The scarcity of adipose tissue over the sacrum is related to the formation of ulcers.

Saito and Tamura (1992) measured subcutaneous fat thickness at 215 different points on the trunks of a

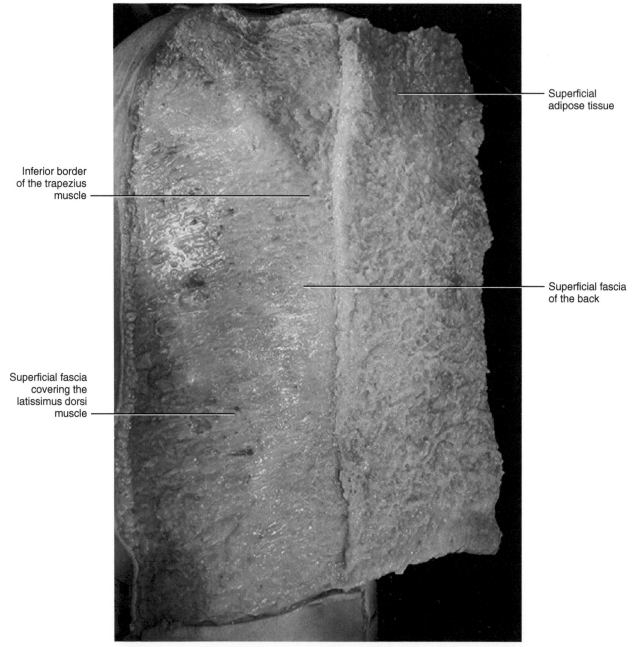

Superficial
adipose tissue

Inferior border
of the trapezius
muscle

Superficial fascia
of the back

Superficial fascia
covering the
latissimus dorsi
muscle

FIGURE 6.1 Superficial fascia of the dorsum. The skin and the SAT are removed on the left. The superficial fascia appears as a fibroelastic layer that covers the whole back.

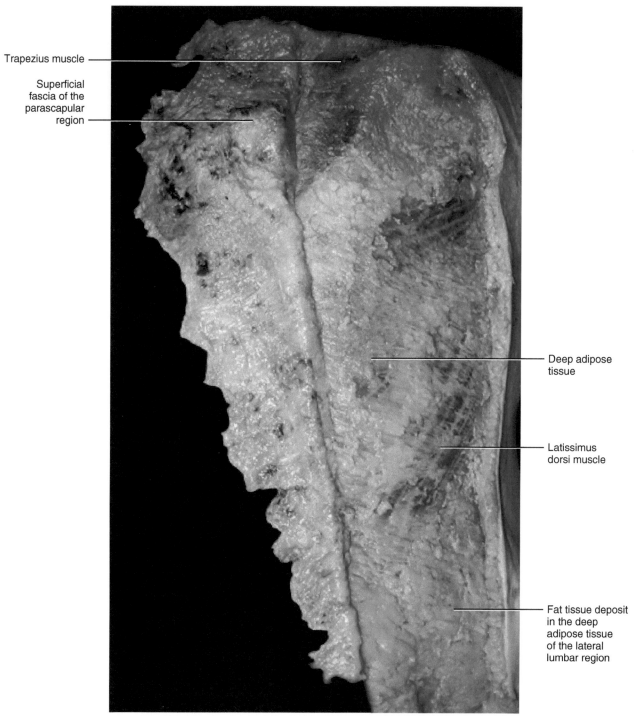

Trapezius muscle

Superficial fascia of the parascapular region

Deep adipose tissue

Latissimus dorsi muscle

Fat tissue deposit in the deep adipose tissue of the lateral lumbar region

FIGURE 6.2 Superficial fascia of the back. The superficial fascia is lifted here to show the DAT. The DAT is scarce and formed mostly by loose connective tissue and some fat lobules. In the lateral lumbar region the DAT thickens, forming an important fat tissue deposit.

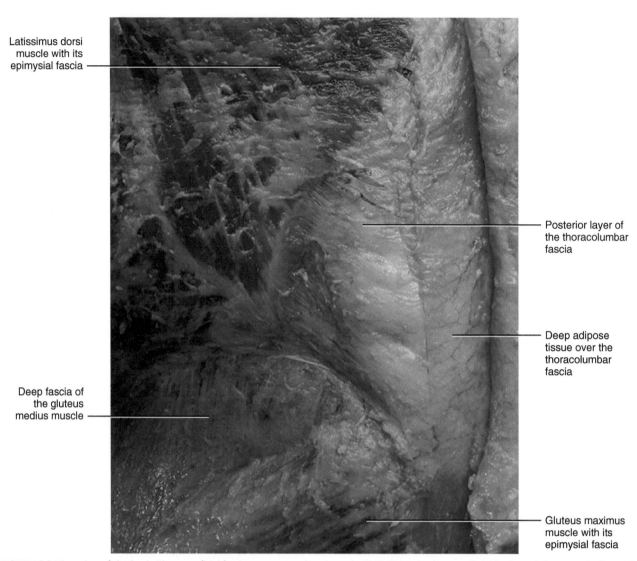

Latissimus dorsi muscle with its epimysial fascia

Posterior layer of the thoracolumbar fascia

Deep adipose tissue over the thoracolumbar fascia

Deep fascia of the gluteus medius muscle

Gluteus maximus muscle with its epimysial fascia

FIGURE 6.3 Dissection of the back. The superficial fascia was removed to show the DAT. Between the superficial fascia and the posterior layer of the TLF, the DAT is just a thin layer of loose connective tissue. It permits a proper gliding between the two fascial layers.

group of young Japanese women. Average subcutaneous fat thickness was 9.8 mm (±1.5 mm). Subcutaneous fat thickness showed higher values at the buttocks, breasts and abdomen and lower values at the back. The difference of fat distribution between obese and lean subjects was observed mainly in the abdominal area but not in the chest or posterior trunk. According to Murakami et al (1999), subcutaneous fat thickness tends to increase with age, especially at lower parts of the trunk, such as the waist and infragluteal region. This could explain why, with age, the circumference of these areas does not change despite weight loss, as the loss of muscular tissue is balanced by increased subcutaneous fat.

The superficial fascia adheres to the deep fascia along the spinous processes (Fig. 6.4). In the thoracic region, the retinaculum cutis profundus is formed by many septa, never separated by more than 1 mm, that insert into the supraspinous ligament. In this way, a connection between superficial and deep fasciae is created. The septa are oblique with a craniocaudal direction. At the level of the first thoracic vertebrae, the superficial fascia crosses the spine and continues into the superficial fascia of the contralateral side (Fig. 6.5). At this point, the superficial fascia is particularly thick and well vascularized. In the lumbar region, fan-shaped thick bundles of the profundus septa originate from the apex of the spinous processes. Distally to L2–L3, the DAT becomes rich in loose connective tissue along the midline and the superficial fasciae of the two sides are connected to form a single layer (Fig. 6.6). Finally, in the sacral region numerous perpendicular, fibrous septa connect the superficial fascia to the midline.

This longitudinal adhesion (along the spinous processes) divides the subcutis of the two halves of the body allowing each to function independently, but at the same time specific points of connection between the two halves exist in the thoracic and lumbar regions. The superficial fascia also partially adheres to

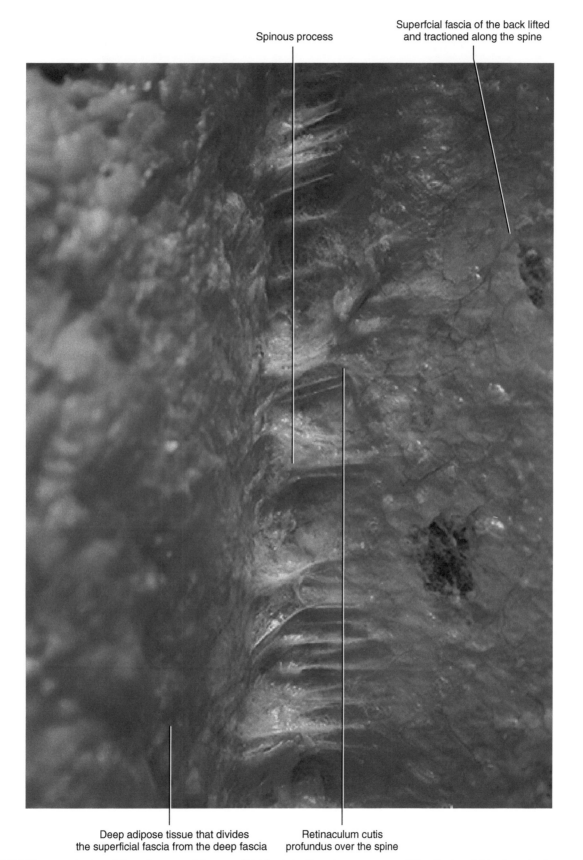

Spinous process

Superfcial fascia of the back lifted and tractioned along the spine

Deep adipose tissue that divides the superficial fascia from the deep fascia

Retinaculum cutis profundus over the spine

FIGURE 6.4 Macroscopic view of the adherence of the superficial fascia to the spinous processes. This adhesion divides the subcutaneous tissue of the two sides of the body.

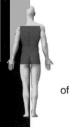

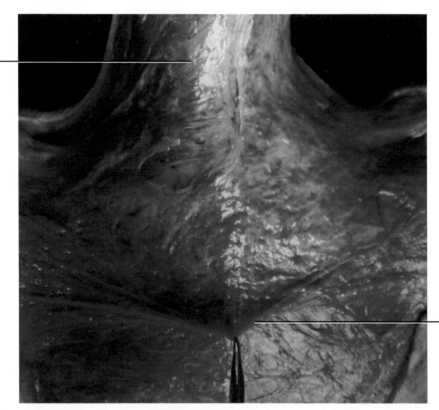

Deep fascia
of the trapezius
muscle —

— Lifted superficial
fascia of the
parascapular region

FIGURE 6.5 Posterior view of the thorax. The skin and the SAT were removed to show the superficial fascia of the parascapular region. The scissors lift the superficial fascia along the midline. The superficial fascia is well vascularized and very elastic, thick and resistant. In the parascapular region, the superficial fascia crosses the midline to connect the two sides of the body.

the deep fascia along the inferior margin of the scapula (Fig. 6.7) and along the iliac crest. These transverse adhesions divide the subcutis to help form cervical, trunk and pelvic sections. These transverse divisions occur in the front and the back.

Due to distinct features of the superficial fascia of the parascapular region, it is called the dorsal thoracic fascia. It is a strong and well-vascularized fibroelastic layer that plays a significant role in the circulation of the overlying skin and subcutaneous tissue. It is used by plastic surgeons as a fasciocutaneous flap. The parascapular subcutaneous region is also important because it is one of the few locations of brown fat in humans. According to Gil et al (2011) functional brown adipose tissue (BAT) in humans has been located in the neck, supraclavicular, mediastinal and interscapular areas. The BAT has intrinsic and beneficial metabolic properties and can dissipate energy directly as heat. For this reason, it is considered important for thermoregulation.

Deep Fasciae

The fascial architecture of the back is complex. Indeed the back contains aponeuroses, aponeurotic fasciae and numerous epimysial fasciae, disposed to form three different myofascial layers. It is important to bear in mind the distinction between fascia and aponeurosis. Aponeurosis is a type of flattened tendon that has

parallel-arranged collagen fibres. This fibre arrangement permits it to resist force in a limited number of planes. An example could be the distal insertion of the erector spinae muscle into the sacrum, which has all the collagen fibres disposed in a longitudinal direction. The deep fasciae have a multilayered structure with collagen fibres in different directions. Therefore, they are able to withstand stress in multiple directions. The epimysial fasciae are thin and adhere to muscles. An example is the fascia covering the trapezius muscle. The aponeurotic fasciae are thicker and could be isolated from the underlying muscles. The best example could be the aponeurotic. Both the epimysial and aponeurotic fascia can transmit forces along myofascial planes. Greater forces are transmitted by the aponeurotic fasciae (some kilos) compared to lighter forces transmitted by the epimysial fasciae (some grams). Where an epimysial fascia is present, it is impossible to separate the action of the muscles from the fascia, as the fascia and muscles are intertwined.

The three muscular–fascial layers that could be recognized in the back are the (Fig. 6.8):

1. superficial layer
2. middle layer
3. deep layer.

Between these muscular–fascial layers, some 'lines of fusion' are present. These are well-defined points where the muscles and fasciae of one layer merge with the muscles and fasciae of an adjacent layer. These

190

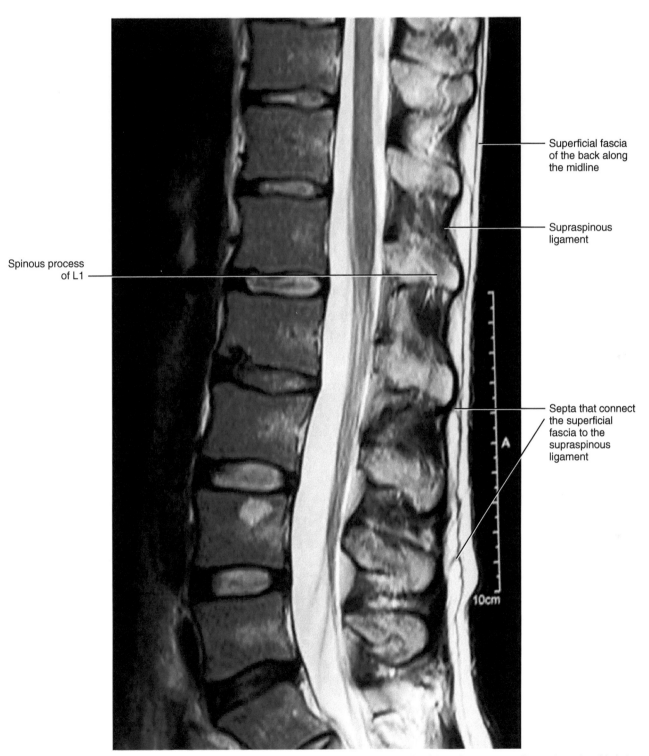

Superficial fascia of the back along the midline

Supraspinous ligament

Spinous process of L1

Septa that connect the superficial fascia to the supraspinous ligament

10cm

FIGURE 6.6 MRI of the spine. The superficial fascia is clearly visible as a black line in the middle of the subcutaneous adipose tissue (in white). See also the septa connecting the superficial fascia with the supraspinous ligament.

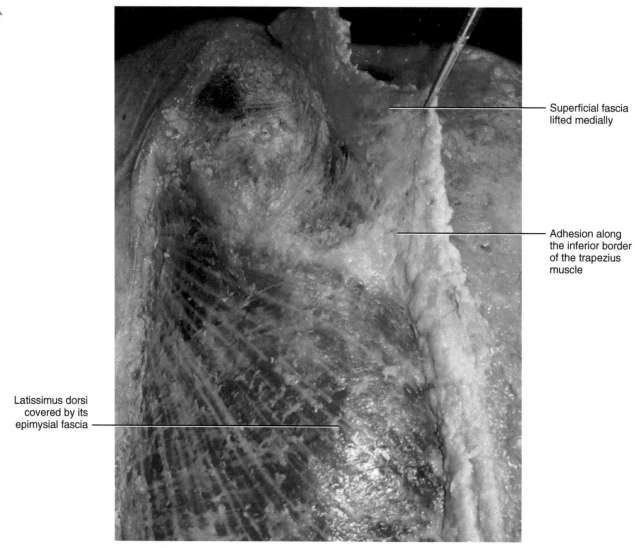

Superficial fascia lifted medially

Adhesion along the inferior border of the trapezius muscle

Latissimus dorsi covered by its epimysial fascia

FIGURE 6.7 Transverse adhesion between the superficial and deep fasciae at the level of the inferior border of the trapezius muscle.

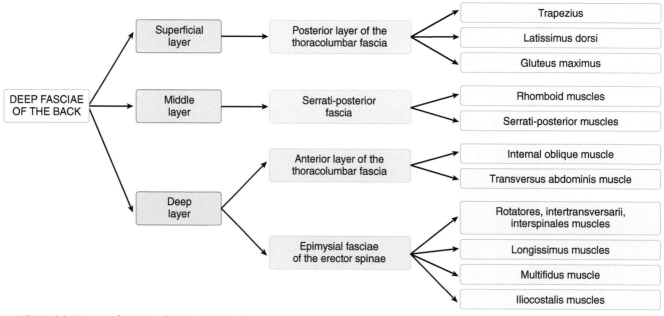

FIGURE 6.8 Diagram of the deep fasciae of the back.

CLINICAL PEARL 6.2 PARASCAPULAR FLAP

In the parascapular region, the superficial fascia becomes thicker and connects the right and left parts of the body. Plastic surgeons call this portion of the fascia the 'parascapular fascia' and use it for fasciocutaneous flaps, due to its strength, adaptability and rich vascularization. Described for the first time by Nassif et al (1982), this flap is vascularized by the cutaneous parascapular artery that is the terminal branch of the circumflex artery of the scapula. This vessel has a mean diameter of 1 mm, and the superficial dorsal fascia is the main component of this flap. Kim et al (1987) proposed that the dorsal thoracic fascia can be transferred as a free flap without its overlying skin and subcutaneous tissue (fascial flap). The rich vascularization of the dorsal thoracic fascia and its elasticity and thickness creates a perfect flap to facilitate wound closure. According to Aharinejad et al (1998) this flap could also be used in patients with chronic venous insufficiency and cutaneous ulcers. Indeed, this flap contains valves in its microvascular bed that facilitate venous return and myofibroblasts are usually present in the valve leaflets. The high number of smaller-sized valves improves the haemodynamics of the leg, thus contributing to the clinical success of free scapular flaps used to treat cutaneous ulcerations in the lower extremities. In addition, the significant thickness of this fascia and its capacity to modify itself with mechanical loading allows the use of this flap in weight bearing zones. In addition, this flap adheres easily to the underlying plane. So, in the heel or in other zones where we need good integration with the underlying structure, this flap is strongly recommended. Sonmez et al (2003) also found significantly less pain and ulceration (P<0.05) in the fasciocutaneous group, compared with the muscle flap group, with regard to the reconstruction of the weight-bearing surfaces of the foot. For this group the only problem was that fasciocutaneous flaps were nonneurosensory, but, according to our histological studies, this superficial fascia is well innervated. These observations may improve the preparation and use of this flap.

lines of fusion allow coordination among the various muscular groups. Later in this chapter the main lines of fusion are described.

Superficial Layer of the Deep Fascia of the Back

The superficial layer of the deep fascia envelops the trapezius, the latissimus dorsi and the gluteus maximus (Figs 6.9 and 6.10). It also includes the posterior layer of the thoracolumbar fascia. The fascia of these muscles is a thin fibrous layer strongly adherent to the underlying muscles via many intramuscular septa (epimysial fascia). This layer attaches to the cranium above the superior nuchal line of the occipital bone. In the midline it is attached to the ligamentum nuchae, supraspinal ligament and spinous processes of all the vertebrae from C7 to L4.

Laterally, in the neck, the superficial layer of the deep fascia of the back is continuous with the superficial layer of the deep cervical fascia of the neck, which envelops the trapezius and sternocleidomastoid muscles. Over the shoulder, it is attached to the spine of the scapula and to the acromion. It continues downwards with the fascia of the deltoid muscle. Anteriorly, it is continuous with the deep fascia of the axilla and the pectoral fascia. On the abdomen, it covers the external oblique muscle, and below it is attached to the crest of the ilium.

Intermediate Layer of the Deep Fascia of the Back

The intermediate layer of the deep fascia of the back is formed by thin muscles: the rhomboids and the serrati posterior muscles with their fasciae (Fig. 6.11). The serrati posterior muscles are deeper with respect to the rhomboid muscles and form a partially separated fascial layer: the serrati fascia (see below). The fascia of rhomboid muscles splits along the medial border of the scapulae: the superficial layer continues into the fascia of the infraspinatus and supraspinatus muscles, the deep layer continues into the fascia of the serratus anterior muscle. Proximally, the rhomboid fascia continues with the fascia of the splenius of the neck and levator scapulae muscles (middle layer of the deep fasciae of the neck) (Fig. 6.12).

Medially, the intermediate layer attaches to the spinous processes and interspinous ligaments and laterally, it extends to the angle of the ribs and continues with the serratus anterior fascia and the clavipectoral fascia. The middle layer is also associated with supraspinatus and infraspinatus fasciae that will be described with the fasciae of the upper limb.

SERRATI FASCIAE

This fascia (Fig. 6.13) is a well-defined fibrous layer that envelops both the serratus posterior inferior and the serratus posterior superior muscles, forming a unique fibromuscular layer. It allows a perfect plane of gliding between the superficial muscles that connect the vertebral column to the extremities and the deeper planes formed by the extensor muscles of the vertebral column. It is impossible to divide the fascia from these muscles because they are completely embedded within the fascia. Testut (1905) considered the inferior serratus posterior muscle more as a fascial tensor than a muscle of force. The muscular fibres of both serrati posterior muscles run in a variety of directions. The superficial fibres are mostly oblique and they coordinate movements between upper and lower limbs and between front and back. The deeper fibres are mostly longitudinally orientated and have more of a role in posture and weight bearing. Laterally, the serrati fascia partially insert into the ribs and partially continue into

Text continued on p. 199

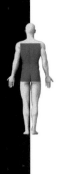

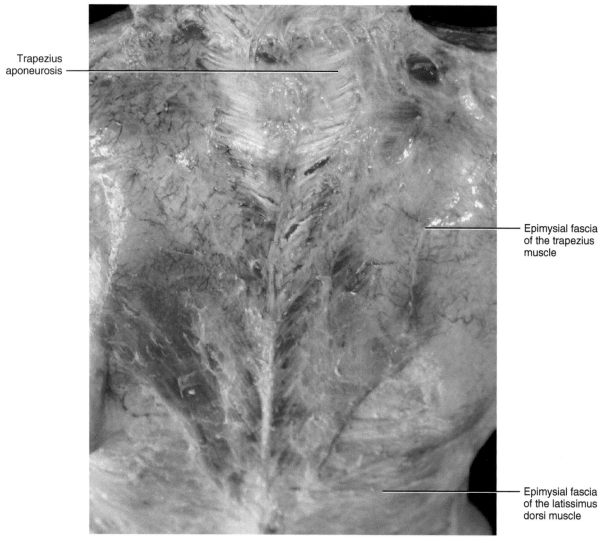

Trapezius aponeurosis

Epimysial fascia of the trapezius muscle

Epimysial fascia of the latissimus dorsi muscle

FIGURE 6.9 Posterior view of the thorax. The trapezius muscles present both an epimysial fascia and an aponeurosis. The aponeurosis connects the trapezius to the spine and it is particularly evident from T1 to T4. The epimysial fascia envelops the trapezius muscle, continues over the aponeurosis and crosses the spine to continue into the epimysial fascia of the contralateral side. Thus a fascial connection between the two trapezii muscles exists, aiding in peripheral motor control during symmetrical contraction of these two muscles.

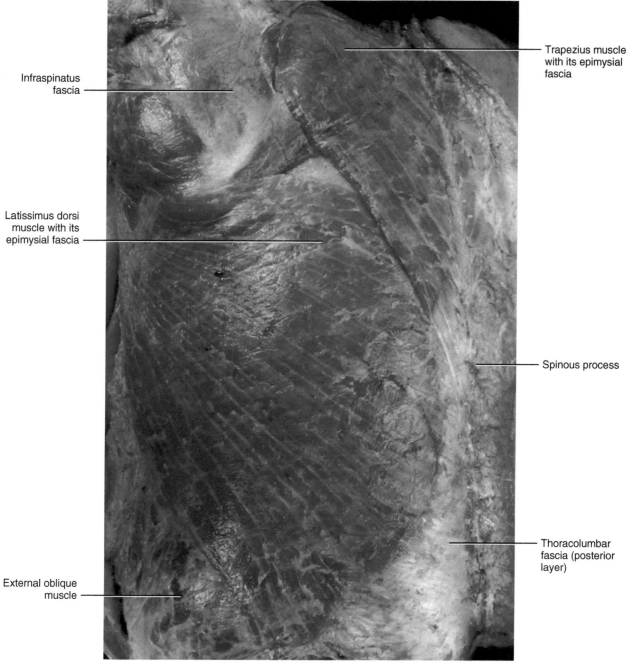

Infraspinatus fascia

Latissimus dorsi muscle with its epimysial fascia

External oblique muscle

Trapezius muscle with its epimysial fascia

Spinous process

Thoracolumbar fascia (posterior layer)

FIGURE 6.10 Dissection of the back. The subcutaneous tissue was removed to show the muscles enveloped by the superficial layer of the deep fascia of the back. This musculofascial layer is formed by the trapezius, latissimus dorsi, external oblique and gluteus maximus muscles and their fasciae.

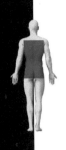

Levator scapulae
muscle

Rhomboid
muscles

Aponeurotic
fascia of the
infraspinatus
muscle

Loose connective
tissue

Fascia of the
serrati posterior
muscles in a
deeper plane

Loose connective
tissue

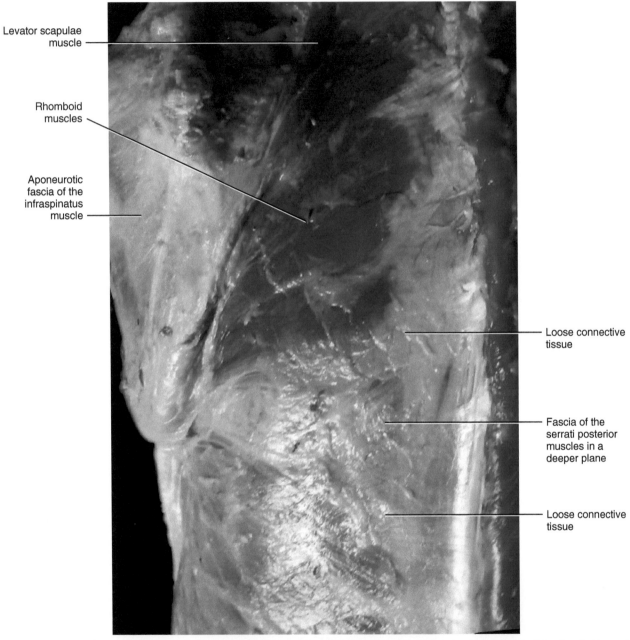

FIGURE 6.11 Dissection of the dorsum. The trapezius muscle was removed to show the intermediate layer. The fascia of the rhomboid muscle continues with the serratus anterior fascia (under the scapula) and with the infraspinatus and supraspinatus fasciae. In the neck, it continues with the middle layer of the deep fascia of the neck enveloping the levator scapulae muscle.

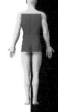

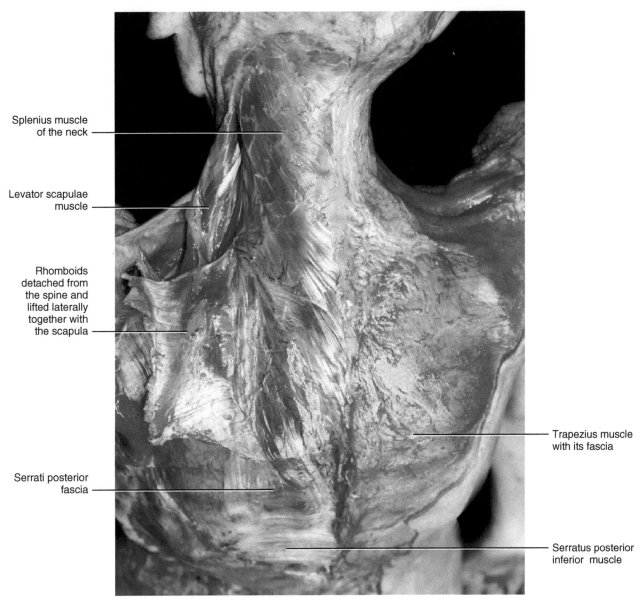

Splenius muscle of the neck

Levator scapulae muscle

Rhomboids detached from the spine and lifted laterally together with the scapula

Serrati posterior fascia

Trapezius muscle with its fascia

Serratus posterior inferior muscle

FIGURE 6.12 Dissection of the posterior region of the neck and thorax. On the right: only the skin and the subcutaneous tissues were removed. On the left: the trapezius muscle was removed and the rhomboids were detached from the spine and lifted laterally to show the continuity among the fascia of the splenii muscles, the rhomboid fascia and the serrati posterior fascia.

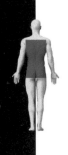

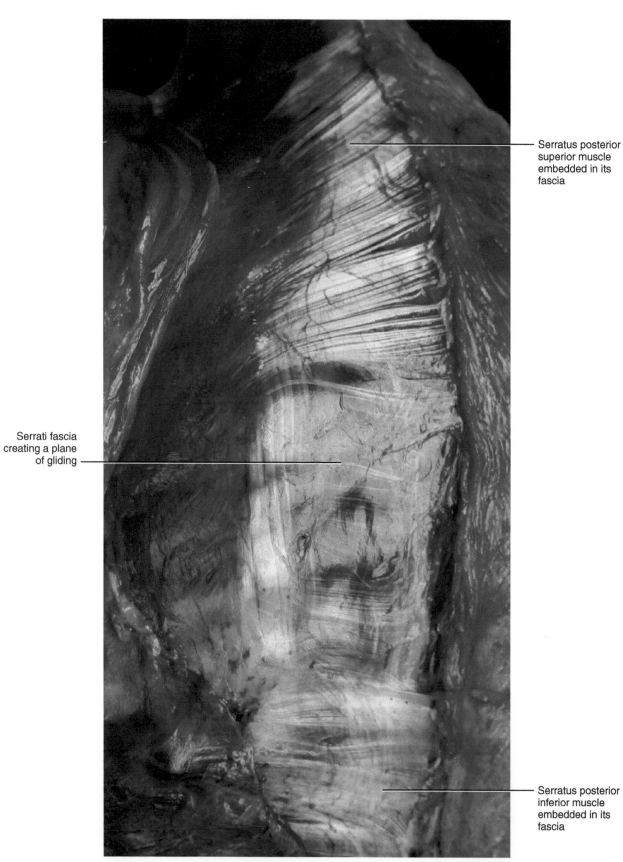

Serratus posterior superior muscle embedded in its fascia

Serrati fascia creating a plane of gliding

Serratus posterior inferior muscle embedded in its fascia

FIGURE 6.13 Dissection of the back. The rhomboid muscles were removed to show the serrati fascia. The serrati fascia envelops the superior and serratus posterior inferior muscles and creates a gliding surface between these superficial muscles, which have the fibres with an oblique direction and the deep muscles that have fibres in a longitudinal direction.

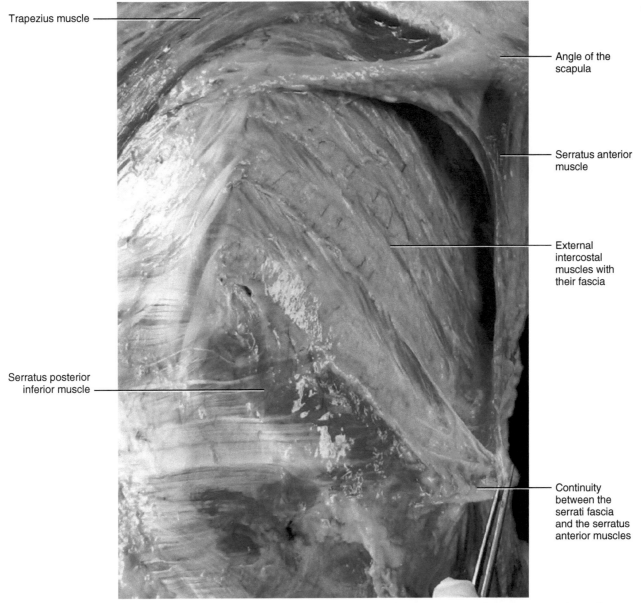

Trapezius muscle

Angle of the scapula

Serratus anterior muscle

External intercostal muscles with their fascia

Serratus posterior inferior muscle

Continuity between the serrati fascia and the serratus anterior muscles

FIGURE 6.14 Posterolateral view of the back, right side. The scissors are stretching the serratus anterior muscle, and consequently creating some lines of forces into the fascia covering the serratus posterior inferior muscle. So, this fascia is stretched laterally every time the serratus anterior muscle contracts.

the fascia of the serratus anterior muscle (Fig. 6.14). Hence, under the scapula a perfect plane of gliding exists between the serratus anterior fascia and serratus posterior fascia (that is deeper), while laterally the two fasciae merge, permitting a better coordination between the anterior and posterior serrati muscles. The gliding under the scapula is necessary to permit the correct movement of the scapula. Distally, the serrati fascia merges with the inner aspect of the posterior layer of the thoracolumbar fascia.

Deep Layer of the Deep Fascia of the Back

This layer includes the anterior layer of the TLF and the fascia surrounding the erector spinae muscles (Figs 6.15 and 6.16). The anterior layer is an aponeurotic

fascia and the erector spinae are covered by epimysial fascia. Examination of the fascial compartment of the erector spinae reveals that only the interspinales and multifidi muscle bellies have their own clearly defined compartment. All the other erector spinae muscles are fused together and it is impossible to clearly divide the respective bellies.

Thoracolumbar Fascia

Numerous descriptions of the TLF exist in the literature and various authors tend to use somewhat different nomenclatures. This makes the interpretation of biomechanical studies difficult. The differences will be touched on where applicable in this section.

Most agree that the TLF is an important structure as forces from the latissimus dorsi and gluteus maximus,

Erector spinae
muscles

Loose connective
tissue between the
posterior layer of
the thoracolumbar
fascia and the
erector spinae
muscles

Posterior layer of
the thoracolumbar
fascia cut along
the midline and
lifted laterally

Superficial
fibres of the
gluteus maximus
inserted into the
thoracolumbar
fascia

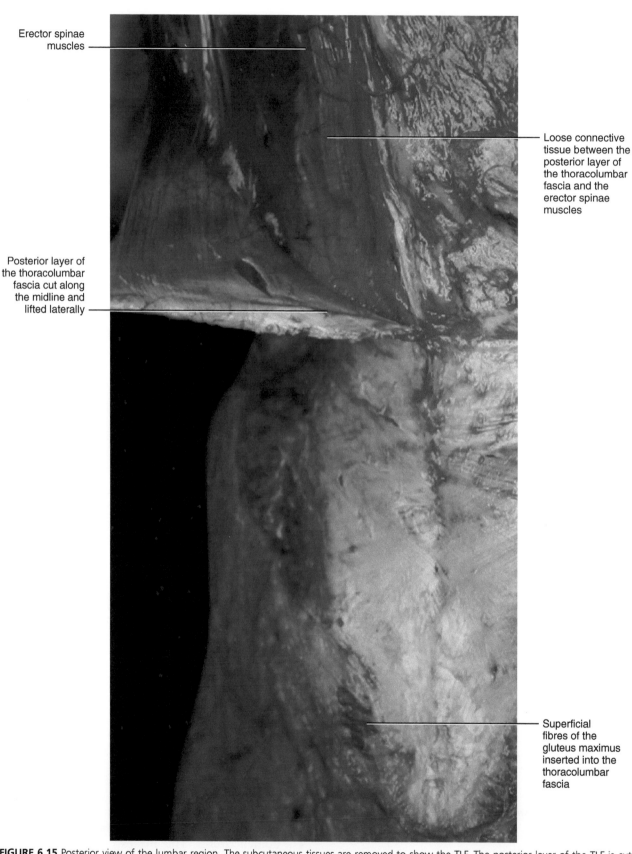

FIGURE 6.15 Posterior view of the lumbar region. The subcutaneous tissues are removed to show the TLF. The posterior layer of the TLF is cut along the midline and lifted laterally. Between the *posterior layer of* the TLF and the erector spinae muscles, loose connective tissue is present. This looseness allows the TLF and the muscles inserted into it (i.e latissimus dorsi, which have fibres with an oblique orientation) to move independently of the erector spinae muscles (with their longitudinal fibre orientation).

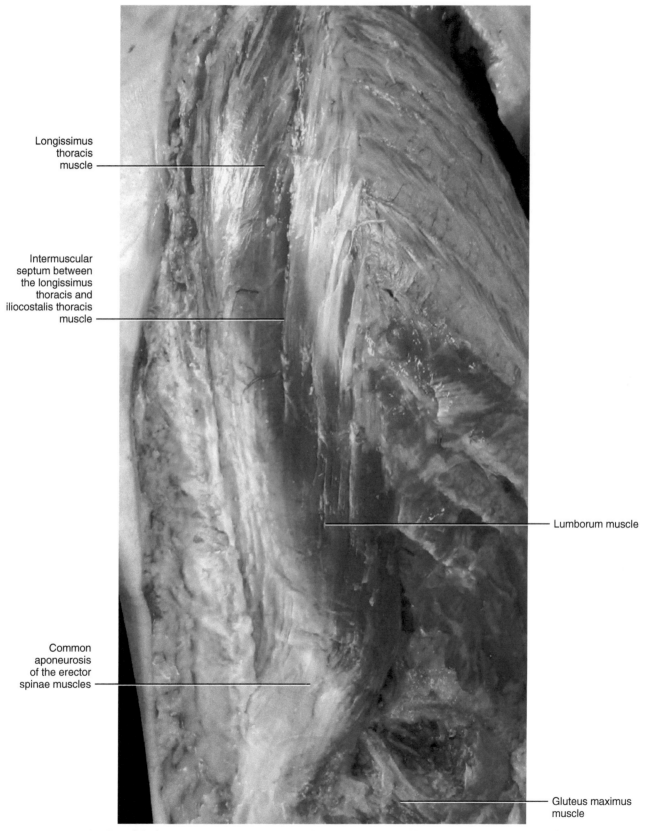

Longissimus thoracis muscle

Intermuscular septum between the longissimus thoracis and iliocostalis thoracis muscle

Lumborum muscle

Common aponeurosis of the erector spinae muscles

Gluteus maximus muscle

FIGURE 6.16 Posterior view of the back. Erector spinae muscles. Over the sacrum it is impossible to separate the aponeurosis of the erector spinae and the thoracolumbar fascia.

the epaxial (paraspinal muscles) and hypaxial (anterior trunk muscles) converge there (Fig. 6.17). However, some authors use a two-layered model of the TLF, and others a three-layered model (Willard et al 2012). The three-layered model resembles the two-layered model, but its anterior layer consists of the fascia passing anterior to the quadratus lumborum muscle. The anterior layer of the two-layered model becomes the middle layer of the three-layered model. The middle layer of the three-layered model consists of the posterior fascia of the quadratus lumborum muscle and the aponeuroses of the abdominal muscles, especially the internal oblique and transversus abdominis muscles (Schuenke et al 2012), which insert into the transverse processes (Fig. 6.18).

The two-layered model of the TLF recognizes a posterior layer surrounding the posterior aspect of the paraspinal muscles and an anterior layer lying between the paraspinal muscles and the quadratus lumborum muscles. In the two-layered model, the fascia on the anterior aspect of the quadratus lumborum muscle is considered to be an extension of the fasciae from the abdominal wall, particularly of the transversus abdominis muscle. The transversus abdominis muscle, together with its fascia, connects the rectus with the quadratus lumborum and psoas muscles. In this way all the hypaxial muscles of the abdomen are joined.

We prefer the two-layered model because the fascia on the anterior aspect of the quadratus lumborum has macroscopic and histological features completely different from the thoracolumbar fascia. The anterior fascia over the quadratus lumborum is thin (0.10 mm, range 0.06–0.14 mm) (Barker & Briggs 1999) and is not able to transmit tension from the various muscles to the thoracolumbar spine, which is the main role of the TLF. From a functional point of view, the anterior fascia is more closely related to the fasciae of the pelvis (iliopsoas fascia) and the abdomen (epimysial fascia of the transversus abdominis muscle), rather than the thoracolumbar fascia.

Based on this analysis, we use the two-layer model for the TLF. Its posterior layer is part of the superficial layer of the deep fascia of the trunk, while its anterior layer is part of the deep layer of the deep fascia of the trunk.

The posterior layer of the TLF is located in the lumbar region just under the subcutaneous tissue (superficial fascia). It connects the latissimus dorsi and the gluteus maximus, and also part of the external oblique muscle and the trapezius through their fasciae (Figs 6.19–6.22). The inner aspect of this lamina fuses with the serrati posterior fascia (middle layer) and with the erector spinae aponeurosis. Distally, this lamina

Text continued on p. 207

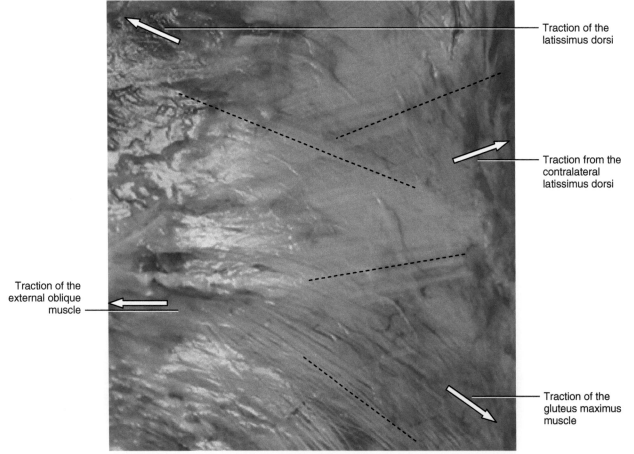

Traction of the latissimus dorsi

Traction from the contralateral latissimus dorsi

Traction of the external oblique muscle

Traction of the gluteus maximus muscle

FIGURE 6.17 A macroscopic view of the posterior layer of thoracolumbar fascia. The multilayered structure is evident. The white arrows show the main direction of muscular contraction and stretching. The dotted lines show the different orientation of the fibrous bundles.

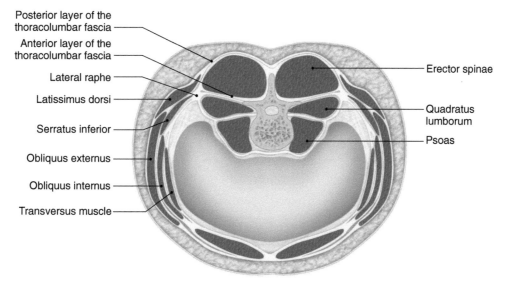

Posterior layer of the
thoracolumbar fascia

Anterior layer of the
thoracolumbar fascia

Lateral raphe

Latissimus dorsi

Serratus inferior

Obliquus externus

Obliquus internus

Transversus muscle

Erector spinae

Quadratus
lumborum

Psoas

FIGURE 6.18 Diagram illustrating the continuity between the TLF (two-layered model) and the fasciae of the abdomen. The posterior layer of the TLF is formed by the fascia of the latissimus dorsi and the fascia of the external oblique muscle (plus the serratus fascia and the fascia of the gluteus maximus muscle). The anterior layer of the TLF is formed by fasciae of the internal oblique muscle and the transversus muscle. Note how the anterior and posterior layers form a fascial compartment for the paraspinal muscles. Part of the fascia of the transversus muscle continues with the fasciae of the quadratus lumborum and psoas muscles, fuses with the anterior longitudinal ligament and joins with the contralateral fascia of the transversus muscle. For some authors this is the anterior layer of the TLF.

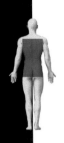

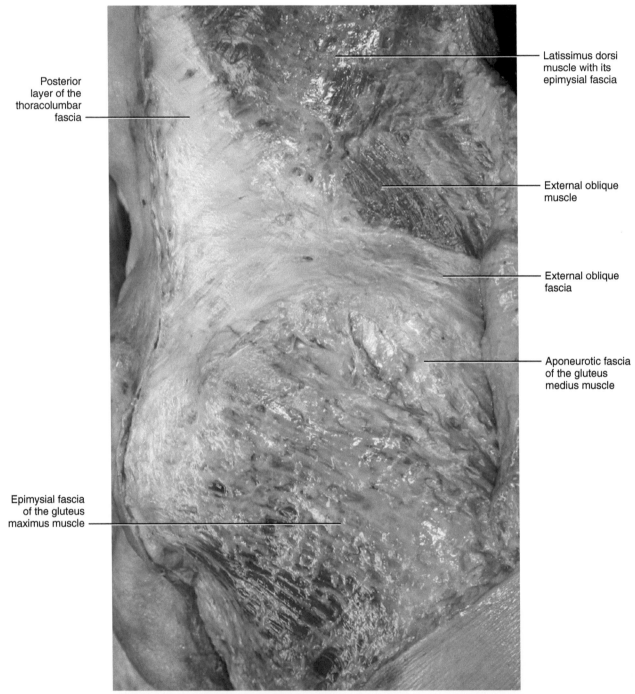

Posterior
layer of the
thoracolumbar
fascia

Latissimus dorsi
muscle with its
epimysial fascia

External oblique
muscle

External oblique
fascia

Aponeurotic fascia
of the gluteus
medius muscle

Epimysial fascia
of the gluteus
maximus muscle

FIGURE 6.19 Posterior layer of the TLF. The gluteus maximus and the latissimus dorsi muscles have many fibres that insert directly into the TLF, while the external oblique muscle is inserted into the TLF by way of its fascia.

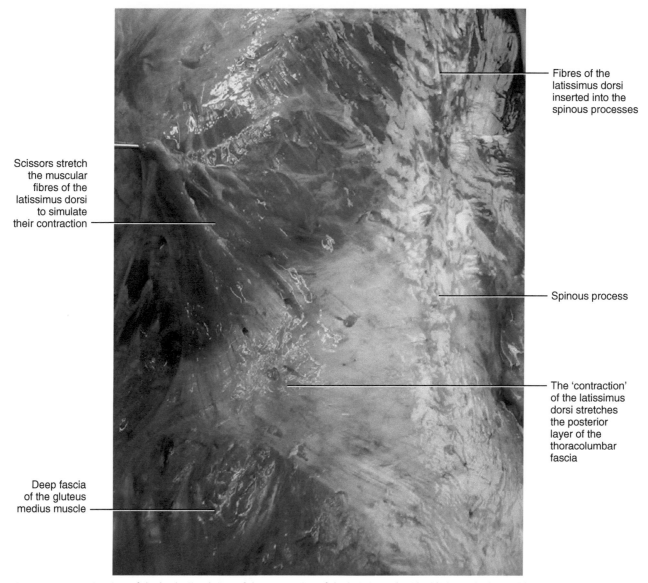

Fibres of the
latissimus dorsi
inserted into the
spinous processes

Scissors stretch
the muscular
fibres of the
latissimus dorsi
to simulate
their contraction

Spinous process

The 'contraction'
of the latissimus
dorsi stretches
the posterior
layer of the
thoracolumbar
fascia

Deep fascia
of the gluteus
medius muscle

FIGURE 6.20 Posterior view of the back. Simulation of the contraction of the latissimus dorsi highlighting the lines of force inside the TLF.

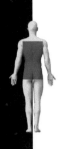

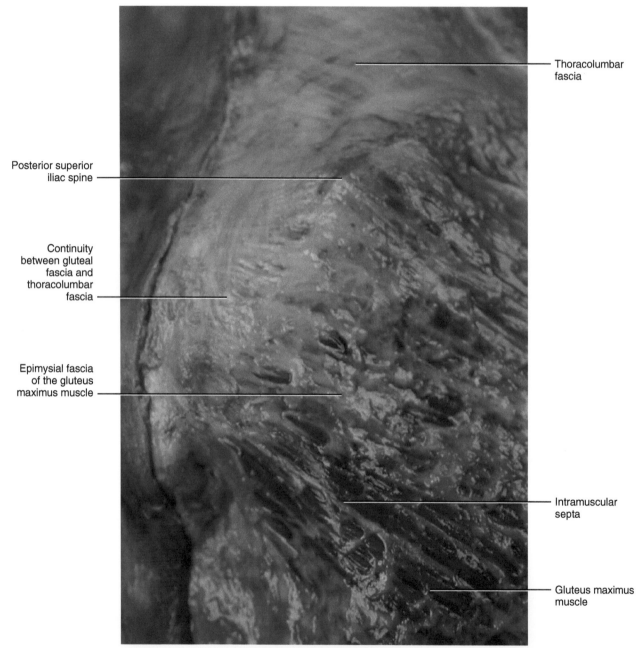

Thoracolumbar fascia

Posterior superior iliac spine

Continuity between gluteal fascia and thoracolumbar fascia

Epimysial fascia of the gluteus maximus muscle

Intramuscular septa

Gluteus maximus muscle

FIGURE 6.21 Posterior view of the right gluteal region. Insertion of the superficial bundles of the gluteus maximus into the thoracolumbar fascia.

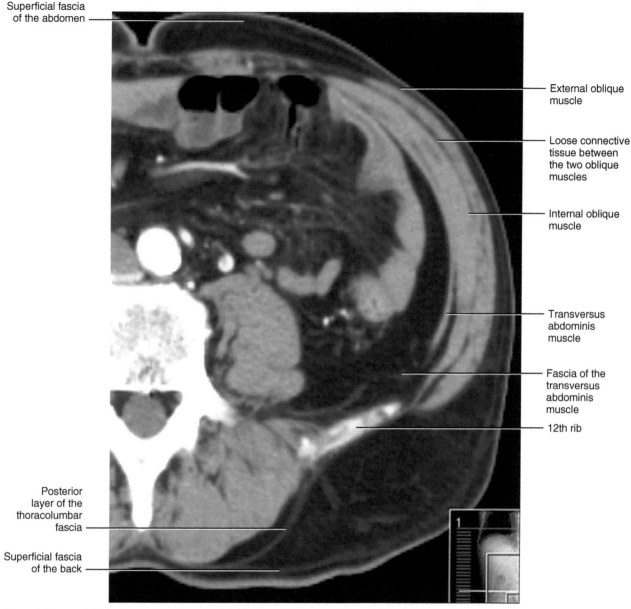

Superficial fascia of the abdomen

External oblique muscle

Loose connective tissue between the two oblique muscles

Internal oblique muscle

Transversus abdominis muscle

Fascia of the transversus abdominis muscle

12th rib

Posterior layer of the thoracolumbar fascia

Superficial fascia of the back

FIGURE 6.22 MRI of the lumbar region. The superficial fascia and the posterior layer of the TLF are clearly evident. Near the spine, the superficial and deep fasciae merge.

attaches to the posterior superior iliac spine, to the iliac crests and to the long dorsal sacroiliac ligament.

The posterior layer of the TLF attaches to the supraspinal ligament and spinous processes to the level of L4. Caudal to L4 its collagen fibrous bundles cross to the contralateral side and attaches to the sacrum, posterior superior iliac spine and iliac crest. There is a definite coupling of the gluteus maximus to the contralateral latissimus dorsi muscle, by way of the posterior layer of the thoracolumbar fascia. Both of these muscles conduct forces contralaterally during movement and tense the TLF. In so doing, they are important in rotation of the trunk and stabilization of the lower lumbar spine and sacroiliac joints. Due to the different fibre directions of the latissimus dorsi and gluteus maximus, the posterior layer of the TLF has a

crosshatched appearance. Therefore, the posterior layer of the TLF can be considered a big retinaculum that connects the two halves of the body with the upper and lower limbs. This structure allows proper balance and distribution of forces that act in the lumbosacral region during movement, notably the pendulum-like actions of the contralateral arms and legs during walking and running.

The role of TLF in the transfer of force among the spine, pelvis and lower limbs was demonstrated, for the first time, by Vleeming et al in 1995. This knowledge emphasizes the fact that local pain (for example) in the sacroiliac joint may be due to any of the structures associated with the transfer of force from the biceps femoris to the sacrotuberous ligament, to the erector spinae, to the thoracolumbar fascia, and to the contralateral latissimus dorsi. Understanding the function of this complex myofascial junction is fundamental to biomechanical analysis and effective rehabilitation of individuals with low back and pelvic girdle pain.

The posterior layer of the TLF has a mean thickness of 680 μm, and could be considered as a multidirectional construct with the same characteristics as the crural fascia. Barker and Briggs (1999) found an average thickness of the posterior layer of the TLF, near the spinous processes, of 0.56 mm.

The posterior layer of the TLF is formed, from a microscopic point of view, by three sublayers, as are all aponeurotic fasciae. These sublayers are named: outer, intermediate and inner (Figs 6.23 and 6.26). The outer sublayer has a mean thickness of 75 μm with parallel undulating collagen fibres and with many elastic fibres. This layer is the continuation of the thin epimysial fascia of the latissimus dorsi and the gluteus maximus muscles. Therefore, it could be considered an epimysial fascia. The intermediate sublayer (152 μm) is made of packed straight collagen bundles, disposed in the same direction without elastic fibres, corresponding to the aponeurosis of the latissimus dorsi muscle. The inner sublayer is made of loose connective tissue (450 μm) and separates the posterior layer of the TLF from the epimysial fascia of the erector spinae muscles. Recently, Tezars et al (2011) demonstrated that the outer layer is the most innervated and provides increased sensitivity.

The anterior layer of the TLF (two-layered model) is attached medially to the tips of the transverse processes of the lumbar vertebrae (Figs 6.24 and 6.25) and inserts laterally into the internal oblique and transversus abdominis muscles. It has features of an aponeurotic fascia. Barker et al (2007) measured its thickness as it approached the tip of the transverse process and found a thickness of approximately 0.62 mm, but elsewhere it varied from 0.11 to 1.34 mm. The attachment of the anterior lamina of the TLF to the transverse process is quite strong. Its strength compares to the force necessary to avulse these processes by strong transversus abdominis contractions. Most of the collagen fibres of this lamina are orientated slightly caudolaterally (10–25 ° below the horizontal) until they reach the transverse processes (Barker et al 2007).

The anatomical continuity between the abdominal muscles and the TLF is important in lumbar segmental control. Barker et al (2004) demonstrated that tension of the TLF caused moderate contraction of the transversus abdominis muscle. From a developmental point of view, the anterior layer of the TLF appears to originate from the intermuscular septum that separates the epaxial muscles (erector spinae) from the hypaxial muscles (abdominal, iliopsoas and quadratus lumborum muscles).

Lateral to the erector spinae muscles, the anterior and posterior lamina of the TLF fuse to form the lateral raphe that extends inferiorly from the iliac crest to the twelfth rib (Bogduk and Macintosh 1984). This lateral raphe is a thickened complex of dense connective tissue and represents the junction of the hypaxial myofascial compartment with the paraspinal sheath of the epaxial muscles. Along this raphe all the forces produced by the muscles, inserted into the anterior and posterior layers of the TLF, converge. The lateral raphe has the role of redistributing these muscular tensions into both the layers of the TLF, assuring that the tension is defuse and not localized to only a few vertebrae. Schuenke et al (2012) have demonstrated, by dissections and MRI studies, a fat-filled lumbar interfascial triangle. This area is defined by the anterior and posterior layers of the thoracolumbar fascia, the lateral border of the paraspinal muscles (from the twelfth rib to the iliac crest) and the lateral raphe. The authors theorize that this triangle 'may function in the distribution of laterally mediated tension to balance different viscoelastic proprieties along either the middle[1] or posterior layers of the TFL'. They also recognize that conversely, tension in the transversus abdominis may be dependent on contraction of muscles inserted into the posterior layer of the TLF. Theobald et al (2007) theorize that another function of the lateral raphe may be to reduce friction of adjacent fasciae under high tension. In other words, tension generated by the abdominal myofascial girdle

---

[1]This author uses the three-layered model for the TLF, and refers to the anterior layer of the TLF as the 'middle layer'.

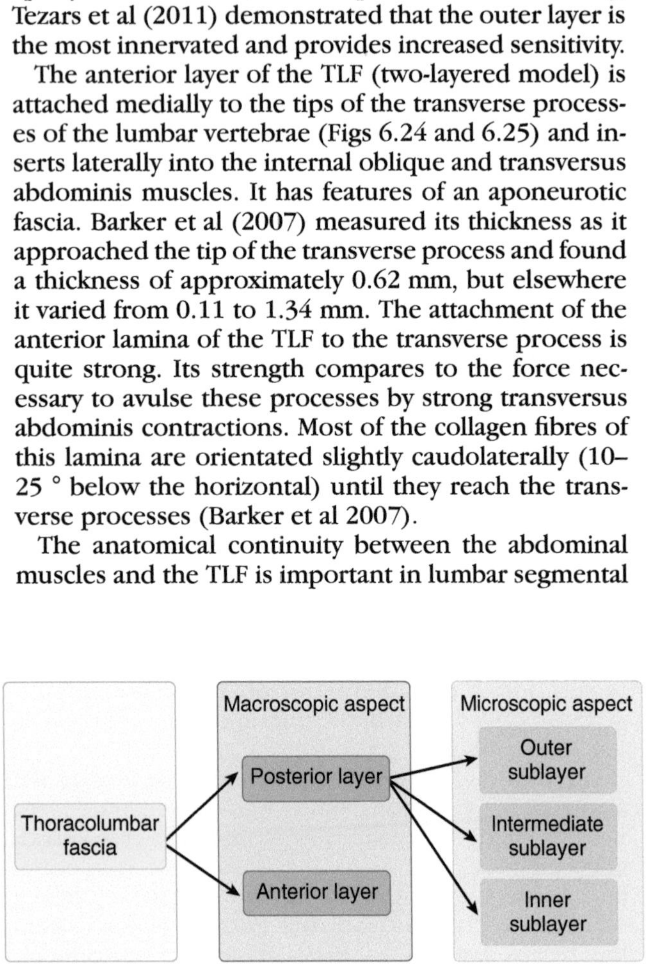

CLINICAL PEARL 6.3 SLUMP TEST

Clinicians have used this test to differentially diagnose and reassess patients thought to have neuromeningeal tension. In this test the sitting patient is asked to flex their head and shoulders forward while extending each leg separately, to create neural tension. According to Barker and Briggs (1999), the fascial continuity from the cervical spine to the lower back and beyond suggests that neural tension may, in reality, be myofascial tension. This myofascial continuity should also be considered when performing a straight-leg raise test.

FIGURE 6.23 Structure of the TLF (two-layered model).

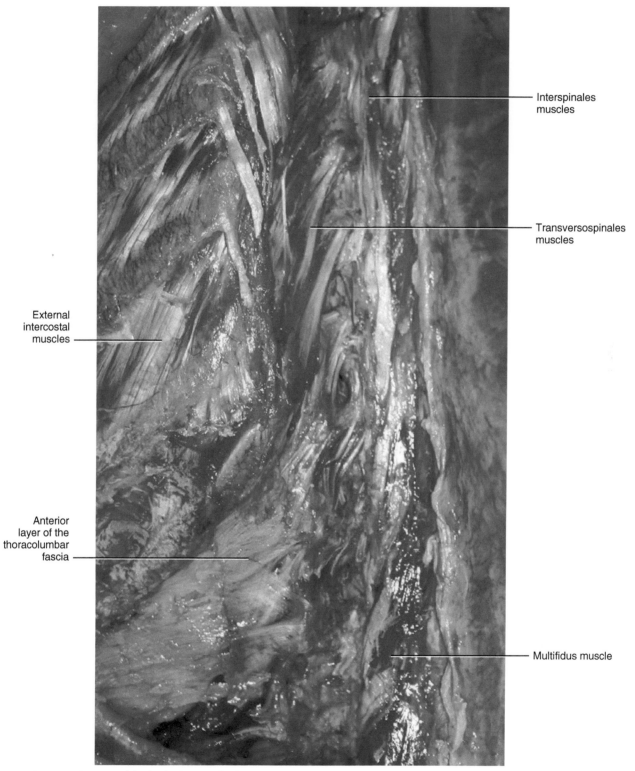

Interspinales
muscles

Transversospinales
muscles

External
intercostal
muscles

Anterior
layer of the
thoracolumbar
fascia

Multifidus muscle

FIGURE 6.24 Posterior view of the back. The superficial and middle myofascial layers were removed to expose the deep layer of the intrinsic back muscles.

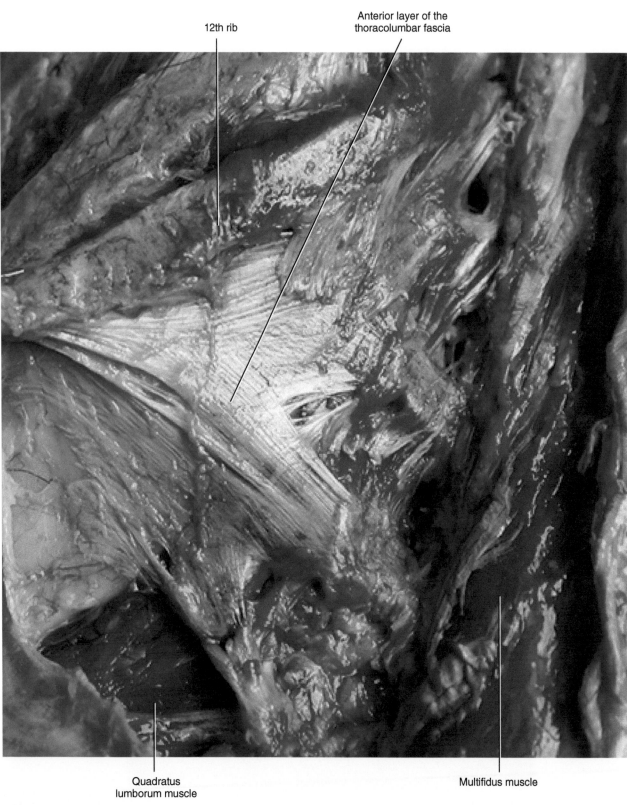

12th rib

Anterior layer of the
thoracolumbar fascia

Quadratus
lumborum muscle

Multifidus muscle

FIGURE 6.25 Posterior view of the lumbar region. All the muscles were removed to show the anterior layer of the TLF (two-layered model). This fibrous layer inserts into the transverse processes of the lumbar vertebra and laterally inserts to the transversus abdominis and internal oblique muscles. The different directions of the fibrous bundles are clearly evident.

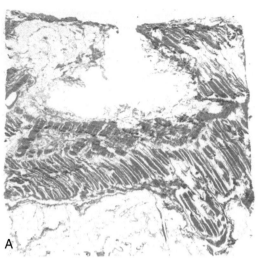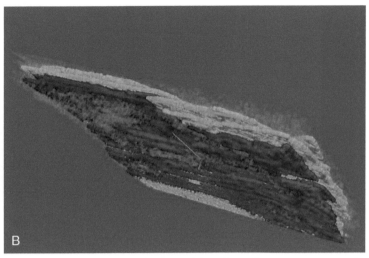

FIGURE 6.26 Posterior layer of the thoracolumbar fascia. **A**: microscopic aspect. Note the cross directions of the collagen fibres. **B**: 3D reconstruction of two sublayer (outer and intermediate). Each colour corresponds to a specific direction of the collagen fibres.

CLINICAL PEARL 6.4 ROLE OF THE TLF IN SPINAL STABILIZATION

When lifting a heavy object, the load is transmitted downwards through the spine to the legs. To stabilize the axial skeleton and minimize compressive loading of the lower lumbar segments, the abdominal muscles contract and the tension in the diaphragm increases. When lifting a heavy object, it is natural for an individual to hold their breath. Wirhed (1984) indicated that this mechanism may decompress the L4 and L5 segments by as much as 40%. Cholewicki et al (1999) used an analogy of a football in the abdominal cavity, stating that the abdominal muscular contraction could increase the abdominal pressure and thus provide mechanical stability to the spine. Gracovetsky (1988) proposed the ineffectiveness of this mechanism as a stabilizer of the spine because, for athletes or workers, generating significant resistance to lifting heavy loads would require pressure so high as to obstruct the abdominal aorta. It is probable that the contraction of the abdominal muscles stretch the TLF and creates a solid structure for the action of the muscles of the back, thus increasing the strength of the back muscles by 30%. This mechanism was called the 'hydraulic amplifier' effect. As the back musculature contracts, within the rigid cylinder created by the anterior and posterior layers of the TLF, a hydraulic effect is created and aids in the extension of the spine. Using a mathematical model, Gracovetsky demonstrated that the extension force produced by expansion of the erector spinae muscles, within the rigid compartment created by the TLF and lamina groove of the spine, is a significant contributor to one's ability to lift a load. This mechanism acts only if the TLF is rigid, permitting the intracompartment pressure to increase. It is therefore probable that lifting a heavy object requires the synergistic activation of the abdominal muscles. Contraction of the abdominal muscles will stretch the two layers of the TLF anteriorly, increase their tension, and create a rigid cylinder. This rigidity will aid contraction of the erector spinae. Thereby adding extra protection to the spine.

across the paraspinal sheath may be dissipated by the dense connective tissue that makes up the lateral raphe (Schuenke et al 2012).

At the base of the lumbar spine, the anterior and posterior layers of the TLF fuse together and insert firmly into the posterior superior iliac spine and the sacrotuberous ligament. In this way they assist in maintaining the integrity of the lower lumbar spine and the sacroiliac joint.

The joining of the anterior and posterior layers of the TLF creates a well-defined fascial compartment for the paraspinal muscles (Fig. 6.18), which are enclosed by the spine and the two layers (two-layer model) of the thoracolumbar fascia. The erector spinae are free to glide inside this space because between their epimysial fascia and the TLF there is loose connective tissue rich in hyaluronic acid (Fig. 6.15). Only in the sacral region does the aponeurosis of the erector spinae and the posterior layer of the TLF adhere. Every time the erector spinae contract, the two layers of the TLF become 'inflated' (hydraulic amplifier mechanism). If these layers are too rigid, they cannot adapt to the variations of muscular volume. The rigidity of these layers could be a possible cause of pain or alteration in muscular activation, and an eventual chronic compartment syndrome.

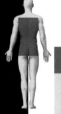
CLINICAL PEARL 6.5 ROLE OF THE TRANSVERSUS ABDOMINIS IN LUMBOPELVIC STABILITY

In the past decade there has been interest in isolated transversus abdominis activation and how it contributes to lumbopelvic stability (Hodges et al 2003). The rationale describing the feed-forward bilateral muscle activation of the transversus abdominis in stabilizing the segmental lumbar spine is unlike that of other trunk muscles. The transversus abdominis maintains an independent action during spinal perturbation. Individuals with low-back pain have altered timing of feed forward onset of the transversus abdominis.

From an evolutionary point of view, the rectus abdominis, transversus abdominis, quadratus lumborum and psoas muscles form the hypaxial muscles (Fig. 6.27). The hypaxial muscles are separated from the epaxial muscles by a septum, which in humans corresponds to the anterior layer of the TLF (two-layered model). The mass of the hypaxial muscles evolved around the visceral cavity of the abdomen, but the fascia maintains the connection among them. In particular, the fascia of the transversus abdominis muscle joins the rectus abdominis with the quadratus lumborum and psoas muscles. From an anatomical point of view, the transversus abdominis muscle is enveloped by epimysial fascia and it is impossible to separate the actions of the fascia from that of the muscle. It is probable that the bilateral activation of the transversus abdominis muscles before movement has the purpose of strengthening the connection among rectus abdominis, quadratus lumborum and psoas muscles.

CLINICAL PEARL 6.6 LUMBAR CHRONIC COMPARTMENT SYNDROME

Styf (1987) demonstrated that during isometric and concentric exercises, the pressure in the erector spinae muscles increases. Intramuscular pressure at rest was 6.1 mmHg (SD=1.4). When the subject experienced muscle fatigue during exercise, the muscle relaxation pressure increased to 14 mmHg. It is possible that if the thoracolumbar fascia is altered, for example becomes more rigid, it cannot adapt to muscle volume variations, causing the internal pressure to become excessive. This situation is called 'compartment syndrome'. The chronic compartment syndrome affecting the erector spinae muscles seems to be an uncommon cause of exercise-induced low-back pain, but subclinical forms could probably explain some chronic low-back pain. Many patients, compared to controls, complain of pain with prolonged lumbar flexion in standing. In this position,

paraspinal muscular pressure has been found to be highly increased and significantly higher in subjects with osteoporosis, degenerative spondylolisthesis and previous lumbar spine surgery (Hammer & Pfefer 2005). Fasciotomy was performed in some of these patients, but the outcomes of this surgery is debated. Indeed a fasciotomy is not necessarily a clinically benign procedure.

In a study on canine leg osteofascial compartments (which correspond closely to humans), fasciotomy resulted in a 15% decrease in muscle force and a 50% decrease in the intracompartmental pressure during muscle contraction (Garfin et al 1981). Improper muscle function also occurs due to the loss of fascial control on muscle pressure and volume. Scar tissue formation might be another complication of fasciotomy (Bermudez et al 1998).

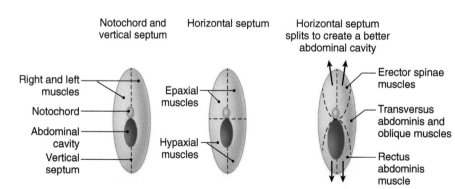

FIGURE 6.27 Scheme of evolution of trunk muscles. At the beginning, only a vertical septum divided the right and left muscles, permitting their separate contraction (for lateroflexion). Next, a horizontal septum divided the epaxial and hypaxial muscles, permitting the flexion and extension of the trunk. The rectus abdominis, quadratus lumborum and psoas muscles form the hypaxial muscles. Finally, the oblique muscles and the transversus abdominis muscle formed inside the horizontal septum. In humans, the horizontal septum corresponds to the anterior layer of the TLF (two-layered model). The mass of the hypaxial muscles evolved around the visceral cavity of the abdomen, but the fascia of the transversus abdominis muscle maintains the connection among them.

Iliopsoas Fascia

The iliopsoas fascia (Fig. 6.28) could be considered a continuation of the fascia of the transversus abdominis muscle[2]. It is separated from the transversalis fascia and from the renal fascia by loose connective tissue. The fascia of the transversus abdominis muscle posteriorly divides into two laminae. The posterior lamina inserts into the transverse processes of the lumbar spine

forming the anterior layer of the TLF. It extends below to the iliolumbar ligament. The anterior lamina covers the iliopsoas and quadratus lumborum muscles, which is why it is called the 'iliopsoas fascia'. It then merges with the anterior longitudinal ligament of the spine to join the fascia of the transversus abdominis muscle on the opposite side. As it passes over the spine, this anterior layer of fascia continues to the periosteum of the body of the spine and attaches to the intervertebral fibrocartilage. Distally, the iliopsoas fascia continues into the pelvis joining with the iliac fascia, and then down to the thigh to merge into the fascia lata. Cranially, this anterior layer of fascia is partially attached to the apex and lower border of the last rib and partially continues with the diaphragmatic fascia. The portion of this fascia that extends from the transverse process of the first lumbar vertebra to the apex and lower

[2]This is an epimysial fascia and has to be distinguished from the transversalis fascia, which is a visceral fascia. These two fasciae are separated by the loose extraperitoneal connective tissue. They are connected only at a few points, such as along the posterior margin of the inguinal ligament.

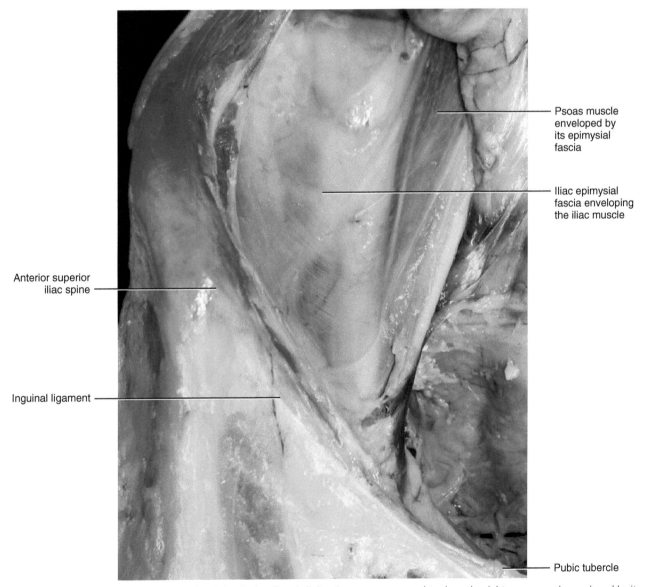

Psoas muscle enveloped by its epimysial fascia

Iliac epimysial fascia enveloping the iliac muscle

Anterior superior iliac spine

Inguinal ligament

Pubic tubercle

FIGURE 6.28 Dissection of the abdomen. The abdominal wall and all the viscera were removed to show the right psoas muscle enveloped by its fascia. The fascia is thin and adheres to the muscle.

213

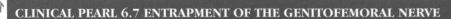

CLINICAL PEARL 6.7 ENTRAPMENT OF THE GENITOFEMORAL NERVE

This entrapment can be responsible for intermittent pain below the inguinal ligament, into the scrotum or labia majora and into the medial thigh (Pecina et al 1997). Hammer (1998) describes a fascial release technique, used over the iliopsoas and adjoining areas, which reduced the compression of the genitofemoral nerve and eliminated the pain. He described a shortened iliopsoas and quadriceps muscle and the palpation of fascial barriers in the iliopsoas and fascia lata. Hammer suggested the application of light pressure against the most evident barrier until it 'melts'. Release of these barriers resulted in reduced tension on the genitofemoral nerve and the elimination of symptoms.

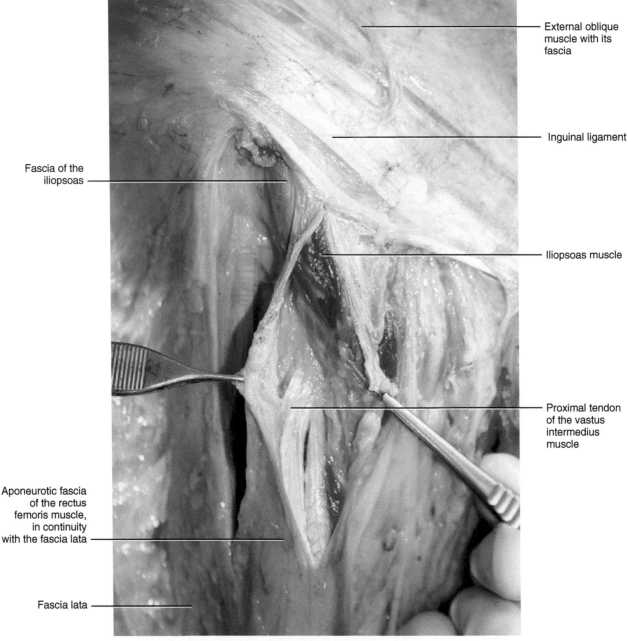

FIGURE 6.29 Anterior view of the thigh. The sartorius muscle and its sheath were removed. Note the distal insertion of the iliopsoas muscle. Here the continuity of the iliopsoas fascia with the sheath of the rectus femoris muscle is seen.

border of the last rib constitutes the lateral lumbocostal arch.

All the branches of the lumbar plexus are behind the iliopsoas fascia and are separated from the peritoneum by a quantity of loose areolar tissue. The branches of the sympathetic trunk pass beneath the tendinous arches of the psoas major. Various nerves of the lumbar plexus also pass through the psoas major and the genital branch of the genitofemoral nerve passes inferiorly within this fascial plane. This explains why increased tension of the psoas fascia might cause muscle weakness or sensory deficits.

The fascia covering the iliacus (fascia iliaca, iliac fascia) is thin above and becomes gradually thicker below as it approaches the inguinal ligament. It is connected laterally to the whole length of the inner lip of the iliac crest and, medially, with the periosteum of the pelvis. The lateral-femoral cutaneous nerve and the femoral nerve course inferiorly in this fascial plane. At the iliopectineal eminence the iliac fascia receives the tendon of insertion of the psoas minor. We suggest that the main role of the psoas minor muscle is to stretch the iliac fascia and to maintain it in a well-defined basal tonus. The psoas minor does not exist in about 40–50% of the human population. When no psoas minor exists, the iliac fascia at the iliopectineal eminence receives some fibres from the psoas major.

Distally, the iliopsoas muscle inserts into the lesser trochanter and its fascia continues with the fascia lata (Fig. 6.29). The iliopsoas muscle is separated from the hip joint by the iliopectineal (or iliopsoas) bursa. This bursa, according to Zilkens et al (2011), communicates with the hip joint in 15% of individuals.

Reference

Abu-Hijleh, M.F., Roshier, A.L., Al-Shboul, Q., Dharap, A.S., Harris, P.F., 2006. The membranous layer of superficial fascia: evidence for its widespread distribution in the body. Surg. Radiol. Anat. 28 (6), 606–619.

Aharinejad, S., Dunn, R.M., Nourani, F., Vernadakis, A.J., Marks, S.C. Jr., 1998. Morphological and clinical aspects of scapular fasciocutaneous free flap transfer for treatment of venous insufficiency in the lower extremity. Clin. Anat. 11 (1), 38–46.

Barker, P.J., Briggs, A., 1999. Attachments of the posterior layer of lumbar fascia. Spine 24 (17), 1757–1764.

Barker, P.J., Briggs, C.A., Bogeski, G., 2004. Tensile transmission across the lumbar fasciae in unembalmed cadavers: effects of tension to various muscular attachments. Spine 29 (2), 129–138.

Barker, P.J., Urquhart, D.M., Story, I.H., Fahrer, M., Briggs, C.A., 2007. The middle layer of lumbar fascia and attachments to lumbar transverse processes: implications for segmental control and fracture. Eur. Spine J. 16 (12), 2232–2237.

Bergstrand, S., Länne, T., Ek, A.C., Lindberg, L.G., Lindén, M., Lindgren, M., 2010. Existence of tissue blood flow in response to external pressure in the sacral region of elderly individuals – using an optical probe prototype. Microcirculation 17 (4), 311–319.

Bermudez, K., Knudson, M., Morabito, D., 1998. Fasciotomy, chronic venous insufficiency and the calf muscle pump. Arch. Surg. 133 (12), 1356–1361.

Bogduk, N., Macintosh, J.E., 1984. The applied anatomy of the thoracolumbar fascia. Spine 9 (2), 164–170.

Cholewicki, J., Juluru, K., Radebold, A., Panjabi, M.M., McGill, S.M., 1999. Lumbar spine stability can be augmented with an abdominal belt and/or increased intra-abdominal pressure. Eur. Spine J. 8 (5), 388–395.

Garfin, S.R., Tipton, C.M., Mubarak, S.J., 1981. Role of fascia in maintenance of muscle tension and pressure. J. Appl. Physiol. 51 (2), 317–320.

Gil, A., Olza, J., Gil-Campos, M., Gomez-Llorente, C., Aguilera, C.M., 2011. Is adipose tissue metabolically different at different sites? Int. J. Pediatr. Obes. 6 (Suppl. 1), 13–20.

Gracovetsky, S., 1988. The Spinal Engine, Springer–Verlag, Wien, New York.

Hammer, W.I., 1998. Genitofemoral entrapment using integrative fascial release. Chiropr. Tech. 10 (4), 169–176.

Hammer, W.I., Pfefer, M.T., 2005. Treatment of a case of subacute lumbar compartment syndrome using the Graston Technique®. J Manipulative Physiol. Ther. 28 (3), 199–204.

Hodges, P., Kaigle Holm, A., Holm, S., Ekström, L., Cresswell, A., Hansson, T., Thorstensson, A., 2003. Intervertebral stiffness of the spine is increased by evoked contraction of transversus abdominis and the diaphragm: in vivo porcine studies. Spine 28 (23), 2594–2601.

Kim, P.S., Gottlieb, J.R., Harris, G.D., Nagle, D.J., Lewis, V.L., 1987. The dorsal thoracic fascia: anatomic significance with clinical applications in reconstructive microsurgery. Plast. Reconstr. Surg. 79 (1), 72–80.

Langer, K., 1862. Zur Anatomie und Physiologie der Haut. II. Uber die Spaltbarkeit der Cutis. Die Spannung der Cutis. Sitzungsberichte der Mathematisch-naturwissenschaftlicher Classe der Kaiserlichen Akademie der Wissenschaften. Wien 45, 133.

Murakami, M., Hikima, R., Arai, S., Yamazaki, K., Iizuka, S., Tochihara, Y., 1999. Short-term longitudinal changes in subcutaneous fat distribution and body size among Japanese women in the third decade of life. Appl. Human Sci. 18 (4), 141–149.

Nassif, T.M., Vidal, L., Bovet, J.L., Baudet, J., 1982. The parascapular flap: a new cutaneous microsurgical free flap. Plast. Reconstr. Surg. 69 (4), 591–600.

Pecina, M.M., Krmpotic-Nemanic, J., Markiewitz, A.D., 1997. Tunnel Syndromes, Peripheral Nerve Compression Syndromes, second ed. CRC Press, New York, pp. 183–185.

Saito, H., Tamura, T., 1992. Subcutaneous fat distribution in Japanese women. Part 1. Fat thickness of the trunk. Ann. Physiol. Anthropol. 11 (5), 495–505.

Schuenke, M.D., Vleeming, A., Van Hoof, T., Willard, F.H., 2012. A description of the lumbar interfascial triangle and its relation with the lateral raphe: anatomical constituents of load transfer through the lateral margin of the thoracolumbar fascia. J. Anat. 221 (6), 568–576.

Sonmez, A., Bayramicli, M., Sonmez, B., Numanoglu, A., 2003. Reconstruction of the weight-bearing surface of the foot with non-neurosensory free flaps. Plast. Reconstr. Surg. 111 (7), 2230–2236.

Sterzi, G., 1910. Il tessuto sottocutaneo (tela subcutanea), Firenze, Niccolai.

Styf, J., 1987. Pressure in the erector spinae muscle during exercise. Spine 12 (7), 675–679.

Tesarz, J., Hoheisel, U., Wiedenhöfer, B., Mense, S., 2011. Sensory innervation of the thoracolumbar fascia in rats and humans. Neuroscience 27 (194), 302–308.

Theobald, P., Byrne, C., Oldfield, S.F., et al., 2007. Lubrication regime of the contact between fat and bone in bovine tissue. Proc. Inst. Mech. Eng. [H] 221 (4), 351–356.

Thorfinn, J., Sjoberg, F., Lidman, D., 2009. Sitting can cause ischaemia in the subcutaneous tissue of the buttocks, which implicates multilayer tissue damage in the development of pressure ulcers. Scand. J. Plast. Reconstr. Surg. Hand Surg. 43 (2), 82–89.

Vleeming, A., Pool-Goudzwaard, A.L., Stoeckart, R., et al., 1995. The posterior layer of the thoracolumbar fascia: its function in load transfer from spine to legs. Spine 20 (7), 753–758.

Willard, F.H., Vleeming, A., Schuenke, M.D., Danneels, L., Schleip, R., 2012. The thoracolumbar fascia: anatomy, function and clinical considerations. J. Anat. 221 (6), 507–536.

Wirhed, R., 1984. Athletic Ability & the Anatomy of Motion, Wolfe Medical Publications Ltd.

Zilkens, C., Miese, F., Jäger, M., Bittersohl, B., Krauspe, R., 2011. Magnetic resonance imaging of hip joint cartilage and labrum. Orthop. Rev. (Pavia) 3 (2), e9.

Bibliography

Barker, P.J., Freeman, A.D., Urquhart, D.M., Anderson, C.R., Briggs, C.A., 2010. The middle layer of lumbar fascia can transmit tensile forces capable of fracturing the lumbar transverse processes: an experimental study. Clin. Biomech. 25 (6), 505–509.

Barker, P.J., Guggenheimer, K.T., Grkovic, I., et al., 2006. Effects of tensioning the lumbar fasciae on segmental stiffness during flexion and extension: Young Investigator Award winner. Spine 31 (4), 397–405.

Hodges, P.W., Richardson, C.A., 1996. Inefficient muscular stabilization of the lumbar spine associated with low back pain. A motor control evaluation of transversus abdominis. Spine 21 (22), 2640–2650.

Hodges, P.W., Richardson, C.A., 1997. Feedforward contraction of transversus abdominis is not influenced by the direction of arm movement. Exp. Brain Res. 114 (2), 362–370.

Hodges, P.W., Richardson, C.A., 1999. Transversus abdominis and the superficial abdominal muscles are controlled independently in a postural task. Neurosci. Lett. 265 (2), 91–94.

Hoheisel, U., Taguchi, T., Treede, R.D., Mense, S., 2011. Nociceptive inbermudezput from the rat thoracolumbar fascia to lumbar dorsal horn neurones. Eur. J. Pain 15 (8), 810–815.

Styf, J., Lysell, E., 1987. Chronic compartment syndrome in the erector spinae muscle. Spine 12 (7), 680–682.

Testut, J.L., Jacob, O., 1905. Précis d'anatomie topographique avec applications medico-chirurgicales, vol. III. Gaston Doin et Cie, Paris, p. 302.

Yahia, H., Rhalmi, S., Newman, N., 1992. Sensory innervation of human thoracolumbar fascia, an immunohistochemical study. Acta Orthop. Scand. 63 (2), 195–197.

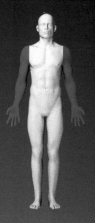

7

Fasciae of the Upper Limb

Superficial Fascia

In the upper limb the superficial fascia is very thin (Figs 7.1 and 7.2) and difficult to isolate from the subcutaneous adipose tissue. It is thicker in the arm and proximal portion of the forearm, while distally it becomes very thin. However, careful dissection reveals that superficial fascia is present in the entire upper limb. The superficial fascia is also thicker on the posterior aspect of the arm compared to the anterior side. It is easier to recognize the lines of force in the deep fascia compared to the superficial fascia, due to the elasticity and adaptability of the superficial fascia.

The superficial fascia of the thorax, upper back and upper limb conjoin in the axilla. The superficial fascia of the pectoral region passes distally over the inferior border of the pectoralis major muscle and continues into the superficial fascia that covers the latissimus dorsi muscle. It continues proximally with the superficial fascia covering the deltoid muscle. It is noteworthy that the superficial fascia of the axilla is a key element that connects the superficial fasciae of the upper limb and trunk. The superficial axillary fascia is not a continuous layer, but presents numerous holes filled with plugs of fibrous tissue and fat (Fig. 7.3). These holes permit the passage of nerves and vessels, contributing to the communication between the deep muscular planes and the subcutaneous tissue. In the axilla the DAT is well represented, particularly in obese people. Many lymph glands are present in the DAT of the axilla.

In the upper limb subcutaneous tissue is scarce, except in the posterior region of the arm where the SAT is usually well represented (Figs 7.4 and 7.5). In thin subjects, the DAT is composed essentially of loose connective tissue with a few scattered adipose cells and thin retinacula cutis profunda. As the DAT is a gliding layer over the deep fascia, it is easy to remove the

Text continued on p. 223

CLINICAL PEARL 7.1 VARIATIONS IN THE SUBCUTANEOUS TISSUE OF THE ARM WITH AGEING

In youth, the posteromedial arm subcutaneous tissue is firmly enmeshed in a tough yet elastic fascial system. With ageing and weight fluctuations, the superficial fascia of the posteromedial arm loses its connections with the axillary fascia, and the retinacula cutis of the superficial adipose tissue (SAT) and the deep adipose tissue (DAT) become less elastic. In addition, there is a relaxation of the superficial fascia itself. This results in significant ptosis of the posteromedial arm. The brachioplasty procedure, according to Lockwood (1995), provides secure anchoring of the superficial fascia to the axillary fascia. Brachioplasty is in less demand than most other body contouring proceudres because of its potential for poor outcomes, including hypertrophic scars, neuropathy and distal lymphoedema. It is possible that many of these problems could be related to superficial fascia damage during this type of surgery.

CLINICAL PEARL 7.2 AXILLARY WEB SYNDROME AFTER BREAST CANCER SURGERY

Arm morbidity after axillary node dissection for primary breast cancer is well described in the literature. Impairment such as upper limb oedema, pain, decreased shoulder mobility, sensory and motor dysfunction can occur. Often present are 'palpable cords' of tissue in the axilla that are made taut and painful by shoulder abduction. Patients often present with lymphoedema and axillary pain that radiates down the arm. In these patients, surgery may alter both the superficial and deep fasciae, damaging the axillary lymphatic flow. In healthy people, loose areolar connective tissue binds the numerous axillary structures together, allowing ample movement by virtue of its extensibility and elasticity. Fat further protects the vital neurovascular structures in this space. Surgical removal or sampling of lymph nodes involves careful dissection of varying numbers of axillary nodes, together with their supporting fat and areolar connective tissue. If this protective axillary connective tissue is damaged, resultant adhesions or scarring can contribute to limited arm/shoulder movement. Newly formed adhesions around lymphatic vessels could cause lymphoedema. Fourie and Robb (2009) proposed a combination of soft tissue mobilizing techniques to modify the tissue gliding in the axilla. Therapists using soft tissue methods can often reduce pain by improving both the range of motion and lymphatic drainage.

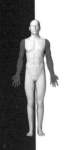

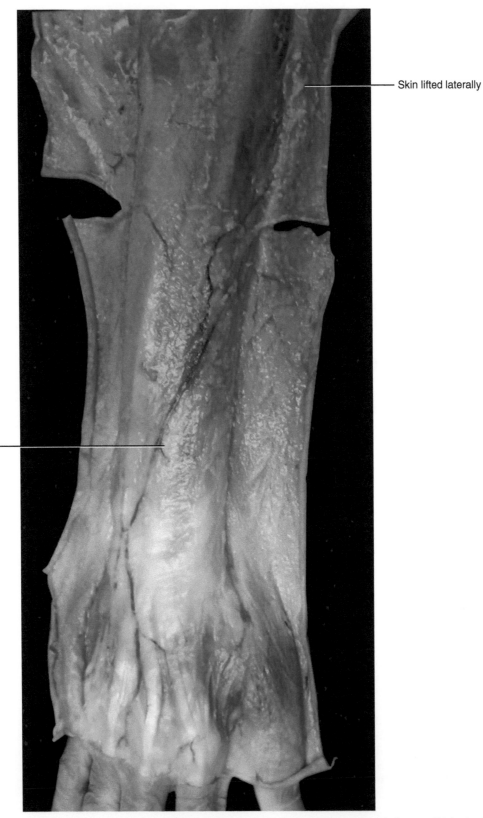

Skin lifted laterally

Superficial veins inside the superficial fascia

FIGURE 7.1 Dorsal region of the forearm. The skin is removed and lifted laterally to show the superficial fascia with the superficial veins (injected with red resin).

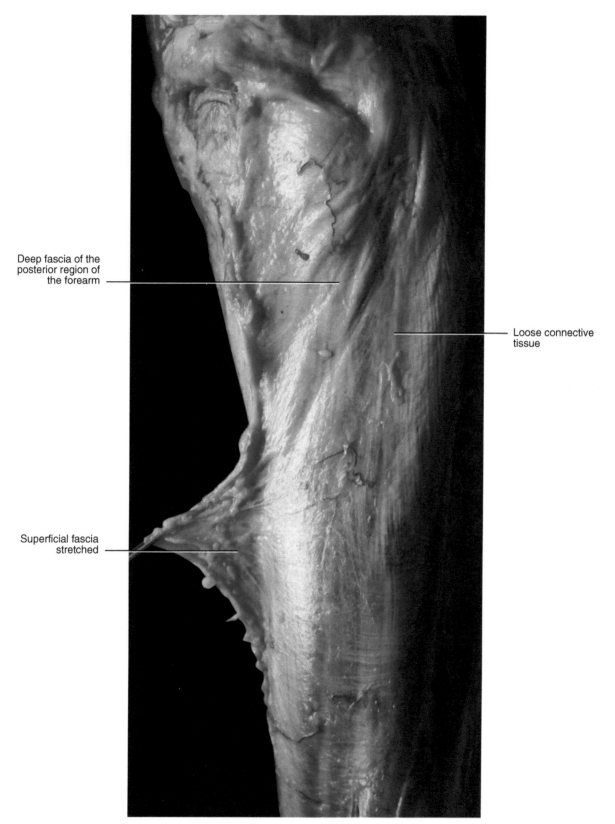

Deep fascia of the
posterior region of
the forearm

Loose connective
tissue

Superficial fascia
stretched

FIGURE 7.2 Dorsal region of the forearm. The superficial fascia is lifted to show the deep aponeurotic fascia. Loose connective tissue is present between the two fascial layers.

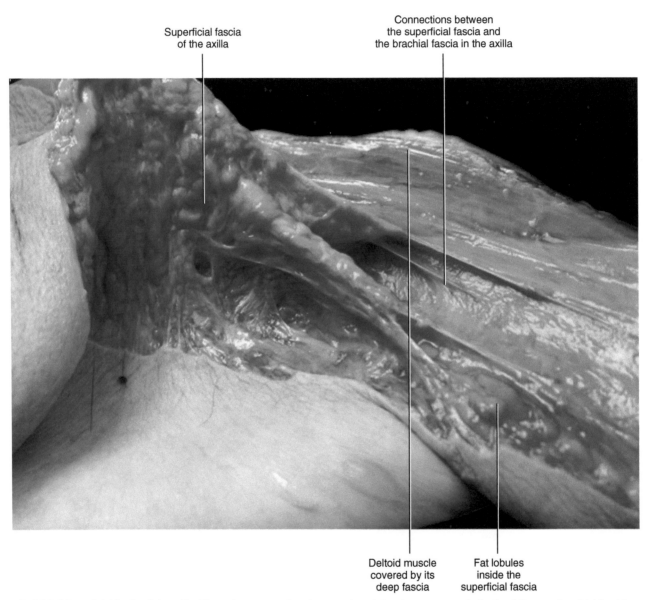

Superficial fascia
of the axilla

Connections between
the superficial fascia and
the brachial fascia in the axilla

Deltoid muscle
covered by its
deep fascia

Fat lobules
inside the
superficial fascia

FIGURE 7.3 Superficial fascia of the axilla. The various connections between it and the deep aponeurotic fascia of the arm (brachial fascia) are evident.

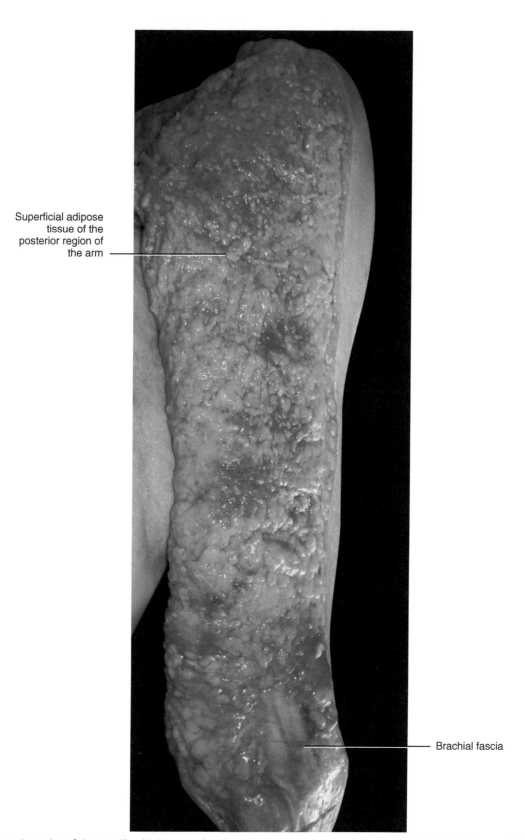

Superficial adipose
tissue of the
posterior region of
the arm

Brachial fascia

FIGURE 7.4 Posterior region of the arm. The skin is removed to show the SAT. The SAT is divided into various lobules by the superficial retinacula cutis. Near the elbow, the superficial fat tissue disappears, and the superficial fascia adheres to the deep fascia.

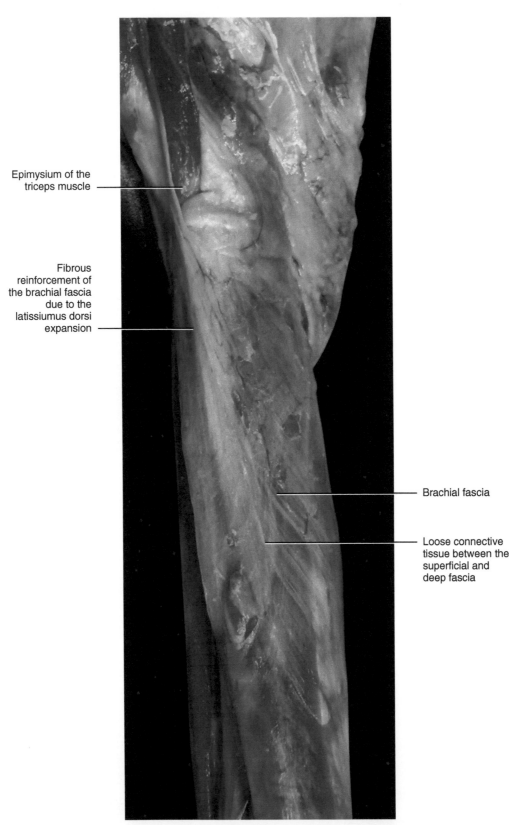

Epimysium of the
triceps muscle

Fibrous
reinforcement of
the brachial fascia
due to the
latissiumus dorsi
expansion

Brachial fascia

Loose connective
tissue between the
superficial and
deep fascia

FIGURE 7.5 Posterior region of the arm. The skin, SAT and superficial fascia are removed to show the deep fascia of the arm. Loose connective tissue with few fat cells is present between the superficial and deep fascia, and permits the gliding between the two fascial layers. Thanks to the loose connective tissue, it is possible to remove the superficial fascia without damaging the deep fascia.

subcutaneous tissue with its superficial fascia without damaging the underlying deep fascia. In the living, this particular aspect of the subcutaneous tissue permits easier movement and lifting of the skin with respect to the muscular planes.

Near the wrist, the DAT becomes more fibrous, causing adhesion of the superficial fascia to the deep fascia. The superficial fascia also adheres to the deep fascia around the elbow. Just over the olecranon, between the superficial and deep fascia is a virtual space called the olecranon bursa. It is a closed compartment created by the fusion of the surrounding superficial and deep fasciae. Also along the inferior margin of the deltoid muscle the DAT disappears, creating an adhesion between superficial and deep fasciae (Fig. 7.6). Thus, the shoulder, arm, forearm and hand subcutaneous compartments are defined.

The superficial fascia can be identified in the dorsum of the hand, although the subcutaneous fat is scarce in this region (Fig. 7.7). Bidic et al (2010) also identified three distinct layers in the dorsum of the hand, using both histology and ultrasound, and showed that all the large dorsal veins and dorsal sensory nerves reside within the intermediate lamina (corresponding to the superficial fascia). The presence of three distinct layers in the dorsum of the hand is important for volumetric hand rejuvenation, with either structural fat grafts or injectable fillers. An injection addressed to the fatty layers that preserves the superficial fascia may improve the results of the various rejuvenation techniques.

In the palm, the DAT is absent and the superficial fascia adheres to the deep fascia to form the palmar aponeurosis (Fig. 7.8). The superficial fascia corresponds to the longitudinal fibrous bundles of

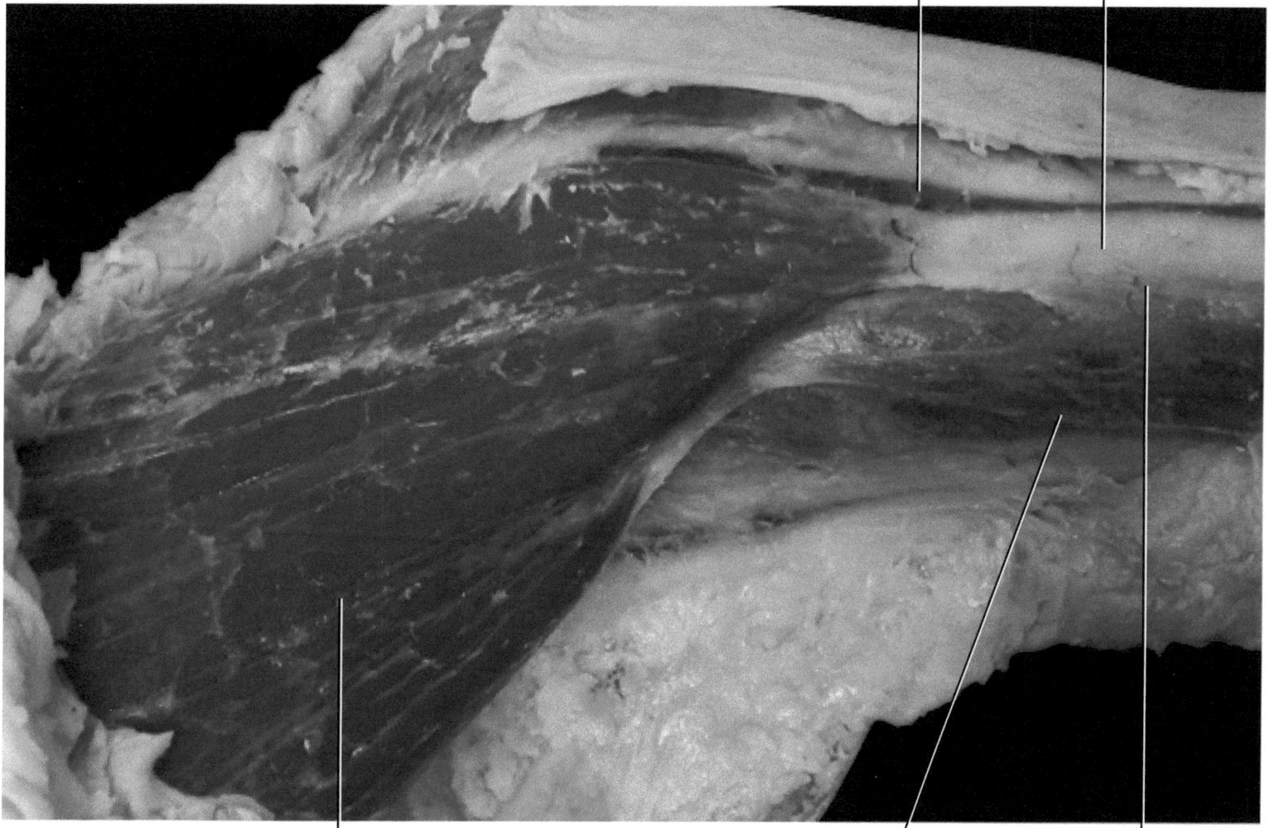

Cephalic vein enveloped by adipose tissue in the deltopectoral groove

Superficial fascia of the forearm

Pectoralis major muscle enveloped by its epimysial fascia

Deep fascia of the arm (brachial fascia)

Adhesion of the superficial fascia to the brachial fascia

FIGURE 7.6 Anterior view of the shoulder. The skin was removed to show the relation of the cephalic vein with the superficial fascia. At the level of the deltopectoral groove it becomes deeper to empty into the axillary vein. Note also the adhesion of the superficial fascia to the brachial fascia along the flow of the cephalic vein.

Extensor tendons under the superficial fascia

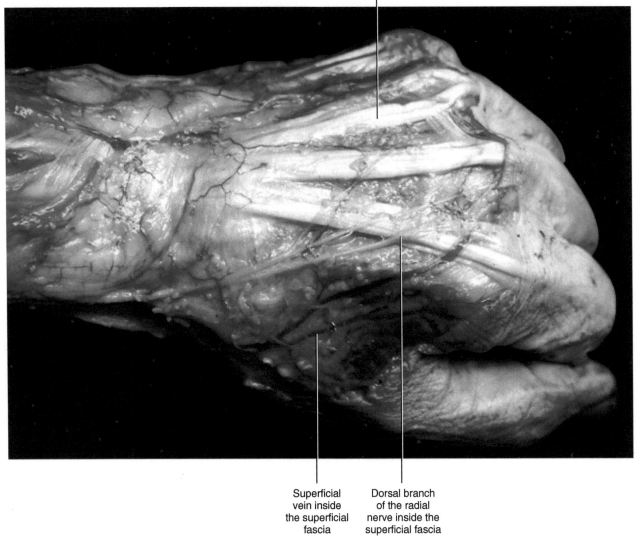

Superficial vein inside the superficial fascia

Dorsal branch of the radial nerve inside the superficial fascia

FIGURE 7.7 Dorsal region of the hand. The skin was removed to show the superficial fascia. Inside the superficial fascia the superficial vessels and nerves are shown.

the palmar aponeurosis, stretched by the palmaris longus muscle. In the palm, the SAT is well represented and has many strong and vertical, fibrous septa which firmly connect the skin with the palmar aponeurosis.

The superficial fascia splits around the subcutaneous veins and nerves forming special compartments (Figs 7.9 and 7.10). According to Abu-Hijleh et al (2006), two sets of veins can be identified in relation to the superficial fascia. One set of 'tributary veins' runs superficial to it and is embedded in SAT, while the 'main veins' run deep to the superficial fascia. Our dissections reveal that the 'main veins' (basilic and cephalic) are enveloped by the superficial fascia, which forms a compartment around each vessel. These compartments resemble the characteristic 'Egyptian eye' sign when viewed by ultrasonography. This relationship of the vessels and superficial fascia is confirmed by Shahnavaz et al (2010). These authors demonstrated

the consistency of the cephalic vein within a double fat plane, suggesting that this double fat plane is a reliable, consistent and helpful guide for the isolation of the cephalic vein in radial forearm free-flap surgery. This consistent relationship between superficial fascia and superficial vessels suggests that the superficial fascia spatially organizes the superficial veins of the upper limbs, so that they can not be displaced during movements or venipucture. The adventitia of the vessels are continuous with the superficial fascial fibrous tissue. Thus, the superficial fascia helps to keep the walls of the veins open.

The superficial fascia also appears to organize superficial nerves such as the medial cutaneous nerve of the arm and of the forearm, the lateral cutaneous nerve of the arm and of the forearm and the posterior cutaneous nerve of the arm and forearm. The distribution of these nerves strongly correlates with the organization of the subcutis.

224

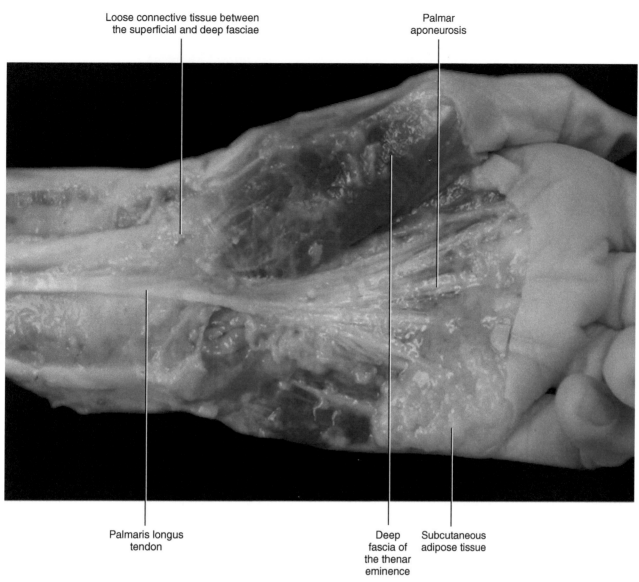

Loose connective tissue between
the superficial and deep fasciae

Palmar
aponeurosis

Palmaris longus
tendon

Deep
fascia of
the thenar
eminence

Subcutaneous
adipose tissue

FIGURE 7.8 Palmar region. In the palm, a true superficial fascia does not exist, but it participates in the formation of the palmar aponeurosis. The tendon of the palmaris muscle crosses the deep fascia in the distal third of the forearm to become subcutaneous and then inserts into the palmar fascia.

CLINICAL PEARL 7.3 COMPRESSION OF CUTANEOUS NERVES CROSSING THE SUPERFICIAL FASCIA

The musculocutaneous nerve can be compressed at different anatomical levels. Proximal compressions are mainly due to coracobrachialis hypertrophy and result in motor and sensory deficits. Distal to the biceps muscle, compression can occur as it emerges laterally to the bicipital tendon at its musculotendinous junction to become the lateral antebrachial cutaneous nerve of the forearm (Davidson et al 1998). This compression can occur below the biceps aponeurosis (lacertus fibrosus). It most often occurs after strenuous elbow extension or forearm pronation. Sometimes it is confused with lateral epicondylopathy. Rarely, the nerve compression can happen more distally, where the lateral antebrachial cutaneous nerve crosses the superficial fascia of the forearm (Belzile & Cloutier 2001). The former entrapment syndrome gives a combined motor and sensory deficit; the latter gives a purely sensory deficit on the radial aspect of the distal volar forearm. It is evident that both the deep and superficial fasciae could be altered and cause entrapment syndromes. Compression due to the superficial fascia causes only sensory deficit, painful dysaesthesia or hyperaesthesia in a well-defined cutaneous territory. Weaknesses and movement limitations are absent, reflexes are normal and the pain is not increased by movement. Often there are skin alterations (trophic changes) and reflex sympathetic dystrophy due to compression of a large amount of autonomic fibres in the area of the cutaneous nerves within the superficial fascia.

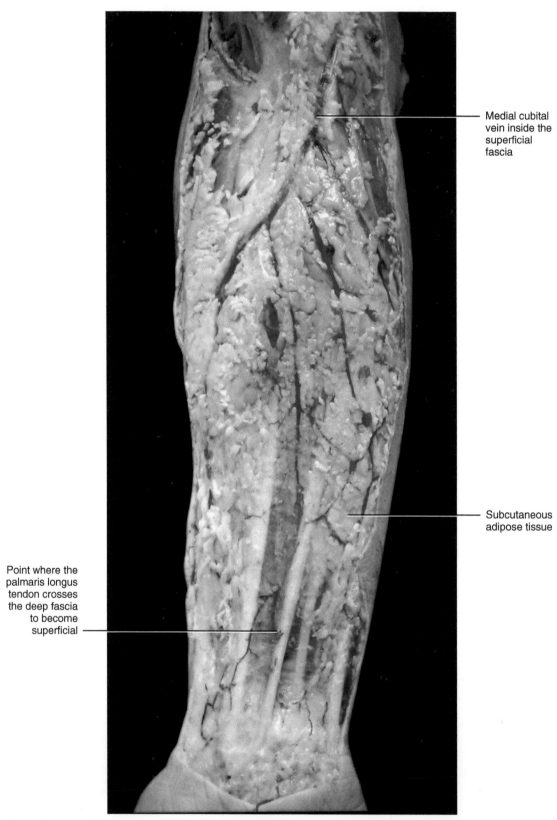

Medial cubital vein inside the superficial fascia

Subcutaneous adipose tissue

Point where the palmaris longus tendon crosses the deep fascia to become superficial

FIGURE 7.9 Anterior region of the forearm. The skin was removed to show the superficial fascia with the superficial veins inside (injected with red resin). In this subject, the subcutaneous adipose tissue is more evident and is located primarily in the SAT.

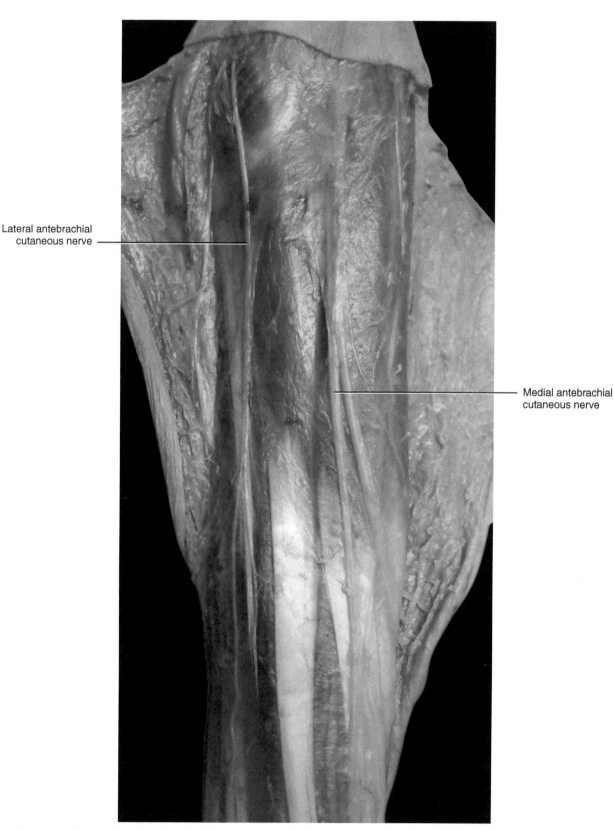

Lateral antebrachial
cutaneous nerve

Medial antebrachial
cutaneous nerve

FIGURE 7.10 Anterior view of the forearm. The skin was removed with the scarce SAT to show the superficial fascia. Inside the superficial fascia, the medial and lateral antebrachial cutaneous nerves are evident.

Deep Fasciae

Deep Fasciae of the Shoulder

Some deep fasciae of the shoulder are aponeurotic fasciae, others are epimysial (see Chapter 3). For example, the fasciae of the pectoralis major, deltoid, trapezius and latissimus dorsi muscles are epymisial fasciae; the supraspinatus and infraspinatus fasciae and all the fasciae of the upper limbs are aponeurotic fasciae.

In the scapular girdle, two well-defined musculofascial planes are described (Fig. 7.11):

- The superficial plane is formed by the trapezius, latissimus dorsi, teres major, deltoid, pectoralis major muscles and the epimysial fascia connecting them. This fascia continues in the neck with the superficial layer of the deep fasciae of the neck that envelops the sternocleidomastoid and trapezius muscles. This fascial layer is formed by epimysial fasciae strongly connected with the underlying muscles, and appears as a clear fascial layer only when it is a bridge between muscles, as in the axillary region where it forms the axillary fascia.

- The deep plane is formed by the supraspinatus and infraspinatus muscles and the fasciae that envelop them. It continues in the neck with the fasciae of the levator scapulae and omohyoideus and medially with the fascia of the rhomboids muscles. Anteriorly, it continues with the clavipectoral fascia, the conjoined tendon of the short head of the biceps and coracobrachialis and the coracoacromial ligament. Laterally, it continues in the trunk with the serratus anterior fascia. All these fasciae are aponeurotic fasciae, but with different thicknesses.

Between these two planes of deep fasciae, the sub-deltoid bursa, that encompasses the anterior, lateral, superior, and variably the posterior aspects of the glenohumeral joint, is present.

All the muscles of the superficial layer have specific myofascial expansions into the brachial fascia, tensioning it in a proximal direction. Where the brachial fascia receives these expansions, longitudinal fibrous bundles are evident, even macroscopically. In particular, the clavicular part of pectoralis major has a myofascial expansion extending in the direction of the anterior brachial fascia, while the costal part of pectoralis major continues with the axillary fascia and then with the medial portion of the brachial fascia (Figs 7.12 and 7.13). Stimulation to contract the pectoralis major, by application of a manual traction, produces lines of force in the following directions:

- If the clavicular part is tensioned, the lines of force spread along the anterior part of the brachial fascia.

- If the costal part of pectoralis major is tensioned, the lines of force propagate towards the axilla and the medial intermuscular septum of the brachial fascia.

The latissimus dorsi muscle sends a fibrous lamina to the triceps brachial fascia, creating a thickening in the posterior portion of the axillary fascia, and, subsequently, to the brachial fascia (Figs 7.14–7.16). This thickening is fan shaped, with the apex directed towards the axilla and the base towards the posteromedial side of the brachial fascia. A fibrous arch extends from the triceps fascia to the tendon of latissimus dorsi (Fig. 7.17), further reinforcing the connection between these two fasciae. By pulling the latissimus dorsi, to simulate its contraction, the lines of force originating in the posterior region of the axilla are clearly seen and continue into the brachial fascia in the following manner:

- Some lines of force are directed posteriorly in the arm towards the centre of the elbow.

- Some lines of force are directed towards the medial intermuscular septum.

The deltoid muscle inserts some muscular fibres into the lateral intermuscular septum and into the associated brachial fascia. Contraction of the deltoid stretches the lateral portion of the brachial fascia.

FIGURE 7.11 Musculofascial planes of the scapular girdle.

Text continued on p. 234

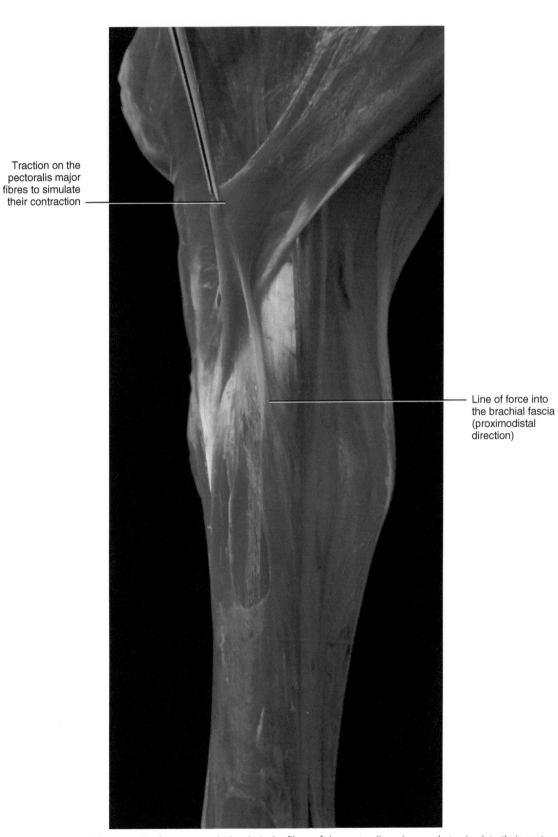

Traction on the
pectoralis major
fibres to simulate
their contraction

Line of force into
the brachial fascia
(proximodistal
direction)

FIGURE 7.12 Anterior view of the arm. The forceps stretch the clavicular fibres of the pectoralis major muscle to simulate their contraction. The lines of force produced along the anterior portion of the brachial fascia are evident.

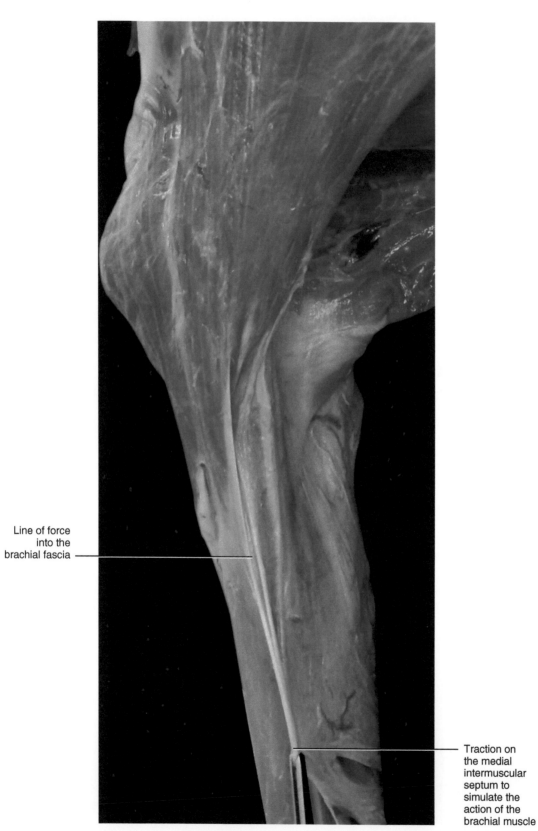

Line of force into the brachial fascia

Traction on the medial intermuscular septum to simulate the action of the brachial muscle

FIGURE 7.13 Anteromedial view of the arm. The forceps stretch the medial intermuscular septum and the brachial fascia in a distal direction to simulate the action of the brachial muscle. In this way, the line of force towards the pectoralis major muscle also appears.

Deltoid fascia

Brachial fascia

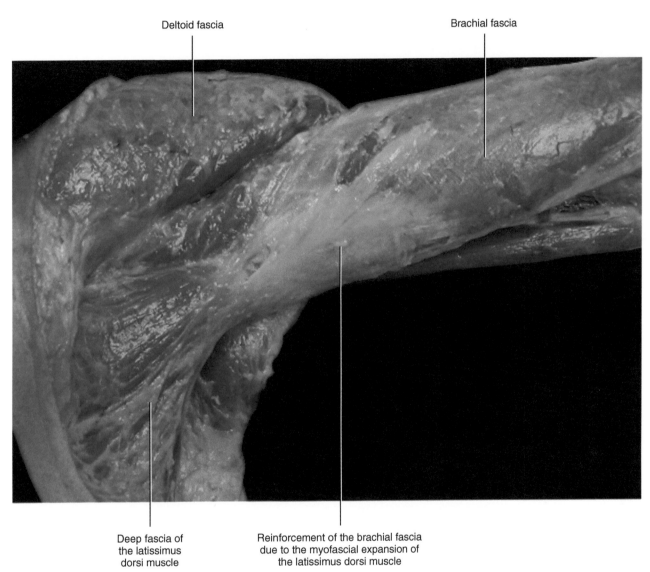

Deep fascia of
the latissimus
dorsi muscle

Reinforcement of the brachial fascia
due to the myofascial expansion of
the latissimus dorsi muscle

FIGURE 7.14 Posterior view of the shoulder region. The reinforcement of the brachial fascia due to the myofascial expansion of the latissimus dorsi muscle is evident.

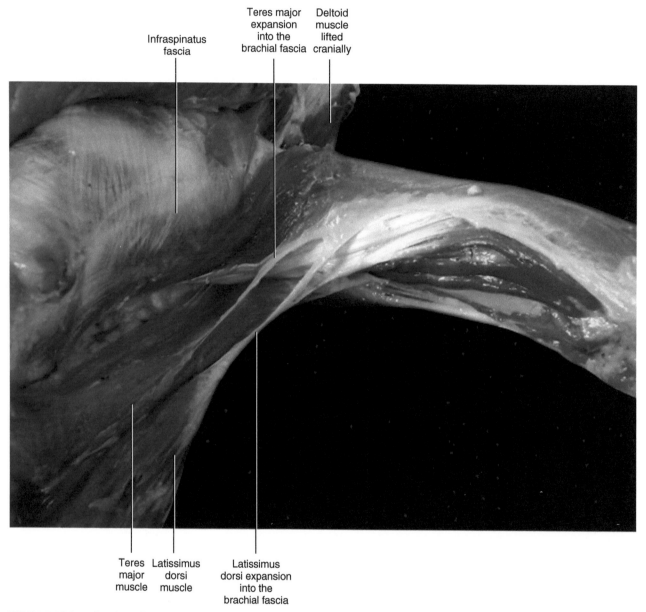

Infraspinatus fascia

Teres major expansion into the brachial fascia

Deltoid muscle lifted cranially

Teres major muscle

Latissimus dorsi muscle

Latissimus dorsi expansion into the brachial fascia

FIGURE 7.15 Posterior view of the shoulder region. The deltoid muscle is detached from its humeral insertion and lifted cranially to show the infraspinatus fascia. Note the aponeurotic aspect of this fascia. The myofascial expansions of the latissimus dorsi and teres major muscles into the posterior portion of the brachial fascia are also evident.

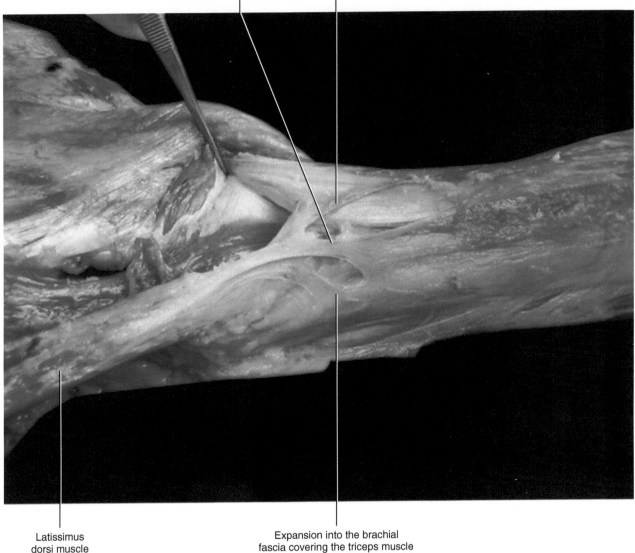

Expansion into
the medial
intermuscular
septum

Oblique expansion
into the anterior
portion of the
brachial fascia

Latissimus
dorsi muscle

Expansion into the brachial
fascia covering the triceps muscle

FIGURE 7.16 Medial view of the arm. The subcutaneous tissue is removed to show the myofascial expansions of the latissimus dorsi into the brachial fascia. There are three primary expansions: one stretches the triceps fascia, one stretches the medial intermuscular septum and one has an oblique direction (anteromedial). The latissimus dorsi requires three myofascial expansions to partcipate in different movements: extension (expansion into the fascia of the triceps), adduction (expansion into the medial intermuscular septum) and intrarotation (oblique expansion).

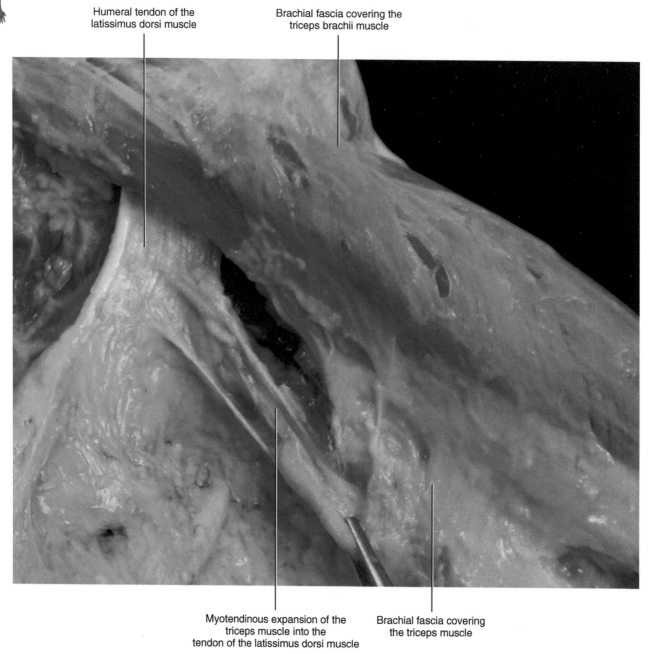

Humeral tendon of the
latissimus dorsi muscle

Brachial fascia covering the
triceps brachii muscle

Myotendinous expansion of the
triceps muscle into the
tendon of the latissimus dorsi muscle

Brachial fascia covering
the triceps muscle

FIGURE 7.17 Posterior view of the proximal portion of the arm. The insertions of the triceps muscle into the latissimus dorsi tendon are evident.

DELTOID FASCIA

The deltoid fascia varies in thickness from subject to subject without any apparent correlation to the size of its underlying muscle mass. It adheres strongly to the muscle and connects the different parts of the deltoid (Figs 7.18 and 7.19). According to Rispoli et al (2009), there are three distinct sections of the deltoid muscle: anterior, lateral and posterior, and each portion continues on with the brachial fascia. The deltoid fascia continues proximally with the fascia covering the trapezius muscle. Over the acromion, scapular spine and clavicle, the deltoid fascia partially adheres to each periosteum.

On histological examination, the deltoid fascia appears to be formed by undulating collagen fibres arranged, more or less, transversely with respect to the underlying muscle. An elevated number of elastic fibres are evident (approximately 15% of all the fibres), forming an irregular mesh. Rare free nerve endings, arranged in a homogenous manner throughout the entire fascia, are also present.

AXILLARY FASCIA

The axillary fascia is a strong fibrous tissue with a quadrilateral shape. It continues laterally with the brachial fascia, medially with the serratus anterior fascia,

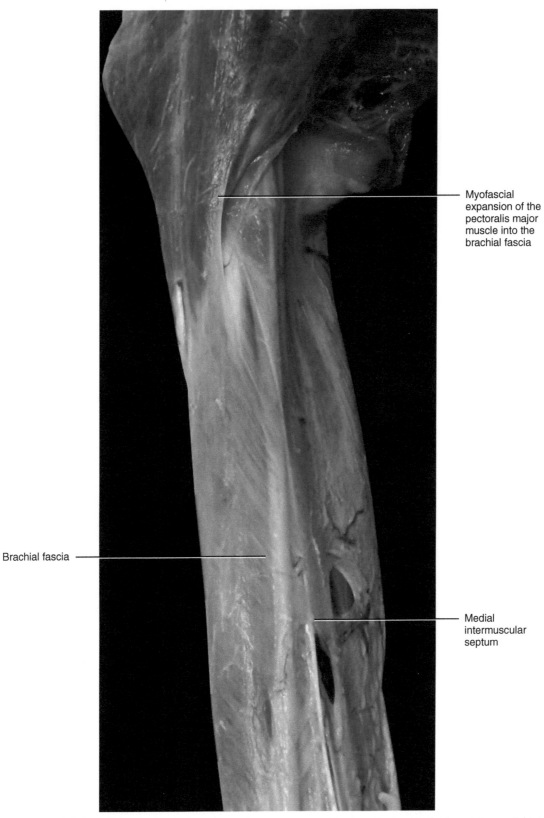

Myofascial expansion of the pectoralis major muscle into the brachial fascia

Brachial fascia

Medial intermuscular septum

FIGURE 7.18 Anteromedial view of the arm. The subcutaneous tissues are removed to show the brachial fascia and the medial intermuscular septum.

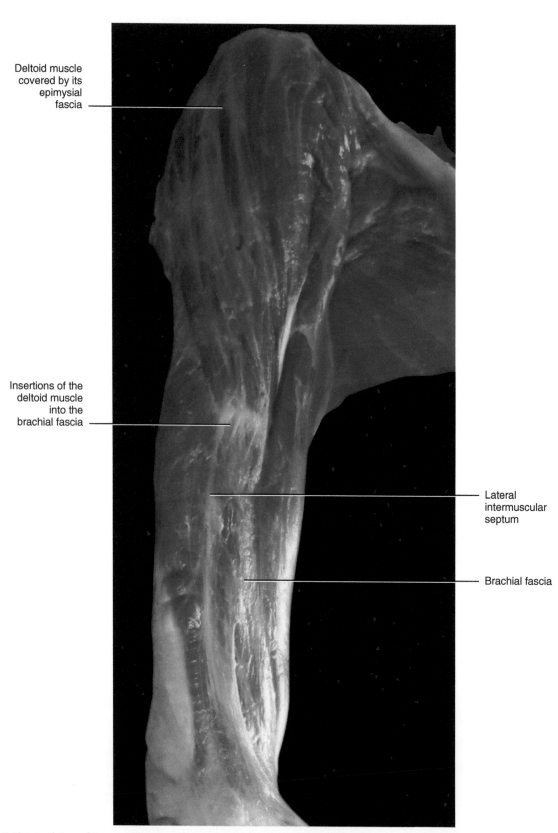

Deltoid muscle covered by its epimysial fascia

Insertions of the deltoid muscle into the brachial fascia

Lateral intermuscular septum

Brachial fascia

FIGURE 7.19 Lateral view of the arm. The subcutaneous tissues are removed to show the brachial fascia and the lateral intermuscular septum.

anteriorly with the pectoralis major fascia and posteriorly with the fascia of latissimus dorsi muscle (Figs 7.20–7.22).

The inner side of this fascia is connected to the suspensory ligament of Gerdy, which, in turn, continues with the clavipectoral fascia and the subscapularis fascia. Thus, in the axilla we have a connection between these two layers of the deep fasciae of the scapular girdle. Many lines of force are recognizable in the axillary fascia due to the actions of the various muscles inserting into this fascia.

SUBSCAPULAR FASCIA (FASCIA SUBSCAPULARIS)

The subscapular fascia is a thin aponeurotic fascia attached to the entire circumference of the subscapular fossa (Fig. 7.23). Some fibres of the subscapularis muscle originate from its deep surface. Singer (1935) describes the subscapular fascia as being the thinnest of the various fasciae surrounding the muscles of the scapula; however, it is a well-defined lamina. Medially, it is continuous with the rhomboid fascia and, laterally, with the glenohumeral joint.

The subscapular fascia is an important element of the scapulothoracic joint. It provides a perfect plane of gliding between the subscapularis and the serratus anterior muscles. In addition, the subscapular fascia strongly connects the subscapularis bursa with the subscapularis muscle, allowing the bursa to follow the course of the muscle exactly. The subscapularis bursa is like a fascial pouch firmly attached to the scapular neck and the adjacent part of the joint capsule. The top of the bursa is also linked to the coracoid process by a fibrous attachment called the suspensory ligament. During movement of the glenohumeral joint, the subscapularis muscle sustains huge changes of orientation, particularly in the upper part of the muscle that

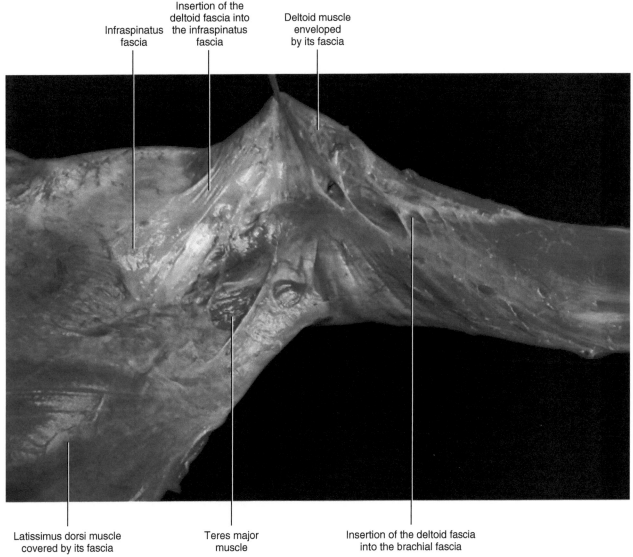

Infraspinatus fascia

Insertion of the deltoid fascia into the infraspinatus fascia

Deltoid muscle enveloped by its fascia

Latissimus dorsi muscle covered by its fascia

Teres major muscle

Insertion of the deltoid fascia into the brachial fascia

FIGURE 7.20 Posterior view of the shoulder region. The deltoid fascia was lifted with forceps and stretched to show its insertion into the infraspinatus fascia and into the brachial fascia. It is evident that the deltoid muscle is in a more superficial plane with respect to the brachial and infraspinatus fasciae.

CLINICAL PEARL 7.4 QUADRILATERAL SPACE SYNDROME

A fracture/dislocation of the humerus could cause adhesions and fibrous bands in the quadrilateral space (bounded superiorly by the teres minor, inferiorly by the teres major, laterally by the surgical humeral neck and medially by the long head of the triceps). This space contains the posterior humeral circumflex artery and the axillary nerve (which supplies the deltoid and teres minor muscles and skin of the posterolateral area of the shoulder and upper arm). The consequences are atypical pain and paraesthesia (which is more common in the lateral aspect of the upper arm). Deltoid atrophy and weakness on resistive deltoid testing are usually present. Symptoms can refer nondermatomally (fascial referral) to the forearm and hand. Muscles and fascia are tender with pinpoint tenderness in the quadrilateral space. There are increased symptoms on active shoulder abduction, lateral rotation and extension at the anterior of the shoulder. The deltoid is affected much more often than the teres minor. These symptoms could also be due to an overuse syndrome, typical of overhead throwers, that causes a densification of the axillary fasciae. Treatment is usually conservative and operative management is reserved for selected patients (Lester 1999). Physical therapy and soft tissue mobilization methods should be attempted, and failure to restore improvement within six months may indicate the need for surgical decompression (Pecina 1997).

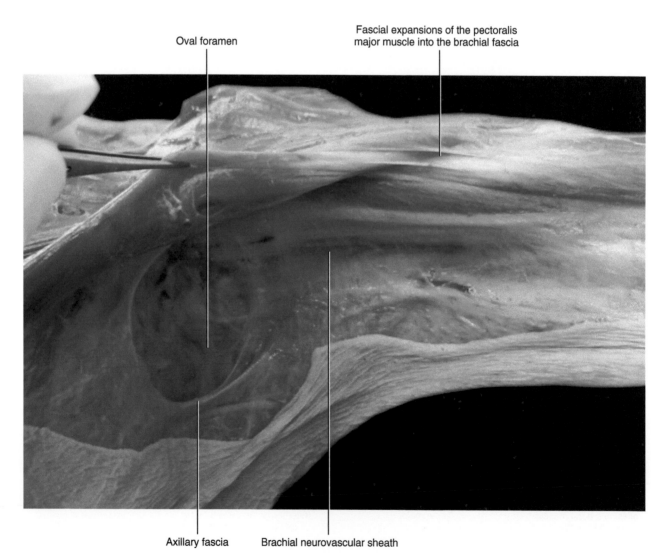

Oval foramen

Fascial expansions of the pectoralis major muscle into the brachial fascia

Axillary fascia   Brachial neurovascular sheath

FIGURE 7.21 Axilla. The superficial fascia and all the subcutaneous fat tissues are removed to show the axillary fascia and its continuation with the brachial fascia and the fascia of pectoralis major muscle (lifted by forceps). The oval foramen of the axilla is clearly evident.

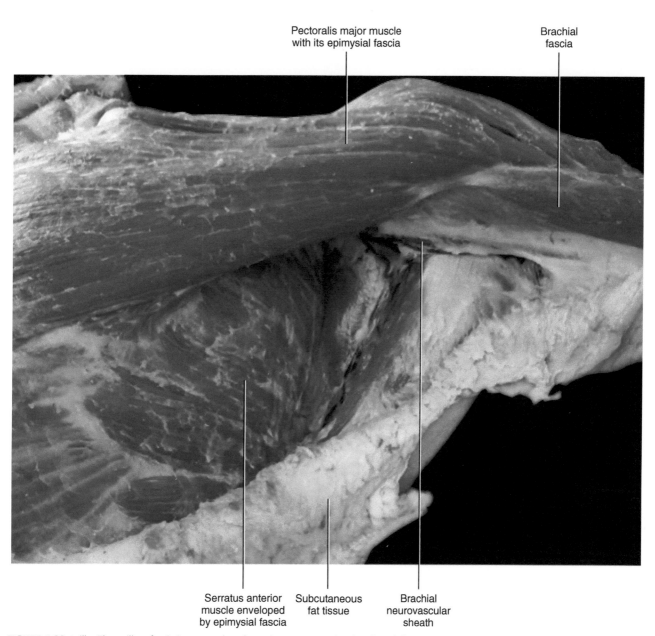

Pectoralis major muscle
with its epimysial fascia

Brachial
fascia

Serratus anterior
muscle enveloped
by epimysial fascia

Subcutaneous
fat tissue

Brachial
neurovascular
sheath

FIGURE 7.22 Axilla. The axillary fascia is removed to show the neurovascular sheath and the serratus anterior muscle. In this cadaver the muscles are well developed. Note that the muscular fasciae are thinner and less evident than in older and hypotrophic subjects.

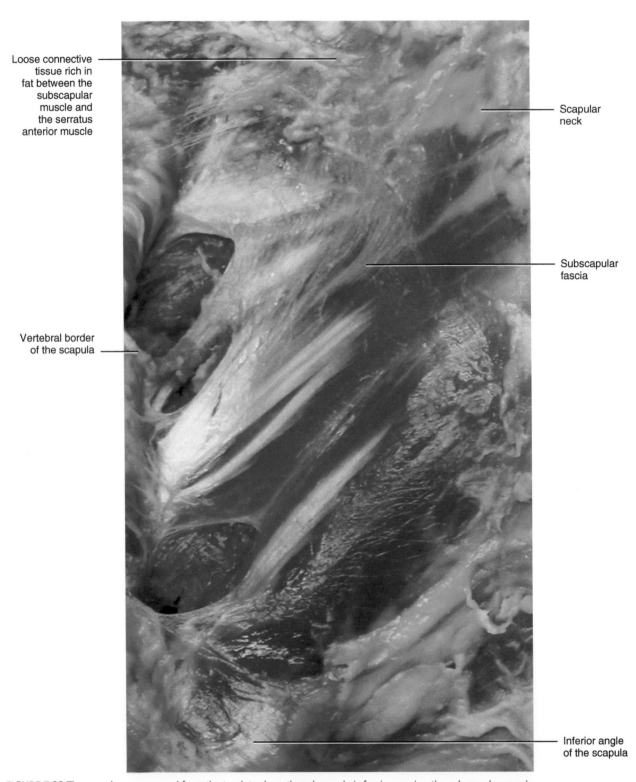

Loose connective tissue rich in fat between the subscapular muscle and the serratus anterior muscle

Scapular neck

Subscapular fascia

Vertebral border of the scapula

Inferior angle of the scapula

FIGURE 7.23 The scapula was removed from the trunk to show the subscapularis fascia covering the subscapular muscle.

coils around the coracoid process. It is the function of the subscapular fascia, subscapularis and subcoracoid bursae to mitigate the friction of the superficial fibres of the subscapularis muscle against the scapular neck, humeral head, and coracoid process.

INFRASPINATUS FASCIA

The infraspinatus fascia is a dense fibrous membrane (aponeurotic fascia), covering the infraspinatus and teres minor muscles and fixed to the circumference of the infraspinatus fossa. Some fibres of these muscles are attached to the deep surface of this fascia. The deltoid, trapezius and latissimus dorsi muscles cover part of the infraspinatus fascia, but between these muscles and the infraspinatus fascia there is loose connective tissue that permits the autonomous gliding of these two myofascial planes. Only in some very specific areas do these muscles adhere to the infraspinatus fascia, creating well-defined lines of forces (Figs 7.24 and 7.25).

Chafik et al (2012) described two distinct and equally common variants in the fascia surrounding the teres minor muscle. One of these is a stout, inflexible fascial compartment enveloping only the teres minor muscle. The other is a continuous fascia enveloping both the infraspinatus and teres minor muscles. In both variants, the primary nerve to the teres minor extends along a fascial sling, becoming subfascial at an average of 44 mm (range 25–68) medially to the teres minor's insertion. These differences suggest that a stout fascial sling may be the potential site of greatest compression and tethering of the primary motor nerve to teres minor. This may explain the symptomatic isolated teres minor muscle atrophy. This syndrome is considered rare, but Friend et al (2010) found it in 3% of patients with shoulder complaints.

SUPRASPINATUS FASCIA

The supraspinatus fascia is a strong fibrous layer that completes the osteofibrous case in which the supraspinatus muscle is contained. It affords attachment by its deep surface to some of the fibres of this muscle. It continues in the neck with the fascia of the levator scapulae muscle, anteriorly with the clavipectoral fascia and medially with the rhomboid fascia. Over the scapular spine it partially adheres and partially joins the infraspinatus fascia (Fig. 7.26).

The supraspinatus fascia varies in thickness (mean thickness 0.7 mm), and occasionally contains some adipose tissue (Singer 1935). For Duparc et al (2010) this fascia is thickened at the level of the spinoglenoid notch which could cause an entrapment of the suprascapular nerve. According to Bektas et al (2003), the spinoglenoid ligament, usually implicated in the compression of the suprascapular nerve, is seen in only 15.6% of cases, while a thickening of the distal third of the supraspinatus fascia is always present.

Deep Fascia of the Arm: Brachial Fascia

In the upper limb, the deep fascia is an aponeurotic fascia that forms a fibrous cuff all around the muscles. It is a strong, almost white laminar sheet of connective tissue that covers the muscles. Collagen fibre bundles arranged in different directions are easily identifiable within this fascia (Stecco et al 2008). Commonly, it is divided into brachial and antebrachial fasciae. The brachial fascia envelops the muscles of the arm, while the antebrachial fascia envelops those of the forearm. The brachial and antebrachial fasciae form a unique sheath that might be compared to an evening glove, proximally tensioned by the various myofascial insertions of the pectoral girdle muscles. This glove is partially free to glide over the underlying muscular plane, but at some points it attaches to bones or inserts into muscular fibres (Figs 7.27 and 7.28). Contraction of these muscular fibres stretches the deep fasciae in specific directions. Where these tensions are stronger or more frequent, the deep fascia becomes thicker. So, specific fibrous reinforcements could be visualized inside the deep fascia. This represents macroscopic evidence of the mechanical action of the muscular insertions.

The brachial fascia has a mean thickness of 863 μm (SD±77 μm), being thinner in the anterior region than the posterior region. It may be easily separated from the underlying muscles (Fig. 7.29), except at the elbow,

Text continued on p. 248

CLINICAL PEARL 7.5 POSSIBLE ROLE OF THE SUBSCAPULARIS MUSCLE IN TENDINOPHATHY OF THE LONG HEAD OF THE BICEPS TENDON

Gleason et al (2006) have demonstrated that there is no separate, identifiable transverse humeral ligament, but rather the fibres covering the intertubercular groove are composed of fibres from the subscapularis and supraspinatus tendons. Magnetic resonance imaging and gross dissection revealed the continuation of superficial fibres of the subscapularis tendon from the tendon body across the intertubercular groove to attach to the greater tuberosity, whereas deeper fibres of the subscapularis tendon inserted on the lesser tuberosity. Longitudinal fibres of the supraspinatus tendon and the coracohumeral ligament were also noted to travel the length of the groove, deep to the other interdigitating fibres but superficial to the biceps tendon. Histological studies confirmed these gross dissection patterns of fibre attachment and also revealed the absence of elastin fibres, which are more commonly seen in ligamentous structures and are typically absent from tendinous structures.

These findings suggest that if the subscapularis muscle is too rigid the 'transverse humeral ligament' could be excessively stretched, with consequent compression of the bicipital groove. This could cause an alteration in the sliding of the tendon of the long head of the biceps. This explains why pain referred to the anterior region of the shoulder may originate from the subscapular region.

CLINICAL PEARL 7.6 DERMATOME OR FASCIATOME?

The superficial fascia is innervated by the cutaneous nerves and the deep fascia by the motor nerves. This means that innervation of the superficial fascia follows the dermatomes and for the deep fascia it follows the peripheral motor nerves.

Symptoms that follow a dermatome (e.g. pain or a rash) indicate a pathology that probably involves the superficial fascia. However, referred pain is not usually associated with a dermatome and only sometimes follows the distribution of a deep nerve. This type of referred pain is typical of the myofascial pain syndrome. The pain may move from one segment to another (e.g. neck to arm) and can radiate proximally or distally. This phenomenon was codified by acupuncture, with its meridian lines distributed according to precise areas, and never physically demonstrated (Lebarbier 1980). More recently, Langevin and Yandow (2002) hypothesized that acupuncture meridians coincide with inter- and intramuscular connective tissue planes and demonstrated that rotation of the acupuncture needle causes 'whorling' of the subcutaneous tissue, extensive fibroblast spreading and the formation of lamellipodia. Langevin et al (2006) later hypothesized that connective tissue functioned as a body-wide mechanosensitive signalling network and communication system. The French school hypothesized the existence of a functional connection between muscle groups with the same motor action, coining the term 'chaînes musculaires' (Busquet 1995). Well-documented myofascial trigger points (Travell & Simons 1983) also indicate the existence of a connection between the location of pain and its origin, often quite a distance away. Stecco (1996) describes a biomechanical model that explains the specific relationships between deep fasciae and muscles (sequences), postulating that these sequences are directly involved in the organization of movement as well as muscular force transmission. Myers (2001) described myofascial connections crossing the entire body, linking the head to the toes and the centre to the periphery (myofascial trains). All these authors, although based on completely different theories, agree in the spatial organization of these 'connections'. Thanks to dissections, we can affirm that the anatomical basis of these 'connections' could be found in the deep fascia and in the specific organization of the myofascial expansions. The myofascial connections create an anatomical continuity between different muscles involved in the same directional movement, and the lines of forces inside the fascia could explain the exact radiation of pain along, for example, the upper limb (fasciatome).

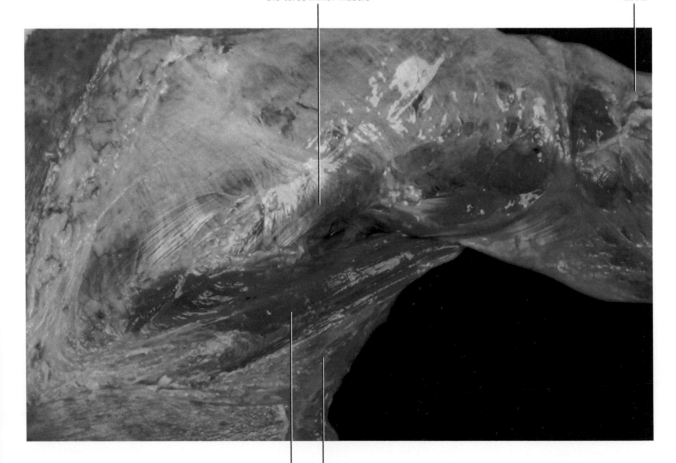

FIGURE 7.24 Posterior view of the shoulder region. The trapezius muscle is removed to show the infraspinatus fascia. This fascia envelops the infraspinatus and teres minor muscles. The teres major muscle has its own separate fascial layer.

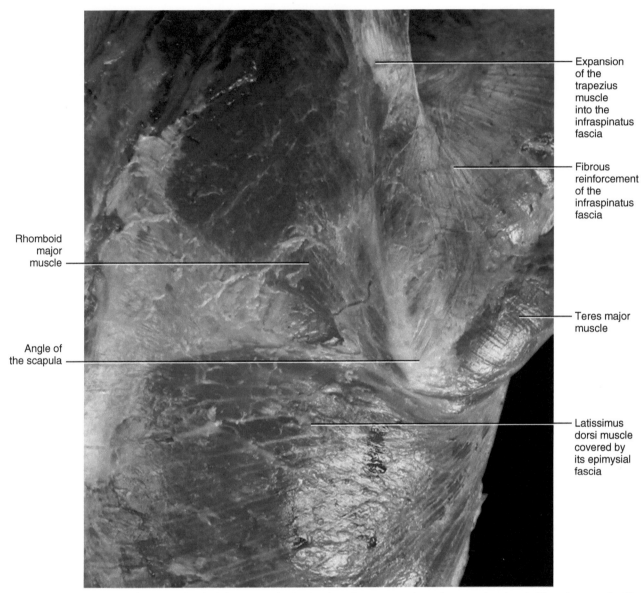

Expansion
of the
trapezius
muscle
into the
infraspinatus
fascia

Fibrous
reinforcement
of the
infraspinatus
fascia

Teres major
muscle

Latissimus
dorsi muscle
covered by
its epimysial
fascia

Rhomboid
major
muscle

Angle of
the scapula

FIGURE 7.25 Posterior view of the scapula. The infraspinatus fascia gives insertions to several muscles: trapezius, rhomboids and teres major. The infraspinatus fascia is, therefore, considered a true aponeurotic fascia whose purpose is to perceive and distribute tensions generated by these muscles acting on the scapula.

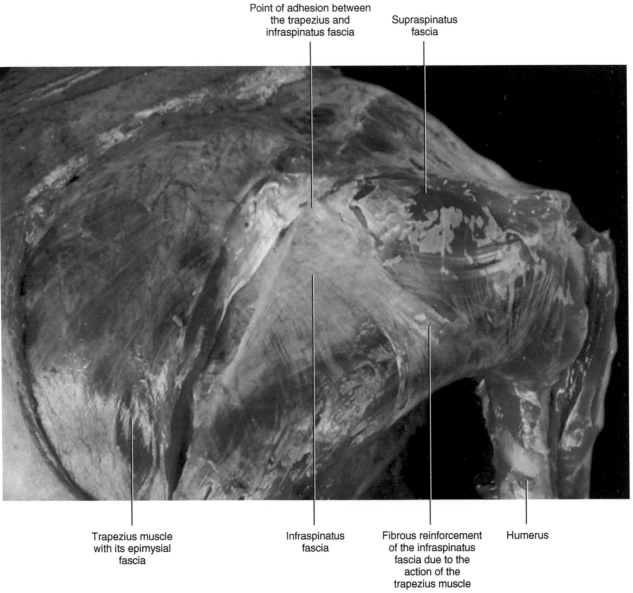

Point of adhesion between
the trapezius and
infraspinatus fascia

Supraspinatus
fascia

Trapezius muscle
with its epimysial
fascia

Infraspinatus
fascia

Fibrous reinforcement
of the infraspinatus
fascia due to the
action of the
trapezius muscle

Humerus

FIGURE 7.26 Posterior view of the shoulder region. Part of the trapezius and deltoid muscles were removed to show the supraspinatus fascia and the adhesion of the trapezius to the infraspinatus fascia. Generally, the trapezius is easily detached from the underlying planes due to the loose connective tissue present between these two structures. Only in the adhesion area does the trapezius and infraspinatus fasciae join. In this way, the traction (stress) of the trapezius muscle on to the infraspinatus fascia causes a fibrous reinforcement of the infraspinatus fascia.

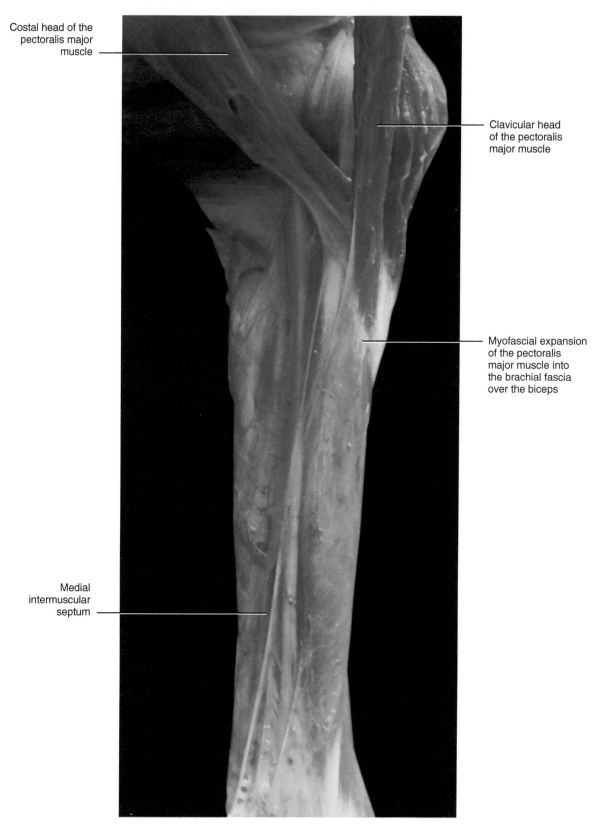

Costal head of the pectoralis major muscle

Clavicular head of the pectoralis major muscle

Myofascial expansion of the pectoralis major muscle into the brachial fascia over the biceps

Medial intermuscular septum

FIGURE 7.27 Anteromedial view of the arm. The clavicular and costal parts of the pectoralis major muscle were isolated from their proximal insertions and stretched to highlight their actions into the anterior portion of the brachial fascia.

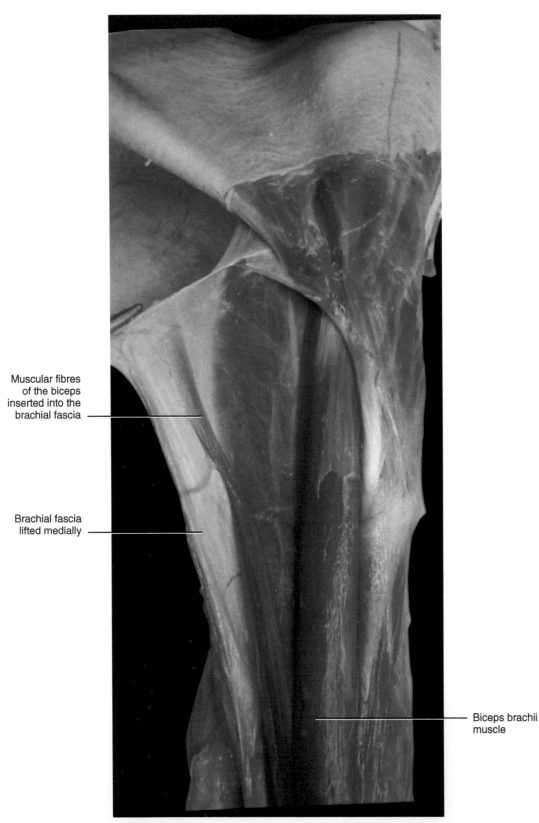

Muscular fibres
of the biceps
inserted into the
brachial fascia

Brachial fascia
lifted medially

Biceps brachii
muscle

FIGURE 7.28 Anterior view of the arm. The brachial fascia is detached from the underlying muscles and lifted medially to show its relation with the biceps brachii muscle. This muscle is generally free to glide under the brachial fascia, thanks to the presence of its epimysium. It also has a myofascial expansion into the brachial fascia. Every time this biceps brachii muscle contracts, it stretches the anteromedial portion of the brachial fascia in a caudal direction.

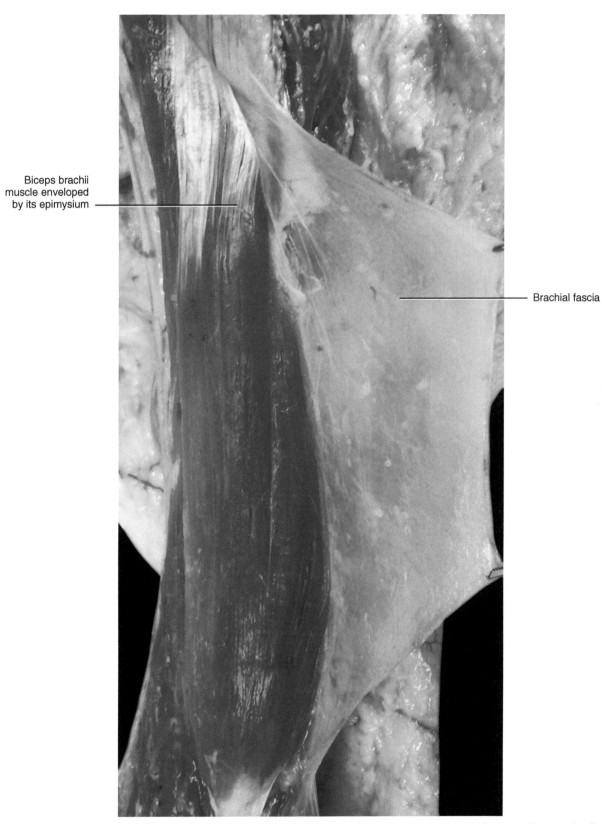

Biceps brachii muscle enveloped by its epimysium

Brachial fascia

FIGURE 7.29 Anterior view of the arm. The brachial fascia is detached from the biceps brachii muscle and lifted laterally. Note the fibrous appearance of the brachial fascia.

where it adheres to the epicondyles. Proximally, it is continuous with the axillary fascia and with the fasciae of the pectoralis major, deltoid and latissimus dorsi muscles. Distally, it is continuous with the antebrachial fascia. The medial and lateral intermuscular septa originate from the brachial fascia, dividing the muscles of the arm into anterior and posterior compartments.

The medial intermuscular septum (Figs 7.30–7.32) is stretched proximally by the coracobrachialis muscle and distally by the epytrochlear muscles (muscles at the medial epicondyle of the humerus), in particular by the pronator teres muscle. Sometimes the pronator teres joins with the distal insertion of the coracobrachialis muscle. The lateral intermuscular septum (Figs 7.33 and 7.34) has a mean thickness of 1.0 mm. This septum is stretched proximally by the deltoid muscle (lateral and posterior portions) and distally by the brachioradialis and extensor carpi radialis longus and brevis muscles which insert into it. Tubbs et al (2009) describe the distal part of this septum as confluent with the annular ligament encircling the head of the radius and with the capsule of the elbow joint. About 10 cm proximal to the elbow, the lateral intermuscular septum is crossed by the radial nerve that passes from the posterior to the anterior compartment of the arm. Both the medial and lateral septa also provide insertions anteriorly to some muscular fibres of the brachialis mucle and posteriorly to some fibres of the triceps muscle.

At the elbow, the brachial fascia is reinforced by the anterior and posterior retinacula (Figs 7.35–7.38). The elbow retinacula have not received much emphasis from researchers, but they are always present. They are fibrous reinforcements of the deep fascia around the elbow, due to the presence of specific myofascial expansions in an oblique direction. In the anterior aspect of the elbow, the main component of the anterior elbow retinaculum is the lacertus fibrosus. The lacertus fibrosus is a fibrous lamina (Figs 7.39 and 7.40) that arises from the distal biceps tendon and blends with the fascia of the forearm. This expansion has two components:

- The main component is formed by a fibrous bundle extending obliquely downwards and medially. These arciform fibres are initially separated but then merge with the forearm fascia. Detaching this fascia from the epitrochlear muscles shows that many muscular fibres and intermuscular septa insert directly into the fascia in this region.

- The second component is formed by collagen fibre bundles arranged longitudinally and running parallel to the median line of the forearm. This component is thinner than the first. This fibrous expansion is initially free to slide over the main biceps tendon and then it extends into the antebrachial fascia between the flexor carpi radialis and the brachioradialis. Numerous fibres of these same muscles originate from this fibrous expansion.

CLINICAL PEARL 7.7 RADIAL NERVE ENTRAPMENT SYNDROME

Radial nerve compression may occur at any point along the anatomical course of the nerve and may have varied aetiologies. The most frequent site of compression is in the proximal forearm in the area of the supinator muscle (arcade of Frohse) and involves the posterior interosseous branch. It has been postulated that repetitive pronation or supination movements may cause fibrosis of the arcade of Frohse, leading to a greater chance of entrapment. However, problems can also occur where the nerve crosses the lateral intermuscular septum, usually related to fractures of the humerus. Entrapment could also occur proximally to the elbow on the lateral portion, between the brachialis and brachioradialis, by the fibrous arcade within the lateral head of the triceps (Cabrera & McCue 1986), as well as distally on the radial aspect of the wrist. Entrapment of a nerve could restrict its movement, placing tension on the nerve during some motions of the upper extremities. Research has demonstrated that nerves normally move in relation to their surrounding connective tissues (Wilgis & Murphy 1986). If there is a densification of this surrounding connective tissue, the nerve conduction could be altered. Butler (1991) believes that the mobility of a nerve that has restricted longitudinal movement can often be restored using what they call 'neural mobilization techniques'. Remembering the strong relation between nerve sheath and deep muscular fasciae (see Chapter 3) we suggest treating the fasciae in connection with the nerve sheath to restore normal nerve mobility and relieve the patient's symptoms.

If the biceps tendon is tractioned proximally to the bicipital aponeurosis (lacertus fibrosus), as to simulate a muscular contraction, two lines of force appear: one in a medial direction, corresponding to the arciform fibres, and one in a longitudinal direction, along the central part of the forearm. Vice versa, traction applied to the flexor carpi radialis muscle to simulate its contraction creates lines of force extending into the brachial fascia via the bicipital aponeurosis.

The main components of the posterior elbow retinaculum are the expansions of the triceps brachii muscle into the antebrachial fascia (Figs 7.41 and 7.42). Windisch et al (2006) described a myofascial expansion that originates from the lateral head of the triceps brachii and crosses the olecranon to reach the posterior border of the ulna and the antebrachial fascia. This expansion measures 2.3–7.2 cm (mean: 4.04 cm). Keener et al (2010) found in all specimens a second distinct myofascial expansion of the lateral head of the triceps that is continuous with the anconeus fascia. This longitudinal expansion has a mean width of

Text continued on p. 262

248

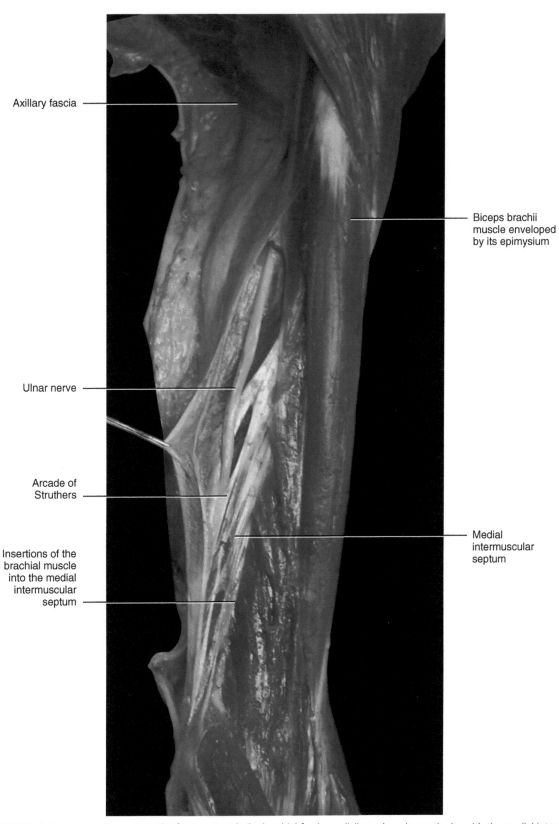

Axillary fascia

Biceps brachii muscle enveloped by its epimysium

Ulnar nerve

Arcade of Struthers

Medial intermuscular septum

Insertions of the brachial muscle into the medial intermuscular septum

FIGURE 7.30 Medial intermuscular septum. The forceps stretch the brachial fascia medially to show its continuity with the medial intermuscular septum. Note the relationship between the ulnar nerve and the medial intermuscular septum.

Coracobrachialis muscle
covered by its fascia.
It is in continuity with
the clavipectoral facia.

Deltoid
muscle

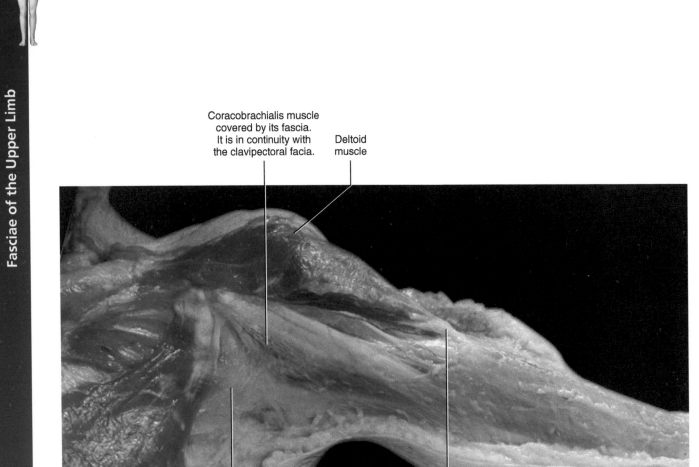

Pectoralis minor
muscle

Clavipectoral
fascia

Insertion of the deltoid fascia
into the brachial fascia

FIGURE 7.31 Anterior view of the shoulder region. The pectoralis major muscle was removed to show the clavipectoral fascia. This fascia continues into the arm with the fascia of the coracobrachialis muscle.

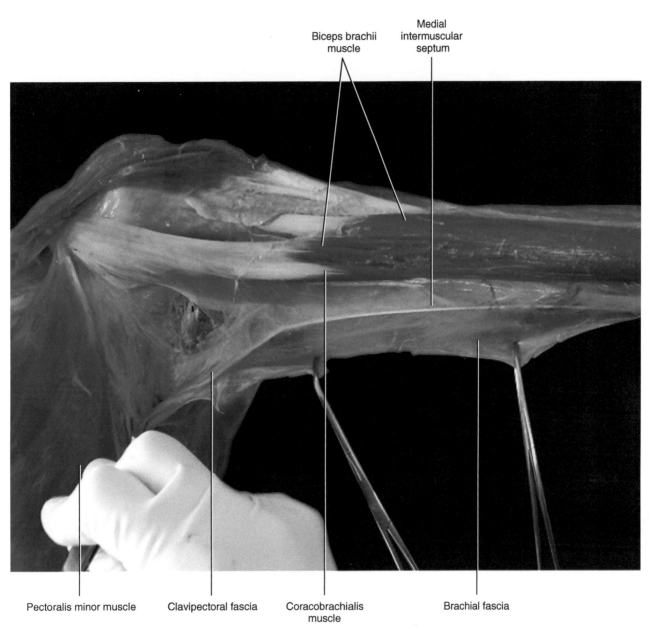

Biceps brachii muscle

Medial intermuscular septum

Pectoralis minor muscle

Clavipectoral fascia

Coracobrachialis muscle

Brachial fascia

FIGURE 7.32 Anterior view of the shoulder region. The clavipectoral fascia is cleared of the adipose tissue and stretched medially. Note its continuity with the brachial fascia and the medial intermuscular septum.

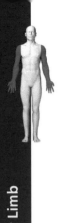
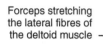

Forceps stretching
the lateral fibres of
the deltoid muscle ——

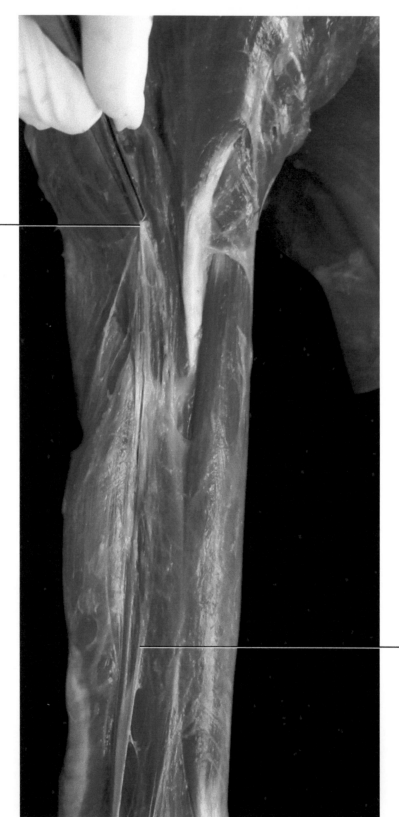

—— Line of force of the
brachial fascia at the
level of the lateral
intermuscular
septum

FIGURE 7.33 Lateral view of the arm. The forceps stretch the lateral portion of the deltoid muscle to simulate its contraction. The line of force into the brachial fascia at the level of the lateral intermuscular septum thus becomes more evident.

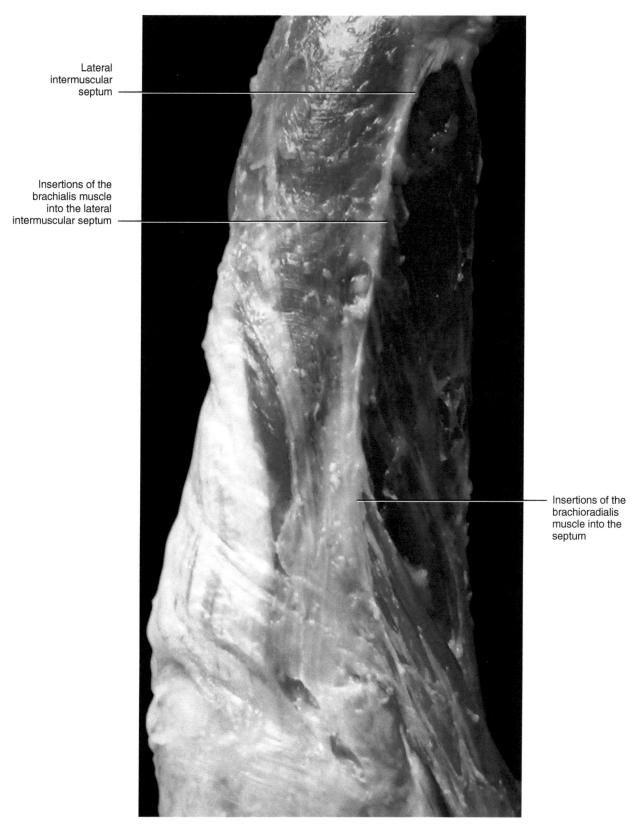

Lateral intermuscular septum

Insertions of the brachialis muscle into the lateral intermuscular septum

Insertions of the brachioradialis muscle into the septum

FIGURE 7.34 Lateral view of the distal part of the arm. The insertions of the brachioradialis and brachialis muscles into the anterior aspect of the lateral intermuscular septum are evident. The intermuscular septum coud be considered an element where different muscular forces converge.

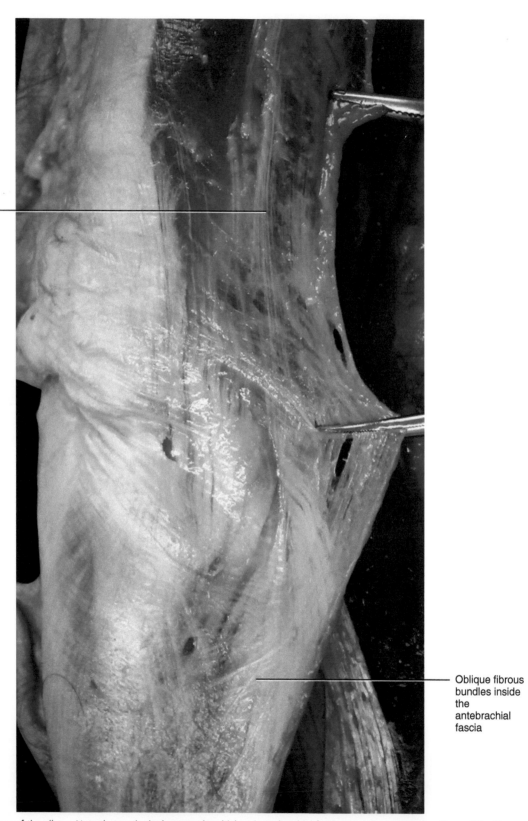

Longitudinal fibrous bundles inside the brachial fascia

Oblique fibrous bundles inside the antebrachial fascia

FIGURE 7.35 Posterior view of the elbow. Note the continuity between brachial and antebrachial fasciae and the various directions of the fibrous bundles inside the fascia. These form the posterior retinaculum of the elbow.

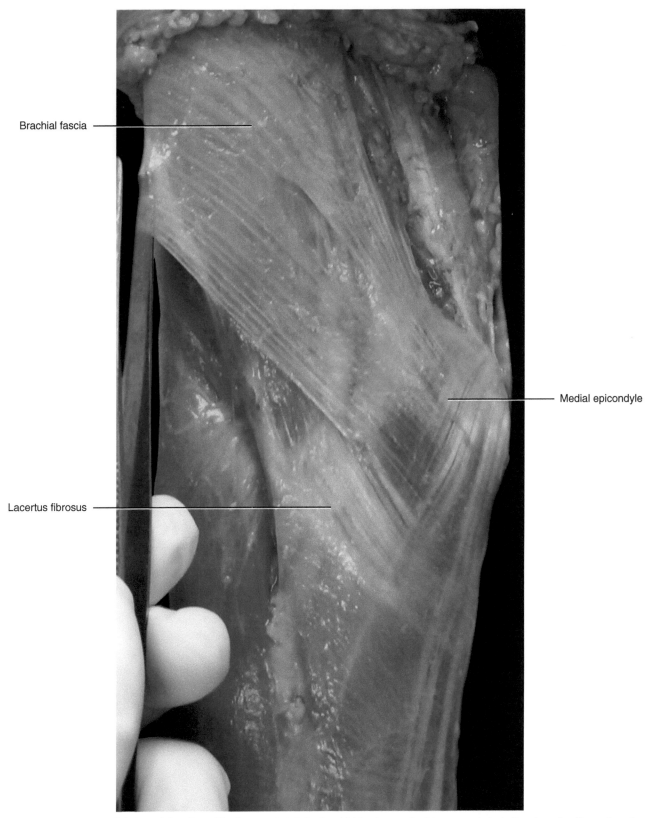

Brachial fascia

Medial epicondyle

Lacertus fibrosus

FIGURE 7.36 Anteromedial view of the elbow. The forceps stretch the brachial fascia over the biceps muscle to better show the fibrous bundles inside the fascia. These form part of the elbow retinaculum. It is evident that the medial epicondyle is a point where different forces converge.

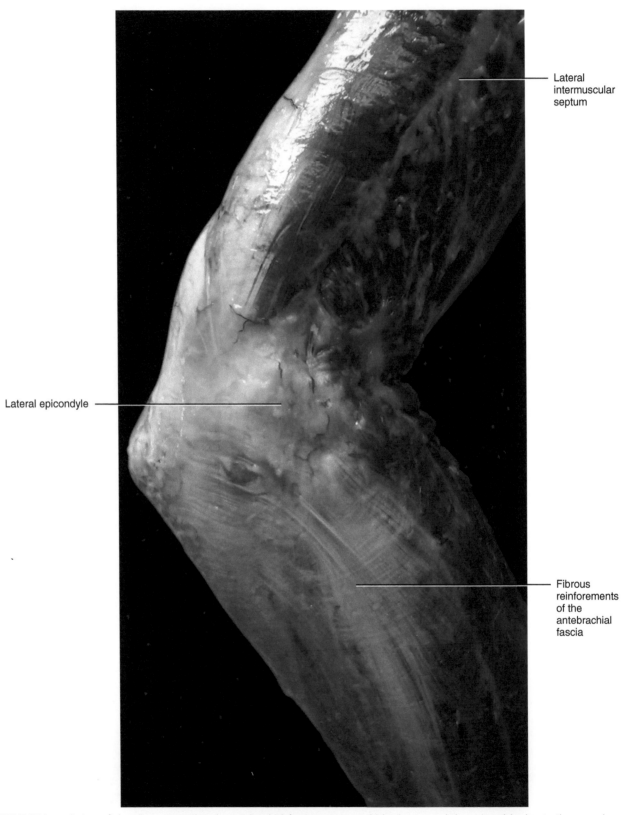

Lateral
intermuscular
septum

Lateral epicondyle

Fibrous
reinforements
of the
antebrachial
fascia

FIGURE 7.37 Lateral view of the elbow. Note that the antebrachial fascia presents a thickening around the epicondyle due to the muscular insertions of the epicondyle muscles into its inner side.

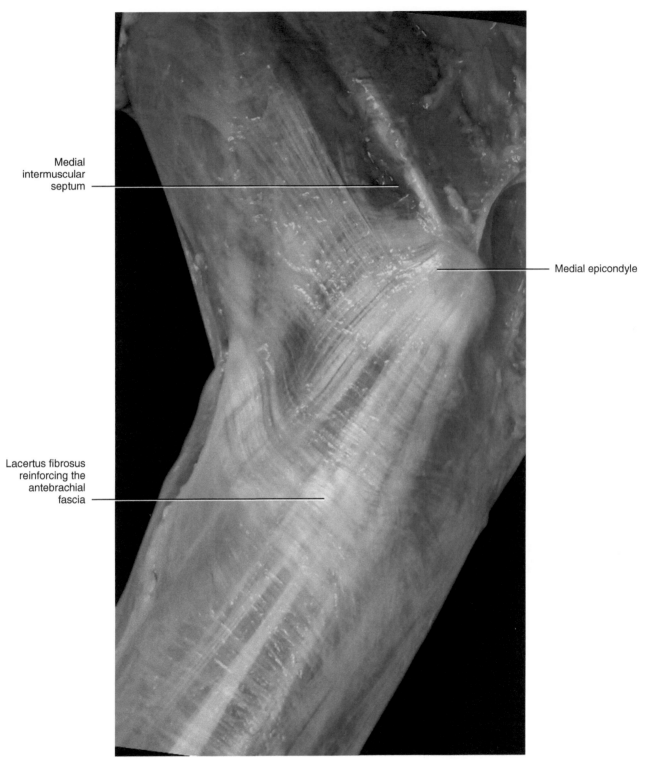

Medial
intermuscular
septum

Medial epicondyle

Lacertus fibrosus
reinforcing the
antebrachial
fascia

FIGURE 7.38 Medial view of the elbow. Note the fibrous reinforcement of the antebrachial fascia due to the lacertus fibrosus.

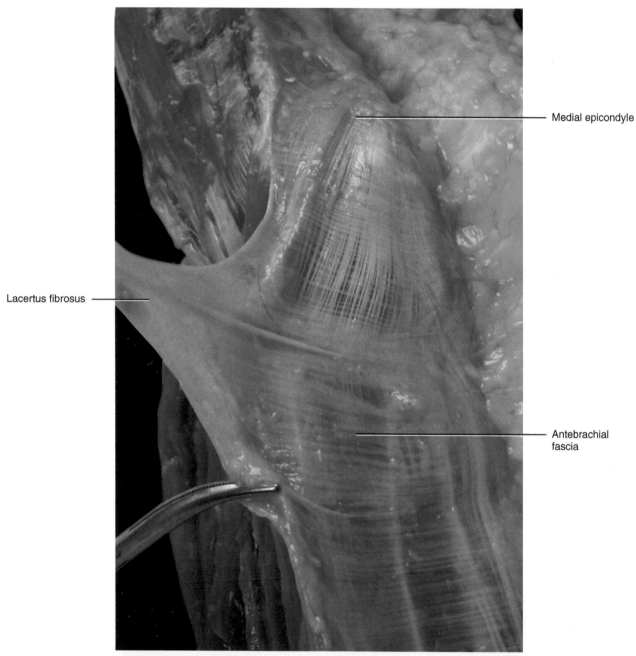

Medial epicondyle

Lacertus fibrosus

Antebrachial fascia

FIGURE 7.39 Medial view of the elbow. The lacertus fibrosus was detached from the biceps muscle and stretched to simulate its action into the medial portion of the antebrachial fascia. From its inner side, the antebrachial fascia gives insertions to many muscle fibres of the pronator teres and flexor carpi radialis muscles.

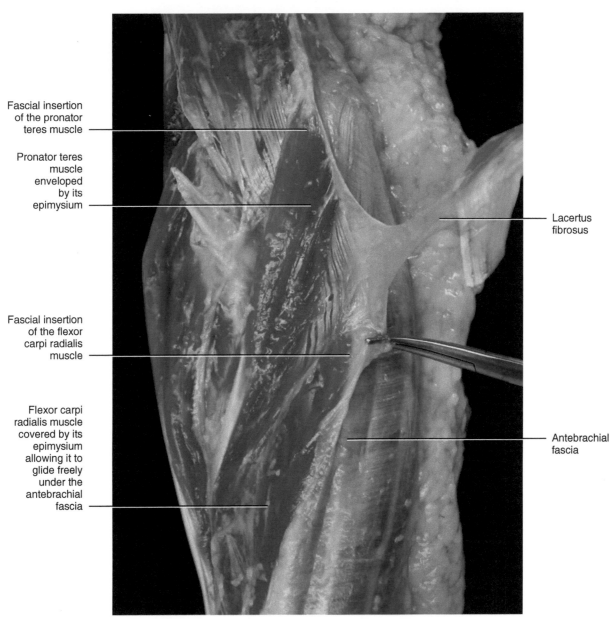

Fascial insertion of the pronator teres muscle

Pronator teres muscle enveloped by its epimysium

Fascial insertion of the flexor carpi radialis muscle

Flexor carpi radialis muscle covered by its epimysium allowing it to glide freely under the antebrachial fascia

Lacertus fibrosus

Antebrachial fascia

FIGURE 7.40 Anteromedial view of the elbow. The antebrachial fascia is lifted laterally to show its relation to the pronator teres and to the flexor carpi radialis. The proximal portion of these muscles is inserted into the inner aspect of the antebrachial fascia, their distal portion is free to glide under the antebrachial fascia due to the presence of their epimysium.

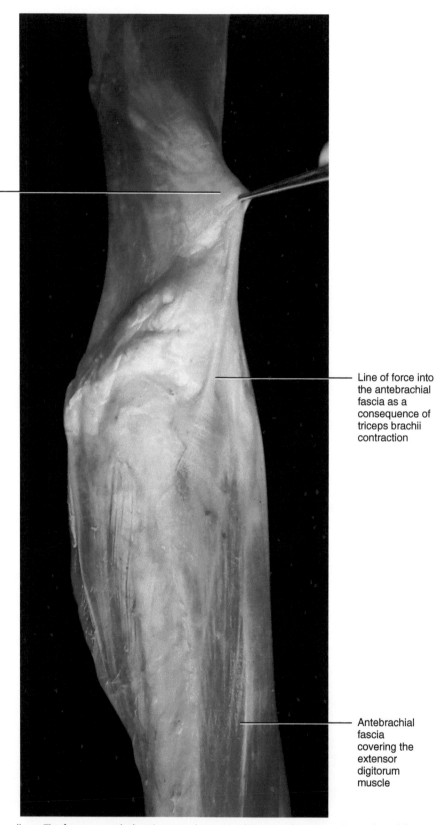

Forceps simulate triceps brachii contraction

Line of force into the antebrachial fascia as a consequence of triceps brachii contraction

Antebrachial fascia covering the extensor digitorum muscle

FIGURE 7.41 Posterior view of the elbow. The forceps stretch the triceps tendon to simulate muscular contraction. A line of force appears up to the antebrachial fascia.

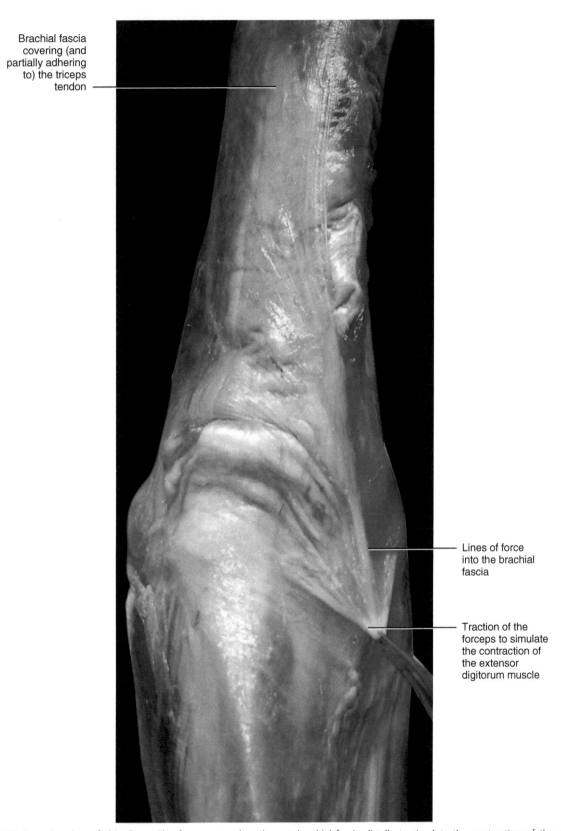

Brachial fascia covering (and partially adhering to) the triceps tendon

Lines of force into the brachial fascia

Traction of the forceps to simulate the contraction of the extensor digitorum muscle

FIGURE 7.42 Posterior view of the elbow. The forceps stretches the antebrachial fascia distally to simulate the contraction of the extensor digitorum muscle. This muscle originates, with many muscular fibres, from the inner aspect of the antebrachial fascia. A line of force appears up to the brachial fascia.

16.8 mm, (approximately 70% of the width of the central tendon). Bolté and Martin (1935) describe another tendinous expansion that originates from the medial head of the triceps and extends distally to unite with the antebrachial fascia. The Osborne's ligament, which goes from medial epicondyle of the humerus to the olecranon, is *also* involved in the formation of the posterior elbow retinaculum. This ligament is more of a wide reinforcement of the deep fascia than a true ligament and it occurs in 80% of cadavers.

If the antebrachial fascia is sectioned and lifted where the lateral triceps expansion merges, then the anconeus, extensor carpi ulnaris and extensor digiti minimi are visible. The two last muscles have numerous insertions into the fascia itself, whereas the anconeus does not have insertions into its overlying fascia (Figs 7.43 and 7.44). The anconeus muscle, however, has many insertions into the elbow capsule. These insertions may serve to stretch the capsule during elbow extension, thus avoiding the stinging of the capsule between the articular surfaces. Between the extensor carpi ulnaris and anconeus on one side and the extensor digiti minimi on the other side, a fibrous septum originates from the internal surface of the posterior antebrachial fascia. This septum is the origin of numerous fibres of the same muscles. If traction is applied to the triceps tendon simulating its contraction, lines of force develop in the posterior antebrachial fascia. These run parallel to the extensor carpi ulnaris. If the fibres of the extensor carpi ulnaris and extensor digiti minimi are tractioned in a distal direction, the lines of force will appear in the posterior brachial fascia.

It is difficult to isolate the different elements surrounding the elbow both from an anatomical and functional point of view. Van der Wal (2009) affirms that the elbow ligaments are created in the minds of the anatomists. For example, there are no actual collateral or annular ligaments as the tissues are all part of a complex connective tissue apparatus. Most anatomy books describe muscle origins and insertions only with respect to their bony insertions. They tend to diminish the importance of their fibrous connections. In 1985 Briggs and Elliott dissected 139 limbs from embalmed specimens to reveal the attachments of extensor muscles in the area of the lateral epicondyle. In only 29 limbs did they find a direct attachment of the extensor carpi radialis brevis muscle to the lateral epicondyle. In all the other limbs, this muscle attached to the extensor carpi radialis longus, extensor digitorum communis, supinator, radial collateral ligament, orbicular ligament (if there are elbow ligaments), the capsule of the elbow joint and the deep fascia. Thus, the connective tissue and the muscle tissue must be considered as one. It is this association that creates the true entheses that keeps bones together in every position of the joint. Van der Wal determined that connective tissue and muscles were not organized in parallel but rather sequentially, allowing so-called ligaments to be functional in all positions. An architectural description of the muscular and connective tissue, that is organized in series and enables the transmission of forces over these dynamic entities, is more appropriate than the classical concept of 'passive' force-guiding structures, such as ligaments organized in parallel to the tendons where connective tissue can transmit forces only in particular joint positions.

Van der Wal also studied the proprioceptors of the elbow region. He found that the discrimination between so-called joint receptors and muscle receptors is an artificial distinction when function is considered. Mechanoreceptors (the so-called muscle receptors) are arranged in the context of force circumstances, i.e. the architecture of muscles and connective tissue rather than of the classical anatomical structures, such as muscles, capsules, and ligaments. In the lateral cubital region of the rat a spectrum of mechanosensitive substrate occurs at the transitional areas between the deep fasciae and their muscle fascicles (that are organized in series with them). The receptors for proprioception are concentrated in those areas where tensile stresses are conveyed over the elbow joint. Structures cannot be divided into either joint receptors or muscle receptors when muscular and collagenous connective tissues function in series to maintain joint integrity and stability.

Deep Fascia of the Forearm: Antebrachial Fascia

The antebrachial fascia appears as a thick (mean thickness 0.75 mm), whitish layer of connective tissue formed by many fibrous bundles running in different directions (Figs 7.45 and 7.46). It covers the flexor and extensor muscle compartments as a 'muff' and sends some septa between them. In this way, this fascia forms three compartments: the anterior, the lateral and the posterior. Two septa separate the deep from the superficial layers of the forearm muscles in the anterior and posterior compartments (Figs 7.47 and 7.48).

In the proximal portion of the forearm, many muscle fibres insert into the deep surface of the antebrachial fascia (Figs 7.49 and 7.50). In the distal portion of the limb, the antebrachial fascia is easily separated from the underlying muscles, but is strongly attached to the radial and ulnar styloids.

The deep fascia of the forearm is well vascularized. Tao et al (2000) found that the number of blood vessels in the deep fascia is greater than that of the superficial fascia. In the forearm, the deep fascial vasculature is the main pathway through which the fasciocutaneous flaps gain their blood supply.

On the volar side, in the lower third of the forearm, the antebrachial fascia is pierced by the tendon of the palmaris longus muscle, which runs distally and superficially to the antebrachial fascia before continuing with the palmar aponeurosis. Distally, the antebrachial fascia continues with the dorsal fascia of the hand and in the palm it continues with the thenar and

Text continued on p. 271

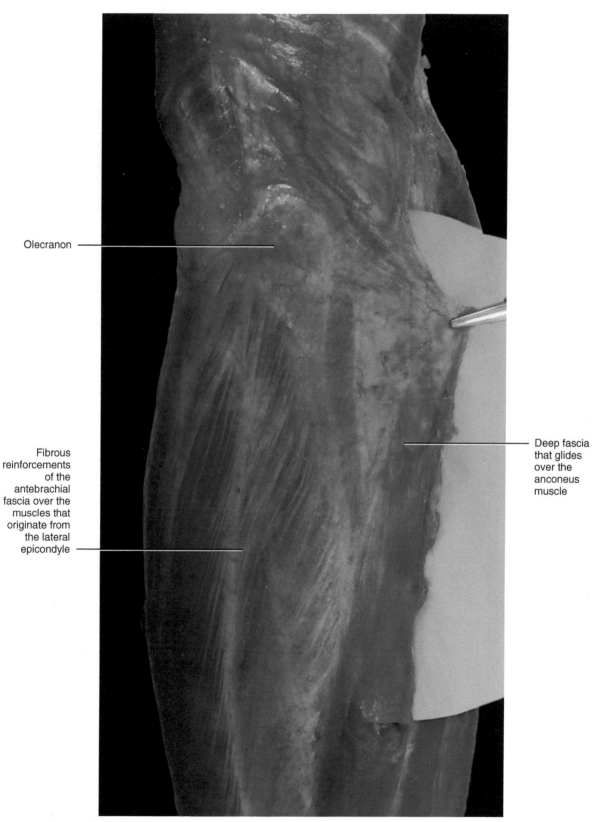

Olecranon

Fibrous
reinforcements
of the
antebrachial
fascia over the
muscles that
originate from
the lateral
epicondyle

Deep fascia
that glides
over the
anconeus
muscle

FIGURE 7.43 Posterior view of the elbow. The deep fascia is a continuous layer from the arm to the forearm, but at the level of the elbow its relationship to the underlying structure changes: it adheres to the olecranon and to the epicondyle. It glides over the anconeus muscle and it gives insertion to many muscle fibres at the epicondyle, adhering to the muscular plane. These muscular attachments, when contracting, stretch the antebrachial fascia allowing its fibrous reinforcement to become clearly visible in this dissection.

Deep fascia
detached
from the
anconeus
muscle and
lifted

Anconeus
muscle with
its epimysial
fascia

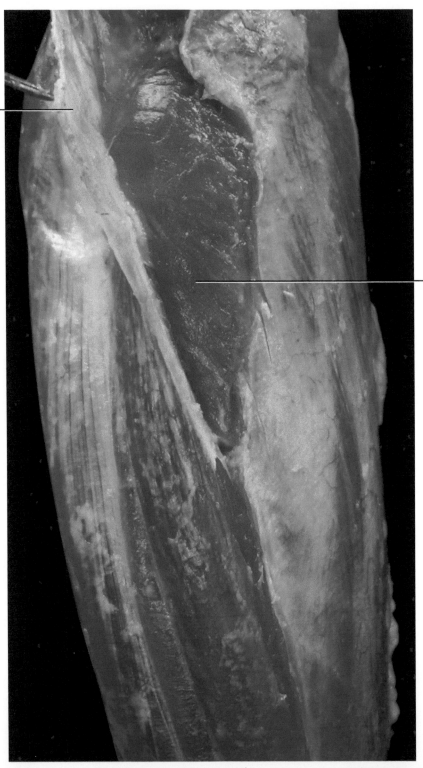

FIGURE 7.44 Posterior view of the elbow. The deep fascia could be detached easily from the anconeus because this muscle is completely enveloped by its epimysial fascia which glides freely under the deep fascia. The deep fascia gliding over the anconeus muscle connects the brachial fascia to the antebrachial fascia.

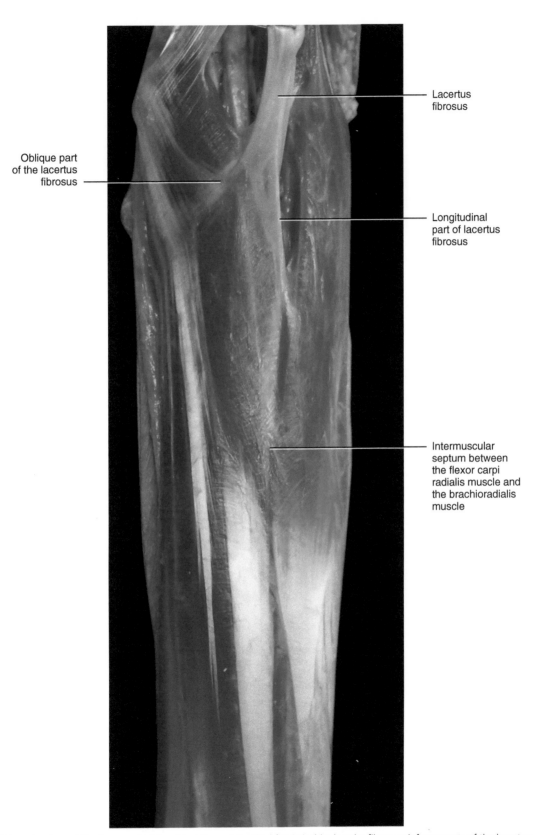

Lacertus
fibrosus

Oblique part
of the lacertus
fibrosus

Longitudinal
part of lacertus
fibrosus

Intermuscular
septum between
the flexor carpi
radialis muscle and
the brachioradialis
muscle

FIGURE 7.45 Anterior view of the forearm. In this subject the antebrachial fascia is thin, but the fibrous reinforcements of the lacertus fibrosus are clearly evident. Note that the lacertus fibrosus presents not only an oblique fibrous bundle, but also a longitudinal one. This longitudinal fibrous bundle stretches the antebrachial fascia over the intermuscular septum between the flexor carpi radialis muscle and the brachioradialis muscle.

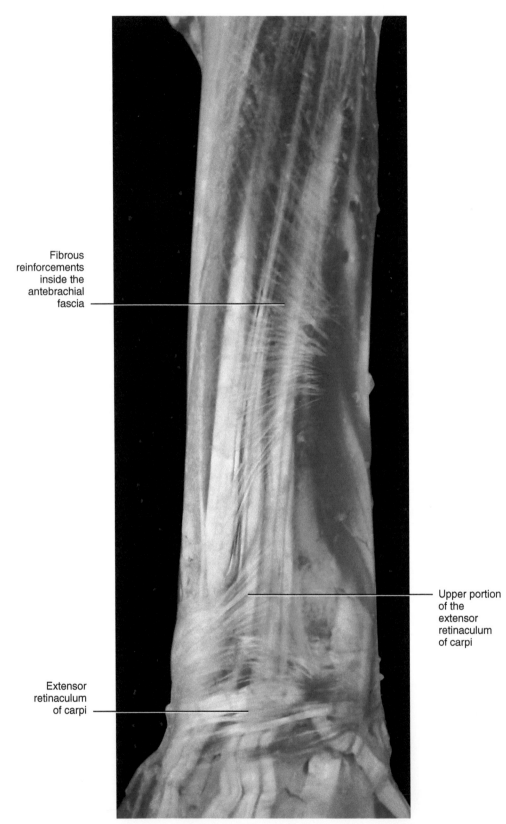

Fibrous
reinforcements
inside the
antebrachial
fascia

Upper portion
of the
extensor
retinaculum
of carpi

Extensor
retinaculum
of carpi

FIGURE 7.46 Posterior view of the forearm. Note the fibrous reinforcements inside the antebrachial fascia. The extensor retinaculum of carpi may be considered a fascial reinforcement, with both transverse and oblique. The latter continues with the oblique fibrous bundles present in the middle of the antebrachial fascia.

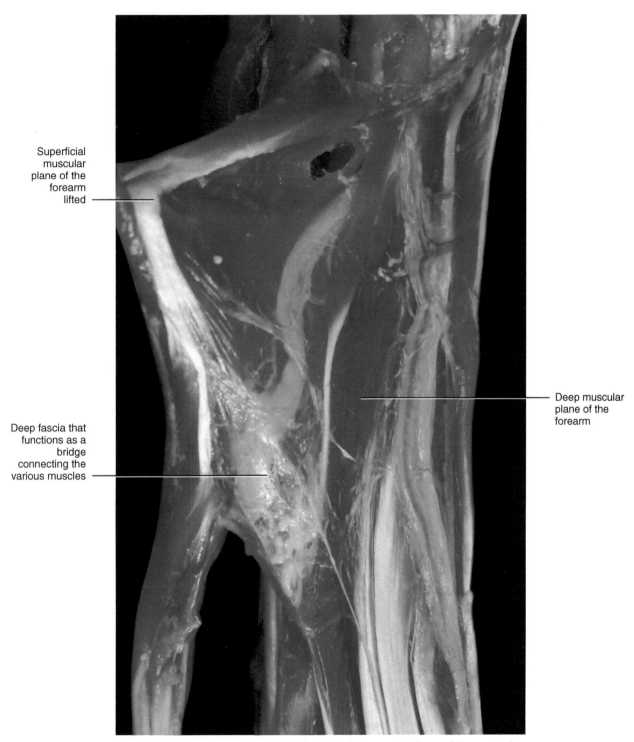

Superficial muscular plane of the forearm lifted

Deep muscular plane of the forearm

Deep fascia that functions as a bridge connecting the various muscles

FIGURE 7.47 View that depicts the deep fascia connecting the superficial and deep muscular planes of the *anterior* forearm.

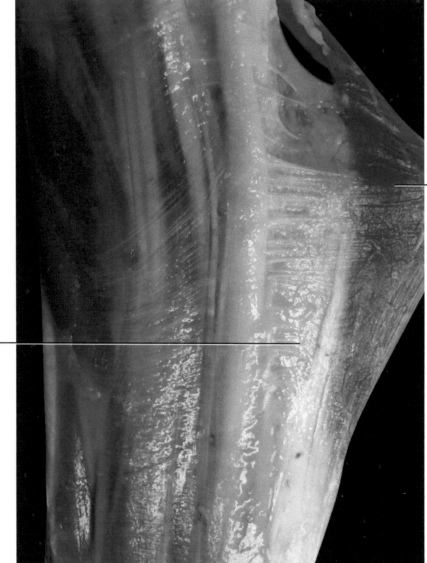

Brachioradialis muscle stretched externally

Deep fascia that functions as a bridge connecting the various muscles

FIGURE 7.48 View showing the deep fascia as the element that connects, like a bridge, the muscles of the lateral and anterior compartments of the forearm.

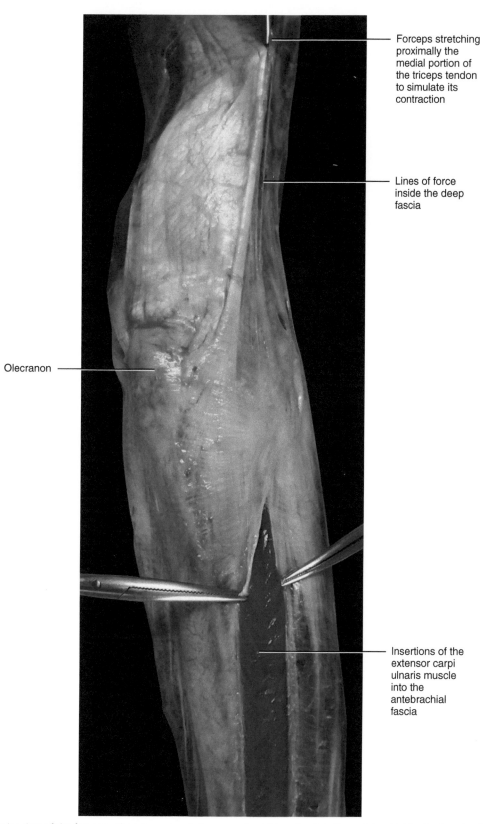

Forceps stretching
proximally the
medial portion of
the triceps tendon
to simulate its
contraction

Lines of force
inside the deep
fascia

Olecranon

Insertions of the
extensor carpi
ulnaris muscle
into the
antebrachial
fascia

FIGURE 7.49 Posterior view of the forearm. The triceps muscle has a myofascial insertion into the antebrachial fascia. It ends where the extensor carpi ulnaris inserts into the inner side of the antebrachial fascia.

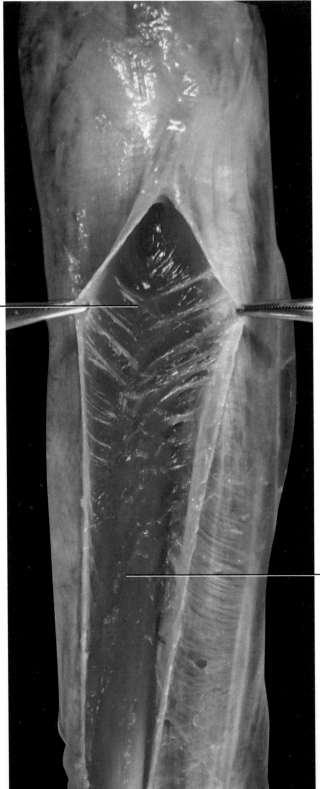

Fascial insertions of the extensor carpi ulnaris muscle into the antebrachial fascia

Extensor carpi ulnaris muscle free to glide under the antebrachial fascia (due to its epimysium)

FIGURE 7.50 Posterior view of the forearm. The antebrachial fascia is cut along the extensor carpi ulnaris muscle to show the relationship of this muscle with the deep fascia. Typical of muscles in this region, there are many muscle fibres inserted proximally into the inner aspect of the antebrachial fascia. In this way the extensor carpi ulnaris muscle stretches the fascia every time it contracts. Distally, it is free to glide under the antebrachial fascia due to the presence of the epimysium that envelops the muscle in its distal part.

CLINICAL PEARL 7.8 LATERAL EPICONDYLOPATHY

Lateral epicondylopathy is commonly diagnosed in patients with pain over the lateral aspect of the elbow, worsened or aggravated by repetitive or excessive movements of the wrist, especially during elbow extension. Patients are usually tender over the lateral epicondyle and resisted wrist extension worsens the pain. It is considered an overuse injury often associated with frequent pronosupination movements. Its prevalence in the general population is approximately 1.0% to 1.5% and affects, more commonly, the dominant arm. The condition reaches 23% in occupational populations (Papa 2012).

This pathology is commonly called tennis elbow or lateral epicondylitis. According to Nirschl & Ashman (2003), the term 'lateral elbow tendinosis' (rather than tendinitis) is preferred because histopathological examination of over 600 cases of chronic epicondylagia revealed a degenerative process consisting of fibroblastic tissue, vascular hyperplasia, disorganized and unstructured collagen and a lack of inflammatory cells.

Intra-articular pathologies, such as chondromalacia of radiocapitellar joint and synovial fringe impingement and those involving the annular ligament, have also been implicated. Other possibilities are compression and/or entrapment of the radial nerve or the anterior cutaneous nerve, traumatic periostitis of extensor carpi radialis brevis, and radiohumeral bursitis. Each of these conditons may appear by itself or in conjunction with epicondylopathy. If we consider the theories of Van der Wal (2009), we can better understand the association with all these other pathological findings. Indeed the muscles, capsule, fascia, ligaments, etc. have to act together to assure a correct movement of the elbow. If one element is altered, all the others follow. Consequently, the treatment of a lateral epicondylopathy might be more effective if it considers all the involved elements and, above all, the deep fascia (which is the anatomical structure that connects them all).

---

hypothenar fascia, on the lateral and medial sides respectively. Centrally it forms the deep layer of the palmar aponeurosis.

The flexor carpi radialis and ulnaris muscles lie beneath the antebrachial fascia but, distally, their paratenons fuse with this fascia, so that the antebrachial fascia appears to envelop them at the wrist. In about 85% of cases studied, the extensor carpi ulnaris sends a tendinous expansion distally to the fascia of the hypothenar eminence (Figs 7.51 and 7.52). This expansion develops in the lateral region of the fifth metacarpal bone and reinforces the fascia overlying the opponens digiti minimi. This expansion presents as a narrow, fibrous band disposed along the distal third of the fifth metacarpal bone and spreads into a fan shape, inserting into the fascia covering the metacarpophalangeal joint. If the tendon of extensor carpi ulnaris is tensioned, the traction is clearly transmitted to this fibrous band.

At the wrist, the antebrachial fascia is reinforced by the flexor and extensor retinacula, called by some authors the annular ligament (Figs 7.53 and 7.54). This fascia is formed by strong fibrous bundles with various cross directions (mediolateral and lateromedial) and arranged in multiple layers. Their mean thickness is 1.19 mm. The flexor retinaculum gives insertions to many muscular fibres of the thenar and hypothenar eminences, that stretch the retinaculum and, consequently, the antebrachial fascia in a caudal direction every time they contract. The wrist retinacula are richly innerved and play an important role in peripheral motor coordination and proprioception (Stecco et al 2010).

The flexor retinaculum of the wrist has to be distinguished from the transverse carpal ligament (Figs 7.55 and 7.56). The retinaculum is a reinforcement of the deep fascia. The transverse carpal ligament is a true

ligament with a width between 22 and 26 mm and a mean thickness of about 2 mm. It connects the hamate and pisiform bones to the scaphoid and trapezium, converting the deep groove on the front of the carpal bones into a fibro-osseous tunnel: the carpal tunnel. The carpal tunnel contains the flexor tendons of the digits and the median nerve. The transverse carpal ligament also forms the floor of Guyon's canal through which the ulnar artery and nerve pass, while its roof is formed by the flexor retinaculum of carpi. This specification is important for clinical practice, as the carpal tunnel syndrome is associated with the transverse ligament and not with the retinaculum. If a mini-invasive surgery cuts only the ligament and preserves the retinaculum, the proprioceptive damage and the diminished force that patients may experience after a carpal tunnel release could be minimized.

Deep Fasciae of the Palm: Palmar Fascial Complex

The palmar fascial complex of the hand has five components: the palmar aponeurosis, the deep palmar fascia, the adductor fascia, the fasciae of the thenar and hypothenar eminences and the septa that connect all these elements.

The palmar aponeurosis[1] is fomed by two sublayers that can be distinguished by histological studies. The superficial layer is formed by collagen fibres all orientated longitudinally. The deep layer is formed by

Text continued on p. 278

---

[1]This is the common name, but this is fascia with aponeurotic features and not just a flat tendon. Indeed, it has fibres disposed in various directions and different muscles insert into it.

CLINICAL PEARL 7.9 ULNAR NERVE ENTRAPMENT

The ulnar nerve could be compressed in many outlets along its course. The most frequent site is at the elbow, where the ulnar nerve could be compressed along its course in the retrocondylar groove (cubital tunnel syndrome). Cubital tunnel syndrome is the second most common peripheral nerve compression syndrome. Patients usually present motor weakness, muscle atrophy and sensory changes in the ulnar region. The clinical diagnosis may be confirmed by nerve conduction studies. The roof of the cubital tunnel is formed by the deep fascia covering the two heads of the flexor carpi ulnaris muscle and by Osborne's ligament (that has to be considered more of a fascial reinforcement than an isolated structure) (Macchi et al 2014). The floor is formed by the elbow capsule and the posterior and transverse portion of the medial collateral ligament. The walls are formed by the medial epicondyle and the olecranon. It is evident that an excessive tension of the deep fascia at this level could reduce the cubital tunnel diameter and cause a cubital tunnel syndrome.

A second site of ulnar compression is the so-called 'arcade of Struthers' (Nakajima et al 2009). Significant controversy exists regarding the existence of this arcade and whether or not this structure is involved in some cases of proximal ulnar nerve entrapment. The arcade of Struthers is a canal whose medial border is formed by the brachial fascia and internal brachial ligament, which is a fascial extension of the coracobrachialis tendon into the brachial fascia. Its anterior border is formed by the medial intermuscular septum and its lateral border by the muscular fibres and fascia of the medial head of the triceps. This arcade occurs 8 cm proximally to the medial epicondyle. Tubbs et al (2011) have dissected 15 cadavers (30 sides) to analyse the course of the ulnar nerve and its relationship to the soft tissues of this region. They identified a thickening in the inferior medial arm that crosses the ulnar nerve and is consistent with the so-called arcade of Struthers in 86.7% of sides. On 57.7% of the sides, the arcade was found to be due to a thickening of the brachial fascia and was classified as a type I arcade. On 19.2% of the sides, the arcade was due to the internal brachial ligament and these were classified as type II arcades. On 23.1% of the sides, the arcade was due to a thickened, medial intermuscular septum and these were classified as type III arcades. Based on this study, we can affirm that the brachial fascia may be thickened in part and this could create a compression of the ulnar nerve.

Finally, the ulnar nerve could be compressed in the Guyon's tunnel (Guyon's ulnar tunnel syndrome). This tunnel is formed by the pisiform, the hook of the hamate, the transverse carpal ligament (which forms the floor) and the flexor carpi retinaculum (which forms the roof). The more important clinical signs are sensory loss to the tip of the little finger and one and a half ulnar digits, and/or motor signs such as weakness on testing of interossei and adductor pollicis muscles. This syndrome is caused by prolonged pressure over the hypothenar eminence (cycling), ganglion, hamate fracture, ulnar artery thrombosis or aneurysm. Excessive tension of the flexor retinaculum of carpi could also cause this syndrome. Many muscular fibres of the thenar and hypothenar eminences originate from the flexor carpi retinaculum and stretch the retinaculum upon contracting. This retinaculum serves as a reinforcement of the antebrachial fascia and also a densification of this fascia could cause Guyon's ulnar tunnel syndrome.

CLINICAL PEARL 7.10 DE QUERVAIN'S SYNDROME

This is a tenosynovitis of the sheath or tunnel that surrounds the tendons of the extensor pollicis brevis and abductor pollicis longus muscles. Evaluation of histological specimens shows a thickening and myxoid degeneration consistent with a chronic degenerative process. Symptoms are pain, tenderness and swelling over the thumb side of the wrist and difficulty in gripping. Finkelstein's test is used for clinical diagnosis. To perform this test, the examining physician grasps the thumb, and the hand is ulnar deviated sharply. If sharp pain occurs along the distal radius, De Quervain's syndrome is likely. The cause of De Quervain's disease remains idiopathic, but generally it is considered an overuse injury more common in persons who make repetitive movements of the thumb. There is limited evidence on the efficacy of glucocorticoid injection in this condition. No other therapeutic modality has shown efficacy or has been assessed in a placebo-controlled clinical trial. The management of De Quervain's disease is determined more by convention than scientific data.

According to Alvarez-Nemegyei (2004), De Quervain's tendinopathy is a tendinous impingement caused by a thickened retinaculum. Due to thickening, the tendon is unable to glide properly and its vascularization could be altered with consequent tendon degeneration. The wrist retinacula is a reinforcement of the antebrachial fascia; therefore, any alteration of the antebrachial fascia could affect the wrist retinacula and cause the tendinous impingement.

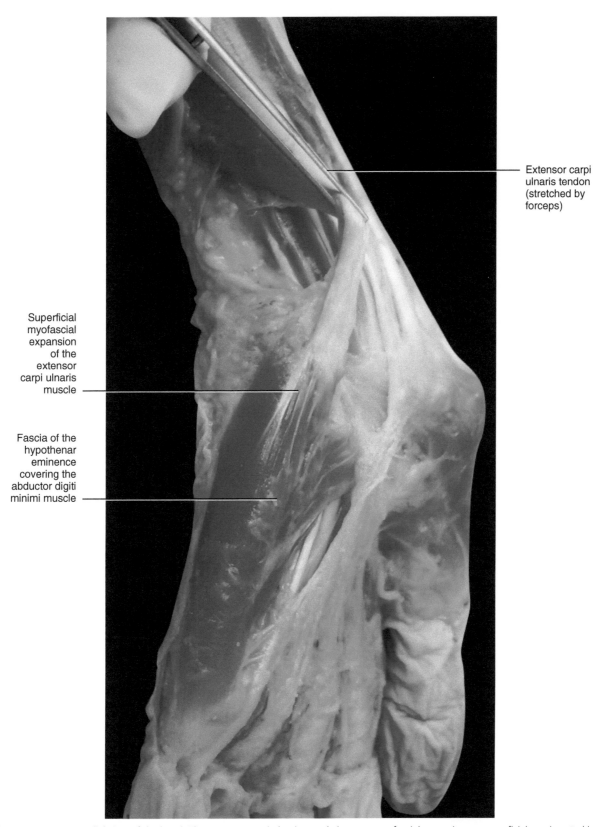

Extensor carpi ulnaris tendon (stretched by forceps)

Superficial myofascial expansion of the extensor carpi ulnaris muscle

Fascia of the hypothenar eminence covering the abductor digiti minimi muscle

FIGURE 7.51 Anteromedial view of the hand. The extensor carpi ulnaris muscle has two myofascial expansions: a superficial one inserted into the fascia covering the abductor digiti minimi muscle and a deeper one into the fascia covering the opponens digiti minimi muscle (Fig. 7.52). This permits the contraction of the extensor carpi ulnaris muscle to stretch all the fascia of the hypothenar eminence.

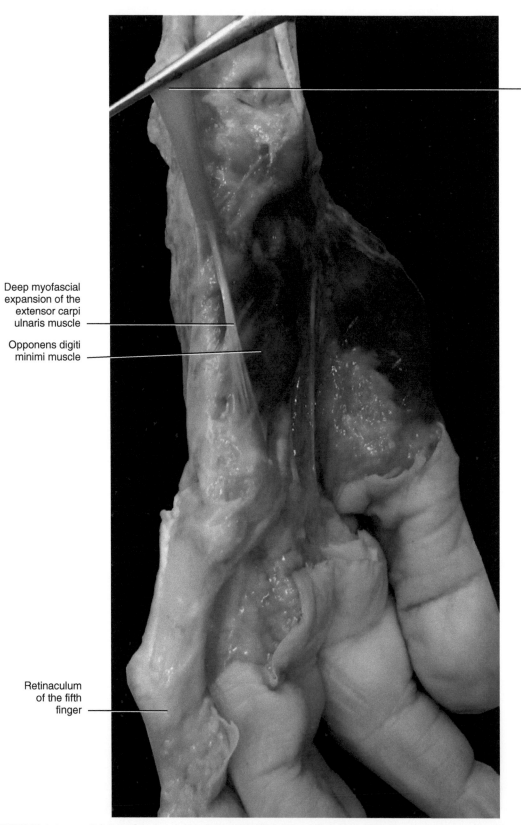

Extensor carpi ulnaris tendon (stretched by forceps)

Deep myofascial expansion of the extensor carpi ulnaris muscle

Opponens digiti minimi muscle

Retinaculum of the fifth finger

FIGURE 7.52 Anteromedial view of the hand. The abductor digiti minimi muscle is removed to show the deep myofascial expansion of the extensor carpi ulnaris muscle into the fascia of the hypothenar eminence covering the opponens digiti minimi muscle.

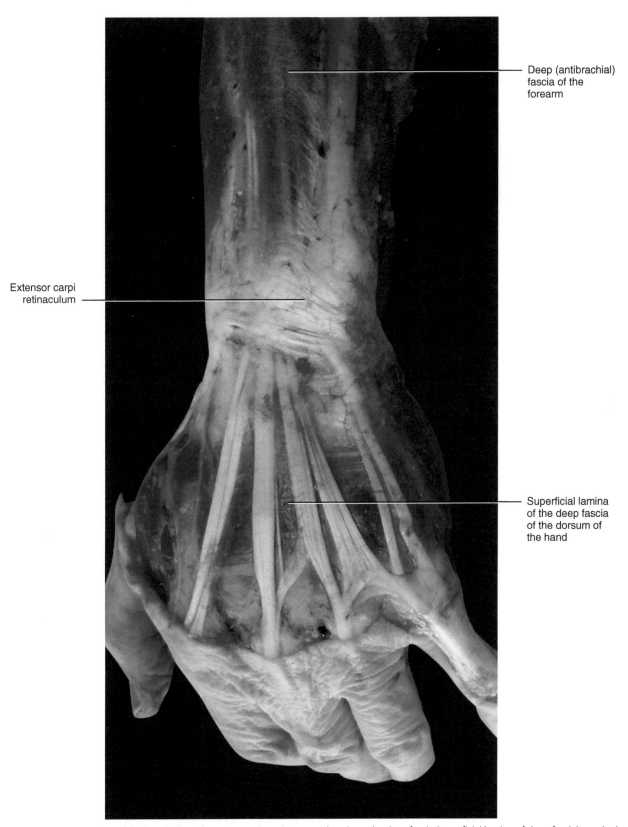

Deep (antibrachial) fascia of the forearm

Extensor carpi retinaculum

Superficial lamina of the deep fascia of the dorsum of the hand

FIGURE 7.53 Posterior view of the hand. The subcutaneous tissue is removed to show the deep fascia (superficial lamina of deep fascia) enveloping the extensor digitorum longus tendons. Note that the extensor carpi retinaculum continues both with the antebrachial fascia and with the deep fascia of the hand.

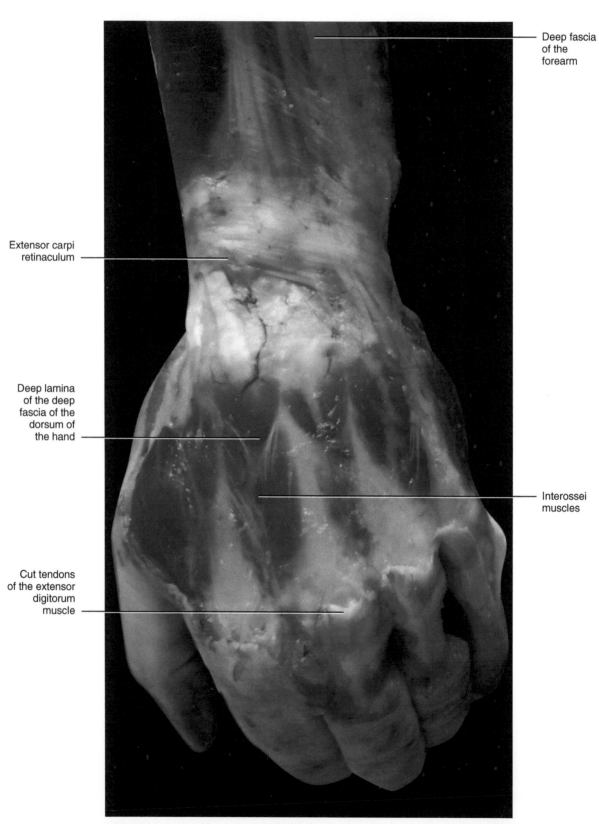

Deep fascia of the forearm

Extensor carpi retinaculum

Deep lamina of the deep fascia of the dorsum of the hand

Interossei muscles

Cut tendons of the extensor digitorum muscle

FIGURE 7.54 Posterior view of the hand. The superficial lamina of the deep fascia and the tendons of the extensor digitorum muscle were removed to show the deep lamina covering the interossei muscles.

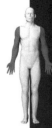

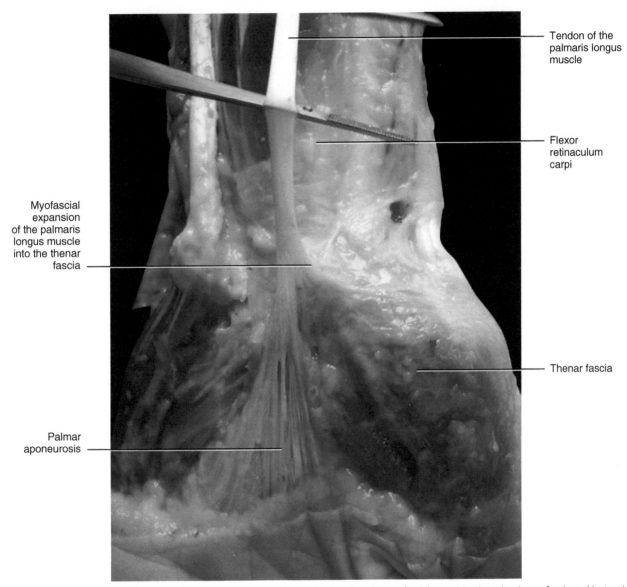

Tendon of the palmaris longus muscle

Flexor retinaculum carpi

Myofascial expansion of the palmaris longus muscle into the thenar fascia

Thenar fascia

Palmar aponeurosis

FIGURE 7.55 Anterior view of the wrist. The palmaris longus tendon is lifted to show its myofascial expansion into the thenar fascia and its tension effect on the longitudinal fibres of the palmar aponeurosis.

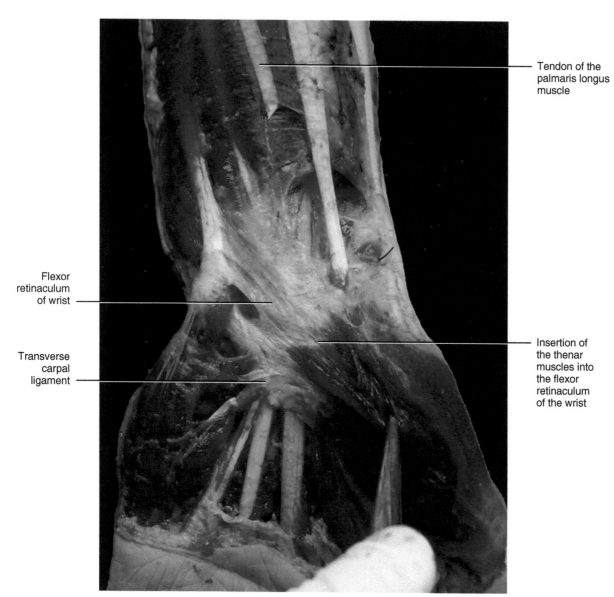

Tendon of the
palmaris longus
muscle

Flexor
retinaculum
of wrist

Insertion of
the thenar
muscles into
the flexor
retinaculum
of the wrist

Transverse
carpal
ligament

FIGURE 7.56 The palmar aponeurosis and the tendon of the palmaris longus muscle were removed to show the insertions of the thenar muscles into the flexor retinaculum of the wrist. Note the difference between the flexor retinaculum and the transverse carpal ligament: the former is composed of oblique fibrous bundles, the latter is deeper and composed of transverse fibrous bundles.

collagen fibres with a transverse orientation. The first layer might be considered a local specialization of the superficial fascia, and the deep transverse layer a local specialization of the deep fascia of the palm and the distal equivalent of the antebrachial fascia. The palmaris longus muscle is a proper tensor of the palmar aponeurosis, and many muscular fibres of the thenar and hypotenar muscles insert into this aponeurosis. The palmaris brevis muscle originates completely from the palmar aponeurosis. In 15% of the population the palmaris longus muscle is absent (Figs 7.57 and 7.58). In these cases the macroscopic appearance of palmar aponeurosis demonstrates decisive disarrangement. This suggests that the mechanical tension of the palmaris longus muscle plays an active role in determining the longitudinal disposition of the fibres of the superficial layer. The longitudinal fibres form

four bands extending towards the second to fifth fingers. At the level of the distal part of the palm a large number of bands pass up to insert into the skin, while others turn aside and continue in the palmar interdigital ligaments. A small number continue distally into the fingers where they terminate in the skin and in the fibrous flexor sheaths above the proximal phalanges. The transverse fibres are thin and are sparse proximally, but distally they increase in number and thickness to finally form a strong transverse ligament.

Under the palmar aponeurosis, the fibrous sheaths of the flexor tendons and another deeper fascial layer, the deep palmar fascia (or interosseous fascia), are found. The deep palmar fascia lies beneath the lumbricalis muscles and above the interossei muscles. Towards the wrist it thins out into the ligaments of the joint capsules of the carpal joints. Towards the fingers

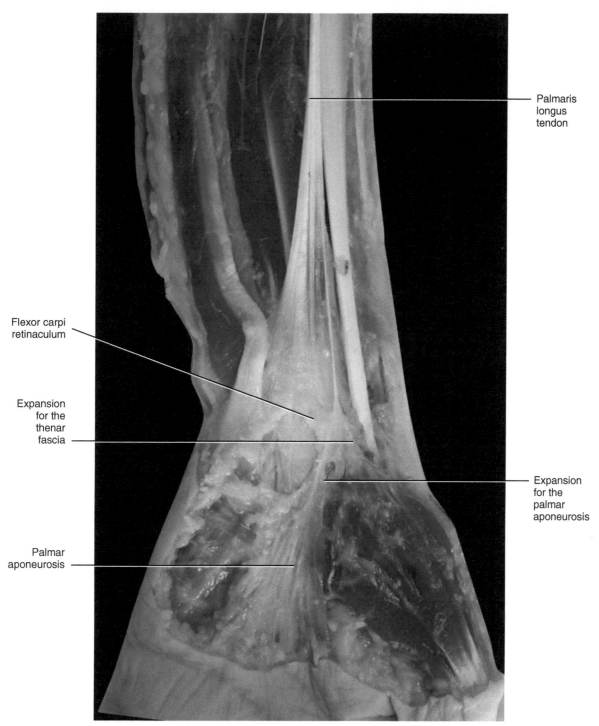

Palmaris
longus
tendon

Flexor carpi
retinaculum

Expansion
for the
thenar
fascia

Expansion
for the
palmar
aponeurosis

Palmar
aponeurosis

FIGURE 7.57 Anterior view of the wrist. In this subject the palmaris longus tendon opens as a fan, having a very thin insertion into the palmar aponeurosis, while the larger portion inserts into the flexor carpi retinaculum.

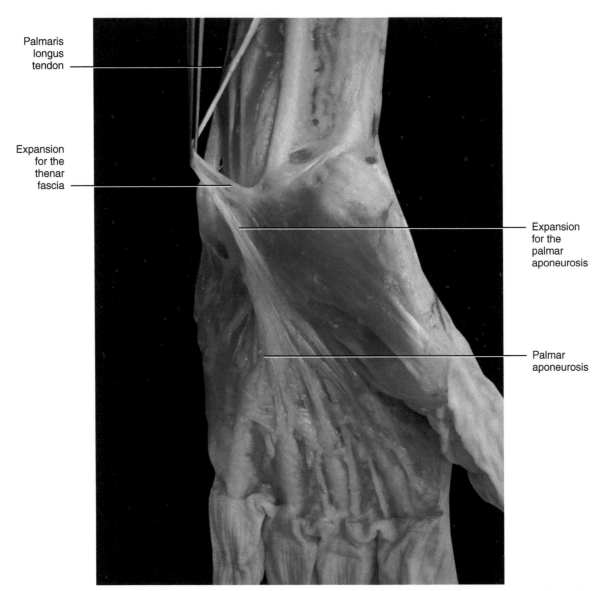

Palmaris
longus
tendon

Expansion
for the
thenar
fascia

Expansion
for the
palmar
aponeurosis

Palmar
aponeurosis

FIGURE 7.58 Anterolateral view of the hand. The palmaris longus tendon was lifted to show the myofascial expansion into the thenar fascia.

it thins out into the capsules of the metacarpophalan-geal joints. The deep palmar fascia is reinforced dis-tally by transverse collagen fibres, forming the deep transverse metacarpal ligament. This ligament occu-pies a central position in the function of the hand. It extends across the hand and attaches to the meta-carpal bones. It is also connected by means of many septa to both the longitudinal and transverse fibres of the palmar aponeurosis. In particular, it is connected to the palmar aponeurosis by two longitudinal septa (marginal septa of the palmar aponeurosis) and, dis-tally, by seven vertical septa, first described by Legueu and Juvara (1892). The intermediate septa are rectan-gular, each with a superficial margin attached to the palmar aponeurosis. The deep margin attaches to the deep palmar fascia, or to the adductor fascia. The septa have proximal free falciform edges and a distal limit where the septum continues into the deep fasciae of the fingers. The septa divide the central compartment

of the hand into eight small compartments. Four of these contain the flexor tendons for the second to fifth fingers, while the other four contain the lumbrical muscles and accompanying digital vessels and nerves.

The palmar aponeurosis is strongly adherent to the skin due to thick, short and vertical retinacula cutis that are spaced closely together in the distal part of the hand. Tangential pressure on the skin, in any direction, transfers force through the retinacula cutis to the palmar aponeurosis and via the septa to the bones of the hand. The system is activated when the palmar aponeurosis is tensed by the contraction of the palmaris longus muscle or by the extension of the metacarpophalangeal joints or both. When the aponeurosis is relaxed, movements of the skin can occur both in a proximodistal direction and from side to side.

The thenar and hypothenar fasciae are epimysial fasciae that are strongly adherent to their underlying muscles. It is impossible to separate a specific fascial layer in this region. Ling and Kumar (2009) noted the absence of a well-defined tough fascia overlying the thenar and hypothenar muscles. Loose connective tissue is present between the individual thenar and hypothenar muscles. These fasciae continue proximally into the flexor retinaculum of the wrist. Many fibres of the thenar and hypothenar muscles insert into the flexor retinaculum of the wrist, stretching it in an oblique–caudal direction. We can affirm that many of the fibrous bundles forming this retinaculum are orientated in the same direction as the muscular fibres of the thenar and hypothenar muscles that insert into it. The thenar and hypothenar fasciae continue laterally and medially with the dorsal fascia of the hand (Figs 7.59 and 7.60). Platzer (1978) and Kanaya et al (2002) describe

the abductor digiti minimi, which sends a tendinous expansion into the dorsal fascia of the fifth finger. This expansion originates from the most dorsal part of the muscle and arches to merge into the dorsal fascia of the fifth finger at the metacarpophalangeal joint, or even more distally towards the phalanges. Tension applied to the abductor digiti minimi is transmitted to this fibrous band and from there to the dorsal fascia of the fifth finger.

The adductor pollicis muscle is covered by its own delicate fascia, the adductor fascia. The adductor fascia extends radially from the third metacarpal bone to insert on the first metacarpal bone, just to the ulnar side of the tendon of the flexor pollicis longus. At the distal border of the adductor pollicis it continues into the fascia covering the first dorsal interosseous muscle.

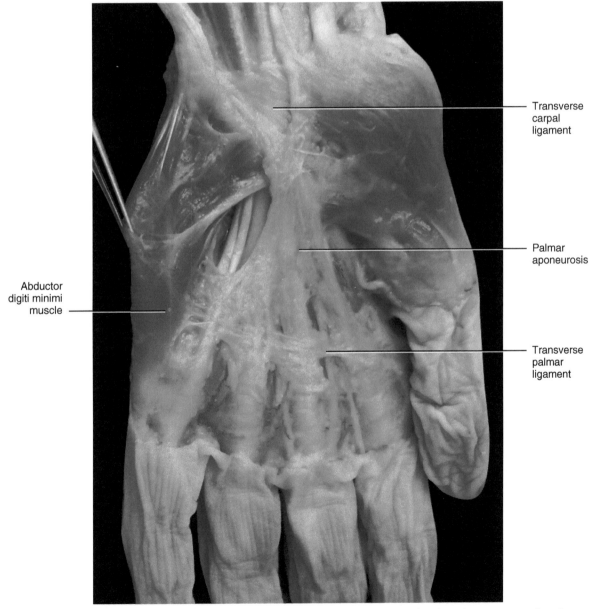

Transverse carpal ligament

Palmar aponeurosis

Transverse palmar ligament

Abductor digiti minimi muscle

FIGURE 7.59 Anterior view of the hand. The superficial layer of the palmar aponeurosis is removed to show the transverse palmar ligament and the insertions of the thenar and hypothenar muscles into the palmar aponeurosis.

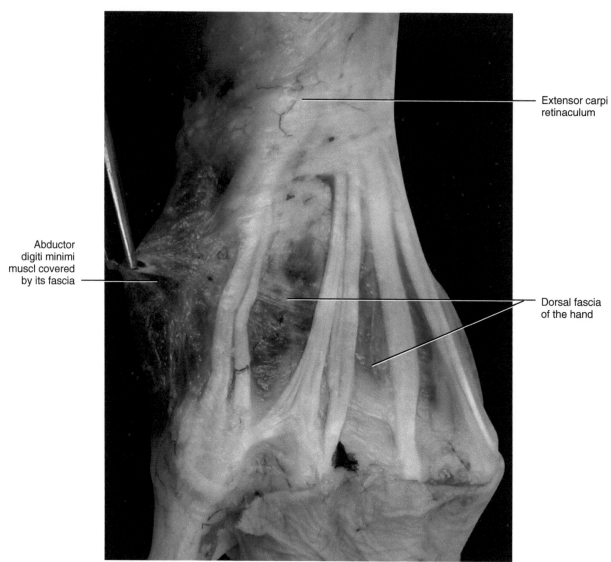

Extensor carpi
retinaculum

Abductor
digiti minimi
muscl covered
by its fascia

Dorsal fascia
of the hand

FIGURE 7.60 Dorsal view of the hand. Note the continuity of the abductor digiti minimi fascia with the dorsal fascia of the hand and with the extensor carpi retinaculum.

Some muscular fibres of the adductor pollicis muscle originate from this fascia.

Dorsal Fasciae of the Hand

In the dorsum of the hand there are two deep fasciae (Figs 7.61 and 7.62). The superficial lamina covers all the extensor tendons and continues proximally with the extensor carpi retinaculum, and distally with the dorsal fascia of the fingers. The deep lamina lies above the interossei dorsalis muscles and fuses with the periosteum of each metacarpal bone. These two fasciae are thin but present aponeurotic features. The presence of loose connective tissue between them permits the gliding of the extensor tendons with respect to the underlying plane. The presence of adhesions between the superficial lamina and the intertendinous connections assure a strong functional correlation between the superficial lamina and the extensor tendons. Landsmeer (1949) explained that the dorsal fascia of

the hand gives the morphological basis for the integration and coordination of the extensor muscles.

Deep Fasciae of the Fingers

Superficial fascia does not exist in the fingers. The skin of the fingers is anchored to the deep fascia by fibrous elements that allow the hand to flex without changing the skin position. The skin is loosely attached to the deeper planes at the prominent creases (skin folds). This contrasts to the skin on the adjacent sides of the crease that possess multiple strong anchor points.

In the fingers, the deep fascia is reinforced around each joint by retinacula. Rayan et al (1997) described the extensor retinacular system that is integrated with the extrinsic and intrinsic musculotendinous structures. It has transverse, sagittal and oblique fibres. The transverse–sagittal fibres form with the palmar plate, a closed cylindrical tube that surrounds the metacarpal head. Sagittal bands envelop the extensor digitorum

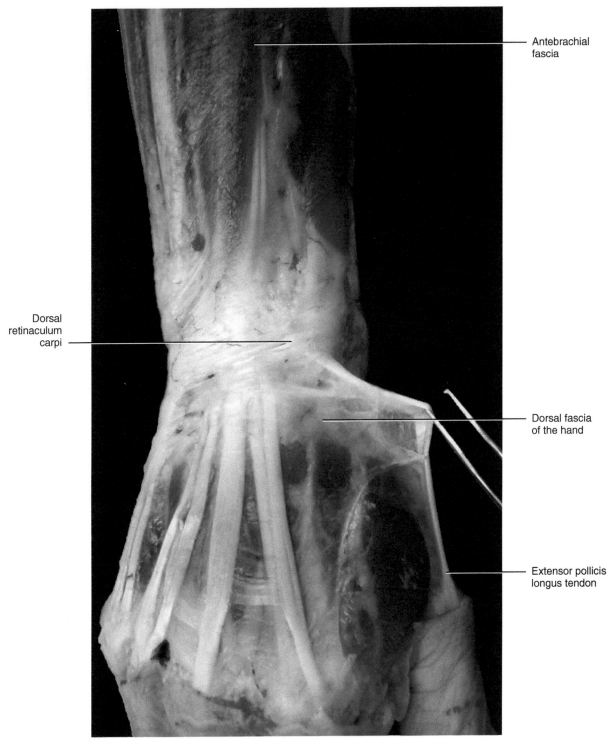

Antebrachial
fascia

Dorsal
retinaculum
carpi

Dorsal fascia
of the hand

Extensor pollicis
longus tendon

FIGURE 7.61 Posterior view of the hand. The extensor pollicis longus tendon is lifted to show that it is enveloped by the dorsal fascia of the hand.

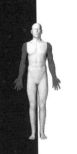

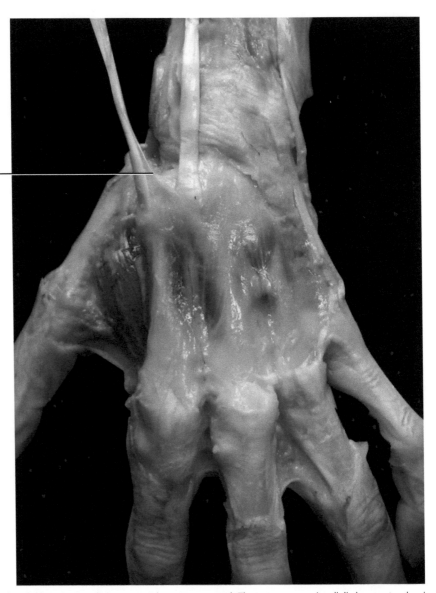

Myofascial
expansion of the
extensor
carpi radialis
longus tendon

FIGURE 7.62 Posterior view of the hand. The extensor digitorum tendons are removed. The extensor carpi radialis longus tendon is stretched to show its myofascial expansion into the deep lamina of the dorsal fascia of the hand.

tendons and the superficial interosseous tendons on both sides. The oblique fibres form the triangular lamina distal to the sagittal band. Any discussion of the role of these retinacular structures must note that they are only part of a tissue complex that meets a variety of functional demands. This three-dimensional complex may be considered a fibrous skeleton designed to assist in the hand's mechanical functions. Landsmeer (Bendz 1985) demonstrated that the oblique ligaments play an important role in synchronizing the movements of the two distal phalanges and they initiate extension of the maximally flexed distal phalanx.

References

Abu-Hijleh, M.F., Roshier, A.L., Al-Shboul, Q., Dharap, A.S., Harris, P.F., 2006. The membranous layer of superficial fascia: Evidence for its widespread distribution in the body. Surg. Radiol. Anat. 28 (6), 606–619.

Alvarez-Nemegyei, J., Canoso, J.J., 2004. Evidence-based soft tissue rheumatology: Epicondylitis and hand stenosing tendinopathy. J. Clin. Rheumatol. 10 (1), 33–40.

Bektas, U., Ay, S., Yilmaz, C., Tekdemir, I., Elhan, A., 2003. Spinoglenoid septum: A new anatomic finding. J. Shoulder Elbow Surg. 12 (5), 491–492.

Belzile, E., Cloutier, D., 2001. Entrapment of the lateral antebrachial cutaneous nerve exiting through the forearm fascia. J. Hand Surg. Am 26 (1), 64–67.

Bendz, P., 1985. The functional significance of the oblique retinacular ligament of Landsmeer. A review and new proposals. J. Hand Surg. Br 10 (1), 25–29.

Bidic, S.M., Hatef, D.A., Rohrich, R.J., 2010. Dorsal hand anatomy relevant to volumetric rejuvenation. Plast. Reconstr. Surg. 126 (1), 163–168.

Bolté, R., Martin, C.R., 1935. Sur quelques faisceaux tenseurs des aponévroses. Ann. Anat. Pathol. 12, 1–8.

Busquet, L., 1995. Les Chaînes Musculaires, Tome II, Frison Roche, Paris.

Butler, D.S., 1991. Mobilisation of the Nervous System, first edition. Churchill Livingstone, Melbourne, Australia.

Cabrera, J.M., McCue, F.C., 1986. Nonosseous athletic injuries of the elbow, forearm and hand. Clin. Sports Med. 5 (4), 681–700.

Chafik, D., Galatz, L.M., Keener, J.D., Kim, H.M., Yamaguchi, K., 2012. Teres minor muscle and related anatomy. J. Shoulder Elbow Surg. 22 (1), 108–114.

Davidson, J.J., Bassett, F.H., 3rd., Nunley, J.A., 1998. Musculocutaneous nerve entrapment revisited. J. Shoulder Elbow Surg. 7 (3), 250–255.

Duparc, F., Coquerel, D., Ozeel, J., Noyon, M., Gerometta, A., Michot, C., 2010. Anatomical basis of the suprascapular nerve entrapment, and clinical relevance of the supraspinatus fascia. Surg. Radiol. Anat. 32 (2), 277–284.

Fourie, W.J., Robb, K.A., 2009. Physiotherapy management of axillary web syndrome following breast cancer treatment: Discussing the use of soft tissue techniques. Physiotherapy 95 (4), 314–320.

Friend, J., Francis, S., McCulloch, J., Ecker, J., Breidahl, W., McMenamin, P., 2010. Teres minor innervation in the context of isolated muscle atrophy. Surg. Radiol. Anat. 32 (3), 243–249.

Gleason, P.D., Beall, D.P., Sanders, T.G., et al., 2006. The transverse humeral ligament: A separate anatomical structure or a continuation of the osseous attachment of the rotator cuff? Am. J. Sports Med. 34 (4), 72–77.

Kanaya, K., Wada, T., Isogai, S., 2002. Variations in insertion of the abductor digiti minimi: An anatomic study. J. Hand Surg. Am 27 (2), 325–328.

Keener, J.D., Chafik, D., Kim, H.M., Galatz, L.M., Yamaguchi, K., 2010. Insertional anatomy of the triceps brachii tendon. J. Shoulder Elbow Surg. 19 (3), 399–405.

Langevin, H.M., 2006. Connective tissue: a body-wide signalling network? Med. Hypotheses 66 (6), 1074–1077.

Langevin, H.M., Yandow, J.A., 2002. Relationship of acupuncture points and meridians to connective tissue planes. Anat. Rec. 269 (6), 257–265.

Lebarbier, A., 1980. Principes élémentaires d'acupuncture, Maisonneuve éd.

Legueu, F., Juvara, E., 1892. Des aponévroses de la paume de la main. Bull Soc. Anat. Paris. 67 (5), 383–400.

Lester, B., Jeong, G.K., Weiland, A.J., Wickiewicz, T.L., 1999. Quadrilateral space syndrome: diagnosis, pathology, and treatment. Am. J. Orthop. 28 (12), 718–725.

Ling, M.Z., Kumar, V.P., 2009. Myofascial compartments of the hand in relation to compartment syndrome: A cadaveric study. Plast. Reconstr. Surg. 123 (2), 613–616.

Lockwood, T., 1995. Brachioplasty with superficial fascial system suspension – variation of the subcutaneous tissue with aging. Plast. Reconstr. Surg. 96 (4), 912–920.

Macchi, V., Tiengo, C., Porzionato, A., et al., 2014. The cubital tunnel: a radiologic and histotopographic study. J. Anat. 225 (2), 262–269.

Myers, T.W., 2001. Anatomy Trains. Churchill Livingstone, Oxford, pp. 171–194.

Nakajima, M., Ono, N., Kojima, T., Kusunose, K., 2009. Ulnar entrapment neuropathy along the medial intermuscular septum in the midarm. Muscle Nerve 39 (5), 707–710.

Nirschl, R.P., Ashman, E.S., 2003. Elbow tendinopathy: tennis elbow. Clin. Sports Med. 22 (4), 813–836.

Papa, J.A., 2012. Two cases of work-related lateral epicondylopathy treated with Graston Technique® and conservative rehabilitation. J. Can. Chiropr. Assoc. 56 (3), 192–200.

Pecina, M.M., Krmpotic-Nemanic, J., Markiewitz, A.D., 1997. Tunnel Syndromes, second ed. CRC Press, Boca Raton, pp. 57–59.

Platzer, W., 1978. Locomotor system. In: Kahle, W., Leonhardt, H., Platzer, W. (Eds.), Color Atlas and Textbook of Human Anatomy, first ed. Georg Thieme Publishers, Stuttgart, pp. 148–164.

Rayan, G.M., Murray, D., Chung, K.W., Rohrer, M., 1997. The extensor retinacular system at the metacarpophalangeal joint: Anatomical and histological study. J. Hand Surg. Br 22 (5), 585–590.

Rispoli, D.M., Athwal, G.S., Sperling, J.W., Cofield, R.H., 2009. The anatomy of the deltoid insertion. J. Shoulder Elbow Surg. 18 (3), 386–390.

Shahnavaz, A., Sader, C., Henry, E., et al., 2010. Double fat plane of the radial forearm free flap and its implications for the microvascular surgeon. J. Otolaryngol. Head. Neck. Surg. 39 (3), 288–291.

Singer, E., 1935. Fasciae of the human body and their relations to the organs they envelop. Williams & Wilkinns Company, Baltimore, pp. 19–21.

Stecco, C., Macchi, V., Lancerotto, L., Tiengo, C., Porzionato, A., De Caro, R., 2010. Comparison of transverse carpal ligament and flexor retinaculum terminology for the wrist. J. Hand Surg. Am 35 (5), 746–753.

Stecco, C., Porzionato, A., Macchi, V., et al., 2008. The expansions of the pectoral girdle muscles onto the brachial fascia: morphological aspects and spatial disposition. Cells Tissues Organs 188 (3), 320–329.

Stecco, L., 1996. La Manipolazione Neuroconnettivale. Marrapese, Roma, pp. 45–62.

Tao, K.Z., Chen, E.Y., Ji, R.M., Dang, R.S., 2000. Anatomical study on arteries of fasciae in the forearm fasciocutaneous flap. Clin. Anat. 13 (1), 1–5.

Travell, J., Simons, D.G., 1983. Myofascial pain and dysfunction. The trigger point manual. Williams & Wilkins, Baltimore, pp. 195–505.

Tubbs, R.S., Apaydin, N., Uz, A., et al., 2009. Anatomy of the lateral intermuscular septum of the arm and its relationships to the radial nerve and its proximal branches. J. Neurosurg. 111 (2), 336–339.

Tubbs, R.S., Deep, A., Shoja, M.M., Mortazavi, M.M., Loukas, M., Cohen-Gadol, A.A., 2011. The arcade of Struthers: An anatomical study with potential neurosurgical significance. Surg. Neurol. Int. 184 (2), 1–10.

Van der Wall, J., 2009. The architecture of the connective tissue in the musculoskeletal system – an often overlooked functional parameter as to proprioception in the locomotor apparatus. In: Huijing, P.A., et al. (Eds.), Fascia Research II. Second International Fascia Research Congress, Elsevier Munich, pp. 21–35.

Wilgis, E.F., Murphy, R., 1986. The significance of longitudinal excursion in peripheral nerves. Hand Clin. 2 (4), 761–766.

Windisch, G., Tesch, N.P., Grechenig, W., Peicha, G., 2006. The triceps brachii muscle and its insertion on the olecranon. Med. Sci. Monit. 12 (8), BR290–BR294.

Bibliography

Assmus, H., Antoniadis, G., Bischoff, C., et al., 2011. Cubital tunnel syndrome: A review and management guidelines. Cent. Eur. Neurosurg. 72 (2), 90–98.

Ay, S., Akinci, M., Sayin, M., Bektas, U., Tekdemir, I., Elhan, A., 2007. The axillary sheath and single-injection axillary block. Clin. Anat. 20 (1), 57–63.

Benninghoff, A., Goerttler, K., 1978. Lehrbuch der Anatomie des Menschen, second ed. Urban & Schwarzenberg, München-Berlin-Wien, pp. 475–477.

Bojsen Moller, F., Schmidt, L., 1974. The palmar aponeurosis and the central spaces of the hand. J. Anat. 117 (1), 55–68.

Briggs, C.A., Elliott, B.G., 1985. Lateral epicondylitis. A review of structures associated with tennis elbow. Anat. Clin. 7 (3), 149–153.

Chiarugi, G., Bucciante, L., 1975. Istituzioni di Anatomia del l'uomo, eleventh ed. Vallardi-Piccin, Padova, pp. 596–599.

Colas, F., Nevoux, J., Gagey, O., 2004. The subscapular and subcoracoid bursae: Descriptive and functional anatomy. J. Shoulder Elbow Surg. 13 (4), 454–458.

Hammer, W.I., 2007. Functional Soft-Tissue Examination and Treatment by Manual Methods, third ed. Jones & Bartlett, Sudbury, MA, pp. 163–211.

Holland, A.J., McGrouther, D.A., 1997. Dupuytren's disease and the relationship between the transverse and longitudinal fibers of the palmar fascia: A dissection study. Clin. Anat. 10 (2), 97–103.

Jelev, L., Surchev, L., 2007. Study of variant anatomical structures (bony canals, fibrous bands, and muscles) in relation to potential supraclavicular nerve entrapment. Clin. Anat. 20 (3), 278–285.

Johson, R.K., Spinner, M., Shrewsbury, M.M., 1979. Median nerve entrapment syndrome in th proximal forearm. J. Hand Surg. Am 4 (1), 48–51.

Landsmeer, J.M., 1949. The anatomy of the dorsal aponeurosis of the human finger and its functional significance. Anat. Rec. 104 (1), 31–44.

Marshall, R., 2001. Living Anatomy: Structure as a Mirror of Function. Melbourne University Press, Melbourne, pp. 274–275.

Martin, S.D., Warren, R.F., Martin, T.L., Kennedy, K., O'Brien, S.J., Wickiewicz, T.L., 1997. Suprascapular neuropathy. Results of non-operative treatment. J. Bone Joint Surg. Am. 79 (8), 1159–1165.

Millesi, H., Schmidhammer, R., 2006. Fascial spaces and recurrent surgery for thoracic outlet syndrome. Handchir. Mikrochir. Plast. Chir. 38 (1), 14–19.

Palmieri, G., Panu, R., Asole, A., Farina, V., Sanna, L., Gabbi, C., 1986. Macroscopic organization and sensitive innervation of the tendinous intersection and the lacertus fibrosus of the biceps brachii muscle in the ass and horse. Arch. Anat. Histol. Embryol. 69, 73–82.

Poirier, P., Charpy, A., 1911. Traité d'Anatomie Humaine. Masson, Paris, pp. 730–733.

Rouvière, H., Delmas, A., 2002. Anatomie humaine, vol. 3, fifteenth ed. Masson, Paris, pp. 92–103.

Sappey, P.C., 1863. Traité d'Anatomie Descriptive. Masson, Paris, p. 62.

Seitz, W.H. Jr., Matsuoka, H., McAdoo, J., Sherman, G., Stickney, D.P., 2007. Acute compression of the median nerve at the elbow by the lacertus fibrosus. J. Shoulder Elbow Surg. 16 (1), 91–94.

Spinner, M., Spinner, R.J., 1998. Management of nerve compression lesions of the upper extremity. In: Omer, G.E., Spinner, M., Van Beek, A.L. (Eds.), Managemen of Peripheral Nerve Problems, second ed. WB Saunders, Philadelphia, pp. 501–533.

Standring, S., Ellis, H., Healy, J., Johnson, D., Williams, A., 2005. Gray's Anatomy, thirty-ninth ed. Churchill Livingstone, London, pp. 851–852.

Stecco, A., Macchi, V., Stecco, C., et al., 2009. Anatomical study of myofascial continuity in the anterior region of the upper limb. J. Bodyw. Mov. Ther. 13 (1), 53–62.

Stecco, C., Gagey, O., Belloni, A., et al., 2007. Anatomy of the deep fascia of the upper limb. Second part : study of innervation. Morphologie 91 (292), 38–43.

Stecco, C., Gagey, O., Macchi, V., et al., 2007. Tendinous muscular insertions onto the deep fascia of the upper limb. First part: anatomical study. Morphologie 91 (292), 29–37.

Stecco, C., Lancerotto, L., Porzionato, A., et al., 2009. The palmaris longus muscle and its relations with the antebrachial fascia and the palmar aponeurosis. Clin. Anat. 22 (2), 221–229.

Stecco, C., Porzionato, A., Macchi, V., et al., 2006. Histological characteristics of the deep fascia of the upper limb. Ital. J. Anat. Embryol. 111 (2), 105–110.

Testut, J.L., Jacob, O., 1905. Précis d'anatomie topographique avec applications medico-chirurgicales, vol. 3. Gaston Doin et Cie, Paris, p. 302.

Tetro, A.M., Evanoff, B.A., Hollstien, S.B., Gelberman, R.H., 1998. A new provocative test for carpal tunnel syndrome: assessment of wrist flexion and nerve compression. J. Bone Joint Surg. Br. 80 (3), 493–498.

Thompson, G.E., Rorie, D.K., 1983. Functional anatomy of the brachial plexus sheaths. Anesthesiology 59 (2), 117–122.

Williams, G.R., Jr., Shakil, M., Klimkiewicz, J., Iannotti, J.P., 1999. Anatomy of the scapulothoracic articulation. Clin. Orthop. Relat. Res. (359), 237–246.

Yazar, F., Kirici, Y., Oran, H., 1998. Accessory insertions of the pectoralis major muscle to the brachial fascia: A case report. Kaibogeku. Zassli. 73 (6), 637–639.

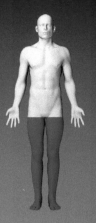

8

Fasciae of the Lower Limb

Superficial Fascia of the Lower Limb

The superficial fascia is present throughout the lower limb as a thin layer of fibroelastic tissue (Figs 8.1 and 8.2). In the gluteal region it is laden with fat, especially in females. It becomes tough and elastic over the tuberosity of the ischium (Fig. 8.3). Around the anus, the superficial fascia contains some muscular fibres that constitute the external anal sphincter. There are muscle fibres inside the superficial fascia in other regions of the lower limb, but they are not organized for specific functions like the anal fibres. Cichowitz et al (2009), for instance, identified some muscular fibres in the subcutaneous tissue of the plantar aspect of the foot.

The superficial fascia adheres to the deep fascia around the joints, over the tibial crest, along the midline of the anterior region of the thigh and over the septum between the gastrocnemii muscles of the leg. In front of the knee, the superficial fascia partially adheres to the deep fascia, creating a virtual space: the prepatellar bursa (Fig. 8.4). Dye et al (2003) analysed the specific relationship between the prepatellar bursa and the fascial layers and found a trilaminar, prepatellar bursa. This bursa is composed of a prepatellar subcutaneous bursa (placed between the skin and the superficial fascia) a prepatellar subfascial bursa (placed between the superficial and deep fasciae) and a prepatellar subaponeurotic bursa (placed between the deep fascia and the quadriceps tendon). In addition, Canoso et al (1983) found no free fluid within any prepatellar bursae, and thus a true synovial lining was not identified. In fact, the knee bursa may be considered a fascial specialization, where the production of hyaluronan (HA) is due to the fasciacytes, rather than a specific anatomical entity with a synovial membrane. This is similar to the bursa at the back of the calcaneus (subcutaneous calcaneal bursa) and over the sacrum (Fig. 8.5). Although these bursae normally contain very little fluid, they can become irritated and fill with fluid.

All the main superficial vessels and nerves flow inside the superficial fascia (Figs 8.6 and 8.7). Caggiati (2000) was the first to describe the long saphenous vein as being enveloped by a fascial layer, which keeps the venous walls open and protects the vessels. He did not identify this 'saphenous fascia' as the superficial fascia. In our dissection we discovered that all the main

superficial vessels and nerves are enveloped by superficial fascia. It is the superficial fascia that forms specific compartments; these are clearly circumscribed and follow the vessels and nerves for their entire course within the subcutaneous tissue. The superficial fascia containing the saphenous veins is connected with the deep fascia by the retinaculum cutis profundus, making it easy to divide the saphenous vein compartment from the deep muscular fascia, except where we have perforantes veins. The saphenous tributaries run in a more superficial plane of the hypodermis, following the various septa of the superficial adipose tissue (SAT), but they are devoid of any fascial sheathing.

Caggiati (2000) described the specific relationship of the long saphenous vein within its fascial compartment:

Stereomicroscopy of cross-sectioned specimens evidences two thick strands originating from the outer adventitia of the long saphenous vein and anchoring it to the opposite faces of the compartment. These strands are also easily recognized by ultrasonography because of their hyperechogenicity. Furthermore, they are composed of interwoven connective fibres emerging directly from the saphenous adventitia. The evaluation of serially sectioned specimens reveals that these strands form two continuous laminae. Such a double-laminar ligament can also be evidenced during anatomic or surgical preparations, especially if care is taken to preserve the planar arrangement of the connective framework of the hypodermis.

Schweighofer et al (2010) described the same structure for the small saphenous vein. This confirms our findings that all the main superficial veins of the lower limbs are enveloped (for their entire length) by a splitting of the superficial fascia.

The SAT is present and relatively thick throughout the lower limbs. Over the tibial crest and in the distal part of the ankle, however, it is thinner. There are numerous fat pads located on the bottom of the foot (Fig. 8.8). These fat pads act as 'cushions' or 'shock absorbers'. The calcaneal fat pad is the largest fat pad in the foot and is located in the heel directly below the calcaneus. This fat pad is a complex structure of adipose and connective tissue. There are strong vertical, fibrous septa that connect the heel and plantar fascia with the

Text continued on p. 297

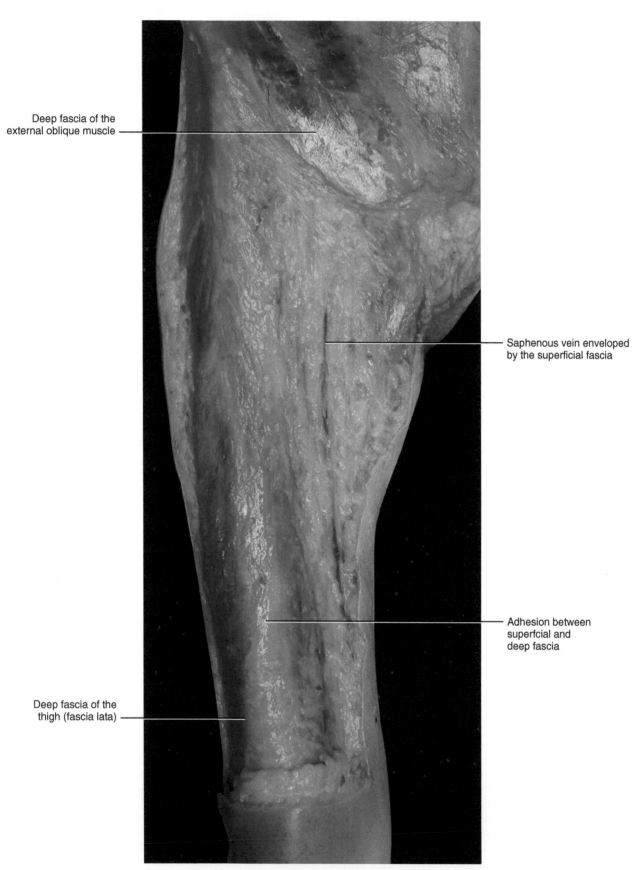

Deep fascia of the
external oblique muscle

Saphenous vein enveloped
by the superficial fascia

Adhesion between
superfcial and
deep fascia

Deep fascia of the
thigh (fascia lata)

FIGURE 8.1 Anterior region of the thigh. The superficial fascia adheres firmly to the deep fascia along the midline and medial part of the thigh, while it can be easily separated from the deep fascia in the lateral portion of the thigh.

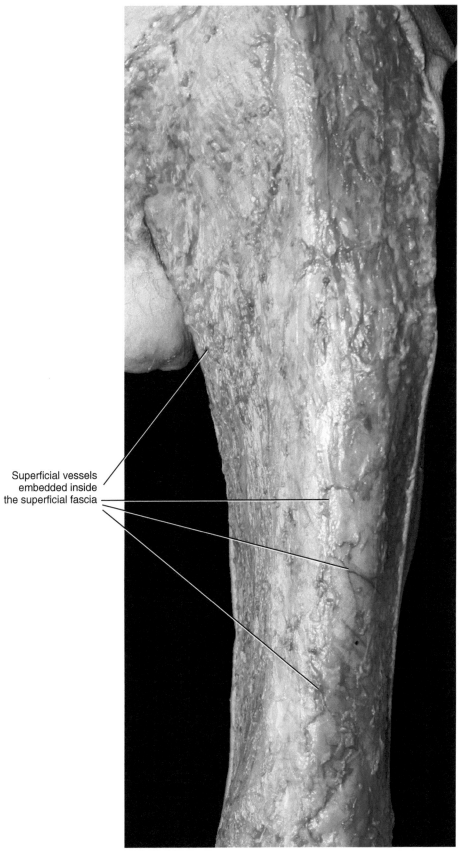

Superficial vessels embedded inside the superficial fascia

FIGURE 8.2 Superficial fascia of the anterior region of the thigh. The SAT is removed and the retinacula cutis superficialis (skin ligaments) were cut to expose the superficial fascia.

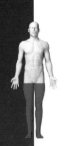

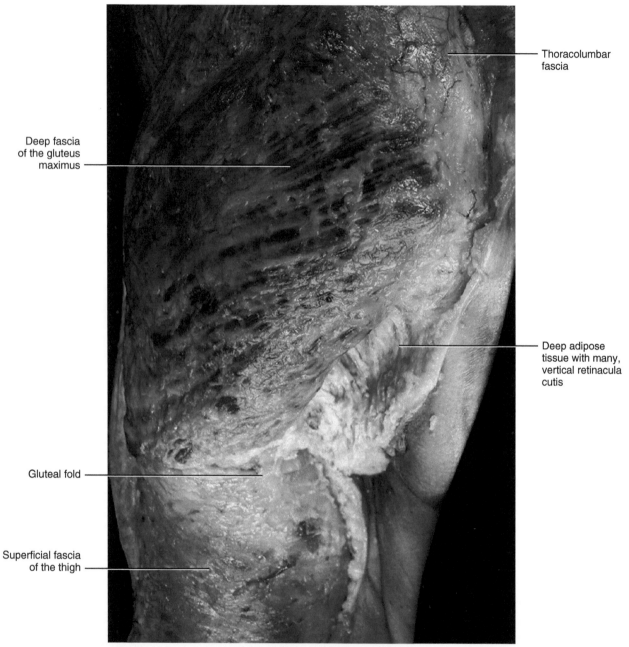

Thoracolumbar fascia

Deep fascia of the gluteus maximus

Deep adipose tissue with many, vertical retinacula cutis

Gluteal fold

Superficial fascia of the thigh

FIGURE 8.3 The gluteal region. Along the line running from the sacrum to the femur femoral trochanter, there are many superficial and deep retinacula cutis. They firmly connect the deep fascia, superficial fascia and skin. This connection circumscribes the distal margin of the gluteal compartment (gluteal fold).

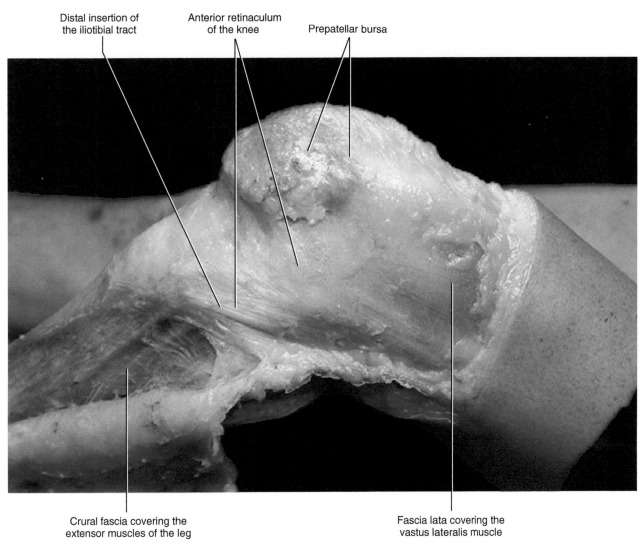

Distal insertion of
the iliotibial tract

Anterior retinaculum
of the knee

Prepatellar bursa

Crural fascia covering the
extensor muscles of the leg

Fascia lata covering the
vastus lateralis muscle

FIGURE 8.4 Prepatellar bursa between the superficial and deep fascia. The bursa was injected with blue resin before the dissection to show it more clearly.

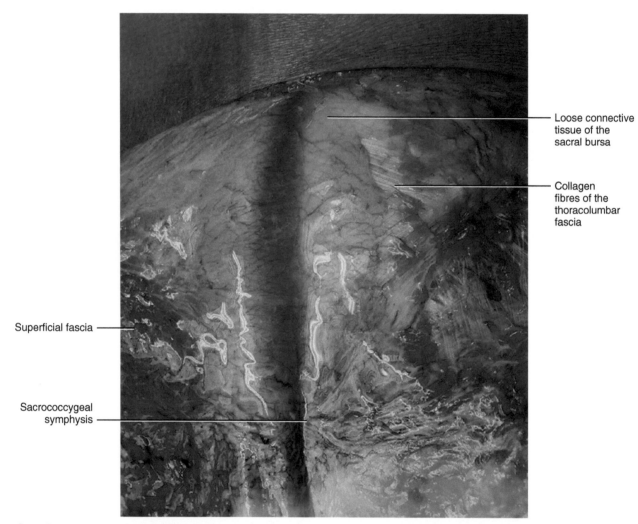

Loose connective
tissue of the
sacral bursa

Collagen
fibres of the
thoracolumbar
fascia

Superficial fascia

Sacrococcygeal
symphysis

FIGURE 8.5 Loose connective tissue between the superficial fascia and the deep fascia over the proximal portion of the sacrum. In appearance, it is similar to a subcutaneous bursa (sacral bursa).

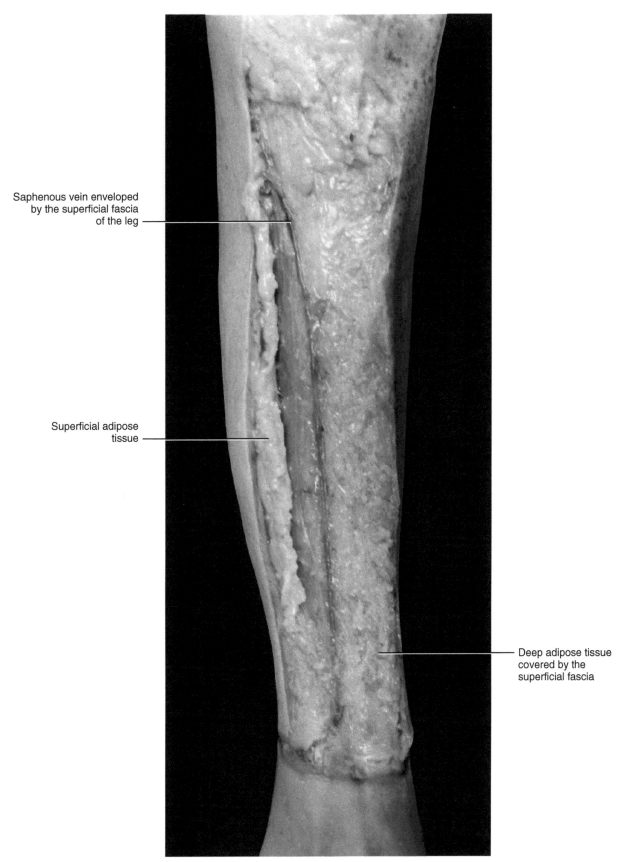

Saphenous vein enveloped
by the superficial fascia
of the leg

Superficial adipose
tissue

Deep adipose tissue
covered by the
superficial fascia

FIGURE 8.6 Superficial fascia of the medial region of the leg. The superficial fascia divides the SAT from the DAT. The saphenous vein is injected with resin to better highlight it.

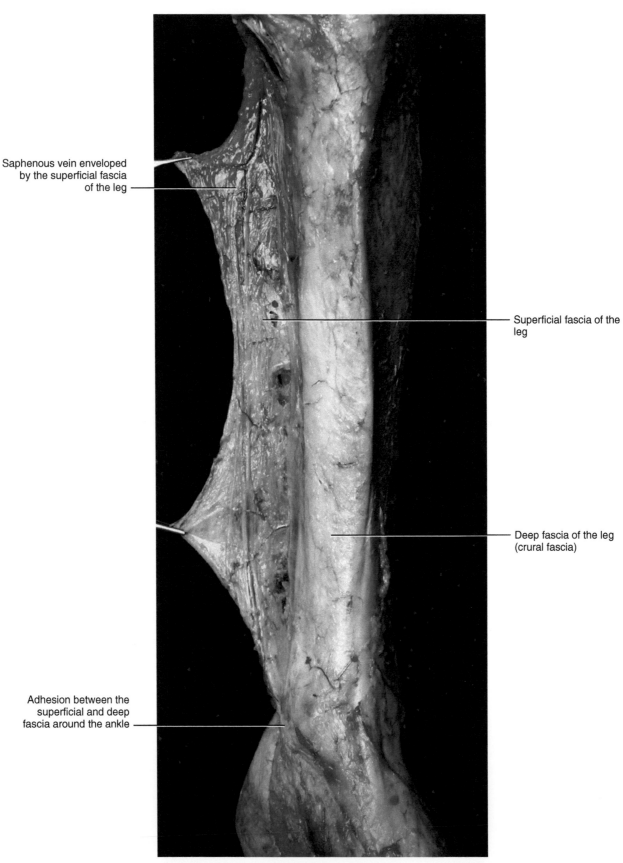

Saphenous vein enveloped
by the superficial fascia
of the leg

Superficial fascia of the
leg

Deep fascia of the leg
(crural fascia)

Adhesion between the
superficial and deep
fascia around the ankle

FIGURE 8.7 Superficial and deep fasciae of the medial region of the leg. The superficial fascia is detached from the deep fascia and lifted medially. The DAT in this subject is scarce but sufficient to permit gliding between the two fascial layers. The saphenous vein is embedded in the superficial fascia.

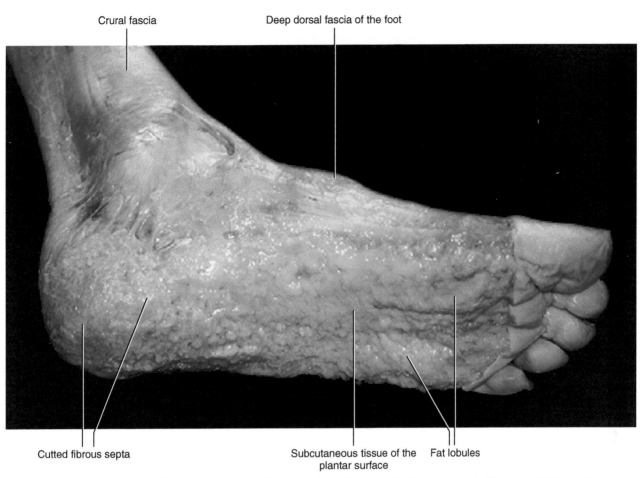

Crural fascia   Deep dorsal fascia of the foot

Cutted fibrous septa   Subcutaneous tissue of the   Fat lobules
plantar surface

FIGURE 8.8 Subcutaneous adipose tissue of the plantar surface of the foot. The plantar fascia is composed of the superficial fascia that adheres to the deep fascia. Therefore, only the SAT is present in the plantar surface and consists of many vertical and strong retinacula cutis that firmly connect the plantar fascia with the skin. The fatty tissue (yellow elements) is placed among these septa (white elements), forming a honeycomb-like structure. This arrangement gives this zone its specific mechanical features.

The anatomical relationships between the saphenous veins and the superficial fascia may have an important role, both in daily clinical practice and in the pathophysiology of varicose disease. First, the tension of the superficial fascia strongly influences the saphenous vein calibre and consequently modulates the blood flow within it. Secondly, the superficial fascia may prevent the saphenous vein from excessive pathological dilatation, acting as a sort of mechanical shield. These anatomical findings could also explain why greater dilatation and tortuosity occur in the saphenous tributaries in primary varicosis. Finally, the superficial fascia could be considered a main marker for the correct identification and stripping of the saphenous vein.

skin. Snow and Bohne (2006) identified two types of retinacula in the SAT of the foot: numerous, small retinacula originating from the plantar fascia and calcaneal tuberosity, and fewer, larger retinacula originating only from the calcaneus. Kimani (1984) demonstrated an abundance of elastic fibres in these retinacula, which suggests that the elastic fibres may modulate the distensibility of the subcutaneous tissues. For example, when subjected to compressive stress and the subsequent return to a normal resting tensile state. Collagen fibres strictly constrain the limit of distension of the subcutis as well as the dermis. They tether the skin to the plantar aponeurosis. These septa divide the subcutaneous fat tissue into isolated compartments, each containing fat. This three-dimensional network of fibroelastic tissue and fat provides a strong anchoring of the skin to the underlying planes while at the same time optimizing its response to load. For example, it mitigates shock generated during the gait or running cycle and makes it possible to achieve a smooth distribution of pressure. The fat pads were found to contain

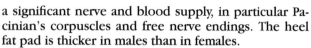

a significant nerve and blood supply, in particular Pacinian's corpuscles and free nerve endings. The heel fat pad is thicker in males than in females.

The deep adipose tissue varies in thickness in the lower limbs. It is almost absent around the sacrum, knee, tibial crest and ankle (Figs 8.9 and 8.10), causing adhesions between the superficial and deep fasciae. For this reason, these bony landmarks are always well palpable even in obese people.

Deep Fascia of the Lower Limb

The deep fascia of the lower limb appears as a strong, white lamina of connective tissue, with a mean thickness of 1 mm. This fascia is thinner only at the level of the anteromedial portion of the thigh, where it covers the adductor muscles (Figs 8.11 and 8.12). It becomes thicker around the knee and ankle, where it is reinforced by the retinacula, and in the lateral region of the thigh, where a longitudinal fibrous band (the iliotibial tract (ITT)) reinforces the fascia lata (Fig. 8.13). The deep fascia of the lower limb could be considered as a support stocking. It envelops the entire foot, leg and thigh as a unique fibrous layer, stretched proximally by the insertions of the pelvis (i.e gluteus maximus and tensor fascia lata muscles) and abdominal muscles external oblique, internal oblique and transversus abdominis. All of these muscles have myofascial insertions into the deep fascia of the lower limb.

Terminology for the deep fasciae of the lower limb varies according to location. In the thigh it is called the 'fascia lata', in the leg the 'crural fascia', in the foot the 'plantar fascia' and 'dorsal fascia of the foot'. All these are just topographical nomenclature, and do not identify defined boundaries of the deep fasciae.

The deep fascia is easily separable from the underlying muscle due to the presence of the epimysial fascia (or epimysium) of the underlying muscles and a thin layer of loose connective tissue, rich in hyaluronic acid, which separates the epimysium from the deep fascia. This loose connective tissue appears as a pliable, gel-like substance, and permits sliding of the muscles under the deep fascia. In some regions, for example in the distal part of the thigh and in the proximal part of the leg, the muscles are connected with the aponeurotic fascia by fibrous expansions or intermuscular septa. The intermuscular septa originate from the inner side of the aponeurotic fasciae and insert into bone. They divide the different muscles into specific compartments and also provide insertions for many muscular fibres.

The deep fasciae around the knee and ankle joints, along the tibial crest and around the heel all present specific adhesions to the deeper structures. In these areas, fascia continues into the periosteum of the bones. These points become areas of great stress concentration, representing the meeting point between hard and soft tissues. For this reason, the fasciae in these areas often assume features similar to the entheses of a tendon or ligament. Sometimes it is also possible to identify fibrocartilage metaplasia, as in the heel insertion of the plantar fascia.

Deep bursae may be present where there is a lot of friction, such as between the iliotibial tract and the lateral condyle of the femur, in the vicinity of the greater trochanter (Fig. 8.14) and between the heel and the Achilles tendon (retrocalcaneal bursa). Dunn et al (2003) and Woodley et al (2008) demonstrated that these deep bursae present many anatomical variations: varing in number, position, and histological appearance. These findings suggest that these bursae could be considered specializations of the deep fascia rather than true synovial structure. The number and form of deep bursae are probably greatly influenced by the amount of mechanical stress on each area. As previously noted, the fasciacytes could produce more HA when subjected to a chronic increase in friction. It is known that HA is a beneficial lubricant and, therefore, it is probable that the increase in HA will aid in reducing the chronic friction that might cause pain.

The deep fascia also forms sheaths for the large vessels and nerves, which protects them from the traction to which surrounding tissues are subjected (Figs 8.15 and 8.16). These fascial sheaths are formed by multiple layers of fibrous and loose connective tissues, and create a telescopic mechanism. If this mechanism is altered, a compressive syndrome could result.

Gluteal Fascia

The gluteal fascia encloses the gluteus maximus and tensor fascia lata muscles (Figs 8.17A–8.21). Over the

Text continued on p. 312

CLINICAL PEARL 8.2 GREATER TROCHANTERIC PAIN SYNDROME

Greater trochanteric pain syndrome (GTPS) is a term used to describe chronic pain overlying the lateral aspect of the hip. The prevalence is higher in women and patients with coexisting low-back pain, osteoarthritis, iliotibial tract (ITT) tenderness and obesity. Patients with greater trochanteric pain syndrome usually suffer from pain radiating to the posterolateral aspect of the thigh, paraesthesiae in the legs and tenderness over the ITT. Previously, the aetiology of the trochanteric pain syndrome was thought to be due to inflammation of the subgluteus maximus bursa (i.e. bursitis). Recently, MRI and ultrasound studies have shown that most cases of GTPS are due to damage of the nearby muscles or fasciae and an inflamed bursa is an uncommon cause (Silva et al 2008). Specifically we suggest that often the GTPS could be due to an excessive tension of the gluteus maximus muscle that compresses the bursa to the bone, and increases friction. The fascial connection among the thoracolumbar fascia, gluteus maximus muscle and ITT could easily explain the radiation of pain in the GTPS.

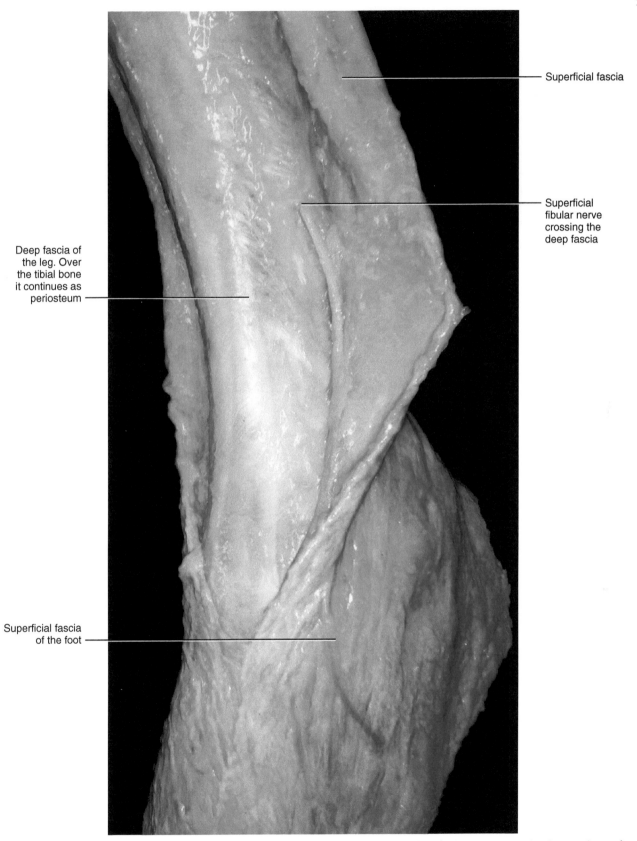

Superficial fascia

Superficial fibular nerve crossing the deep fascia

Deep fascia of the leg. Over the tibial bone it continues as periosteum

Superficial fascia of the foot

FIGURE 8.9 Anterolateral view of the leg and ankle. The superficial fascia is detached from the deep fascia. Loose connective tissue and some fat lobules are present between the two fascial layers. In this subject, the deep fascia is very fibrous.

Deep fascia of
the leg. Over
the tibial bone
it continues as
periosteum

Adhesion
between superficial
and deep fasciae
around the ankle

Superficial fascia
of the foot

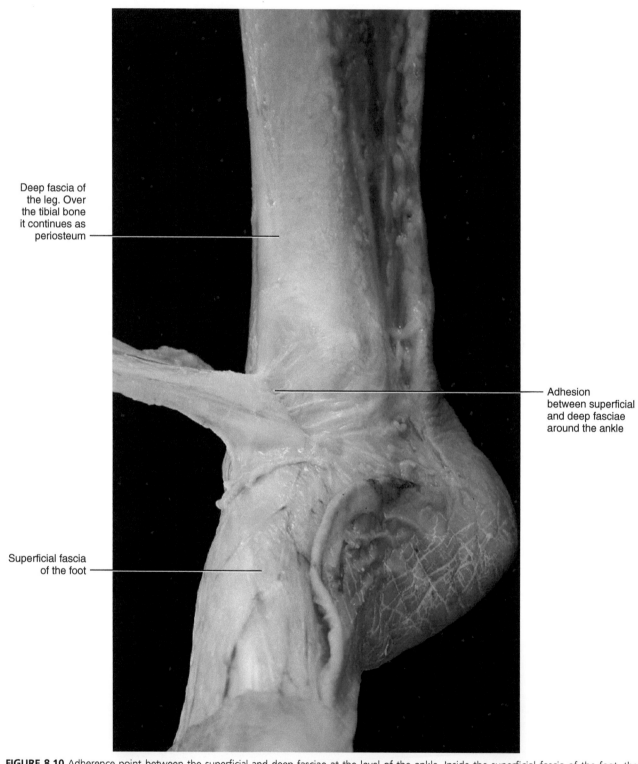

FIGURE 8.10 Adherence point between the superficial and deep fasciae at the level of the ankle. Inside the superficial fascia of the foot, the superficial vessels are evident (injected in red).

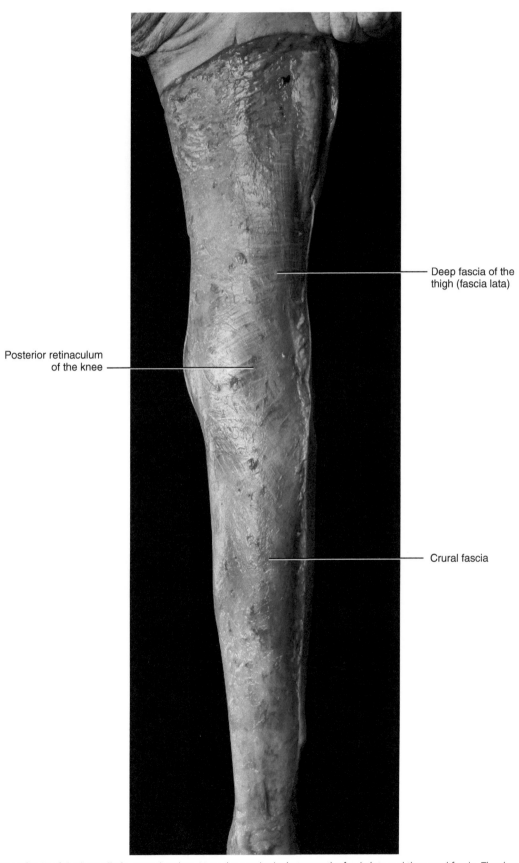

Deep fascia of the
thigh (fascia lata)

Posterior retinaculum
of the knee

Crural fascia

FIGURE 8.11 Deep fascia of the lower limb, posterior view. Note the continuity between the fascia lata and the crural fascia. The deep fascia is not a homogeneous structure. It is formed by numerous fibrous bundles with various directions, particularly evident in the popliteal region (posterior retinaculum of the knee).

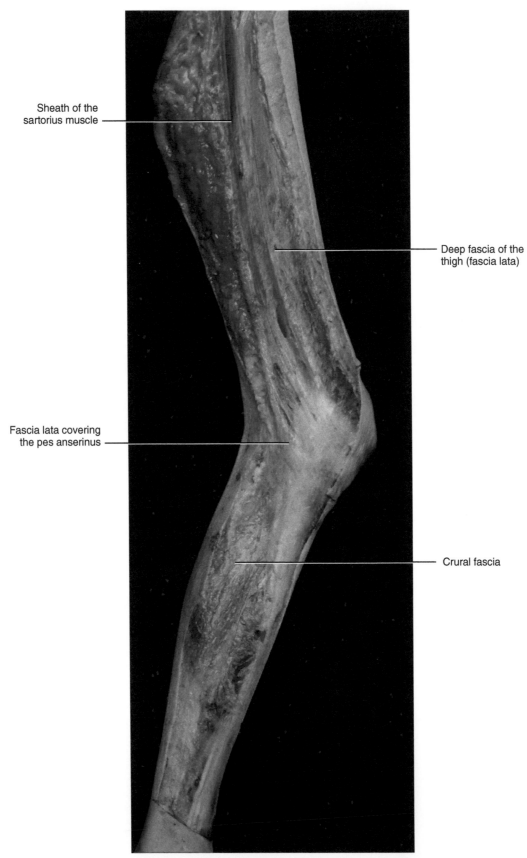

Sheath of the
sartorius muscle

Deep fascia of the
thigh (fascia lata)

Fascia lata covering
the pes anserinus

Crural fascia

FIGURE 8.12 Deep fascia of the lower limb, medial view. The sartorius sheath is continuous with the fascia lata, but at the same time it creates a specific compartment for the sartorius muscle. The crural fascia is stretched proximally by the myofascial expansions of the pes anserinus muscles.

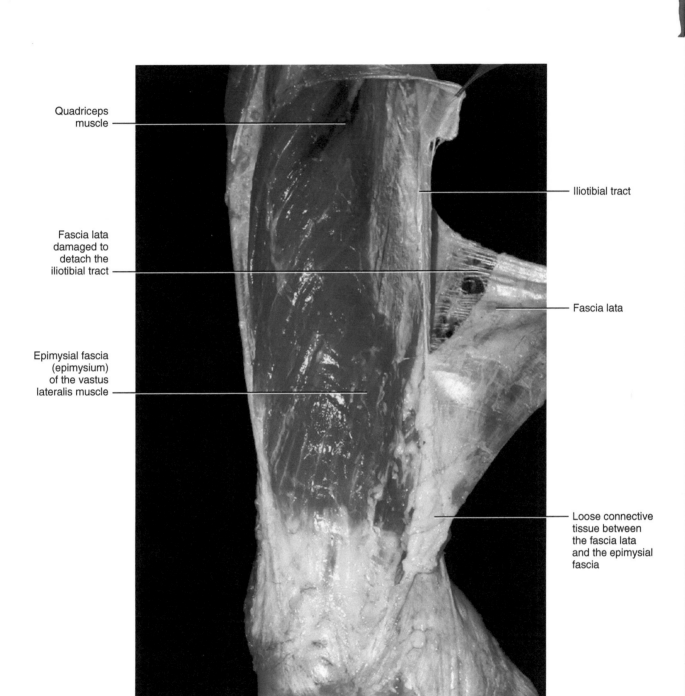

Quadriceps muscle

Iliotibial tract

Fascia lata damaged to detach the iliotibial tract

Fascia lata

Epimysial fascia (epimysium) of the vastus lateralis muscle

Loose connective tissue between the fascia lata and the epimysial fascia

FIGURE 8.13 Antero-lateral view of the left thigh. The aponeurotic fascia of the thigh (fascia lata) is lifted laterally to show the epimysial fascia of the quadriceps muscle. The fascia lata appears as a white fibrous layer very resistant to traction. The fascia lata is easily separated from the underlying muscle due to the presence of loose connective tissue between the fascia and epimysium of the quadriceps muscle. The loose connective tissue appears as a pliable, gel-like substance. In order to isolate the ITT, the fascia lata had to be damaged. The ITT is just a reinforcement of the fascia lata.

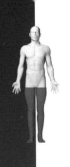

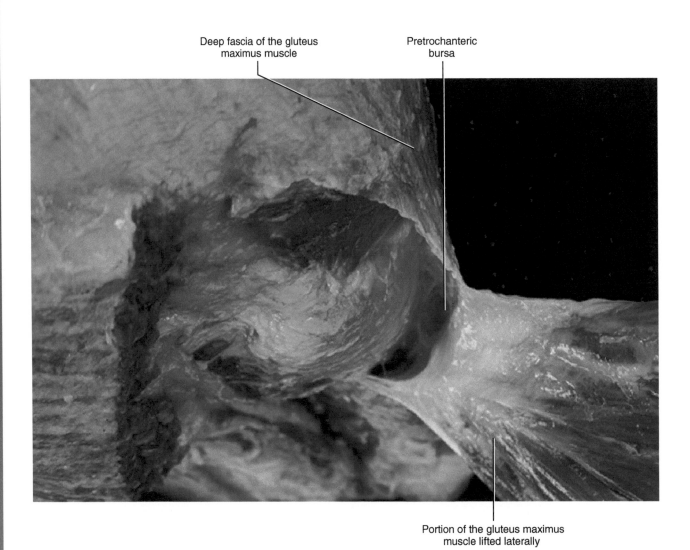

Deep fascia of the gluteus maximus muscle

Pretrochanteric bursa

Portion of the gluteus maximus muscle lifted laterally

FIGURE 8.14 Trochanteric bursa. This bursa is situated adjacent to the femur, between the insertion of the gluteus maximus and gluteus medius muscles into the greater trochanter of the femur and the femoral shaft. It works as a shock absorber and as a lubricant for the movement of the muscles adjacent to it.

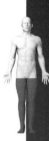

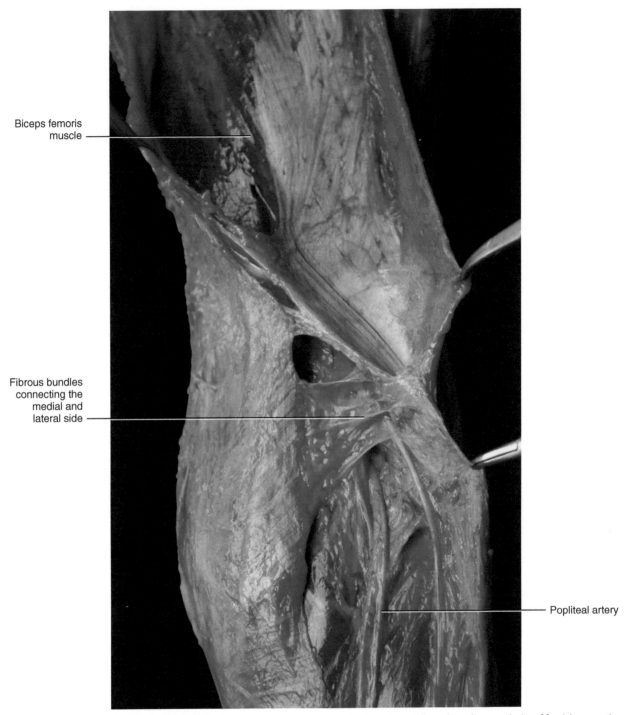

Biceps femoris muscle

Fibrous bundles connecting the medial and lateral side

Popliteal artery

FIGURE 8.15 Fascial network of the popliteal region. The fascia lata was cut and is tractioned medially to show the complexity of fascial connections. Some fibrous bundles connect the fasciae of the medial and lateral heads of the gastrocnemius muscle, and create a roof for the popliteal vessels. These bundles may cause a compression syndrome.

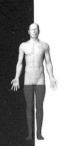

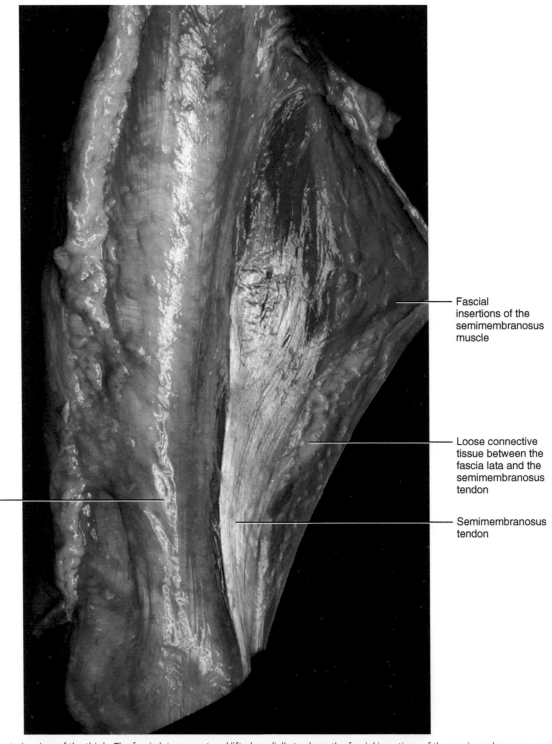

Fascial insertions of the semimembranosus muscle

Loose connective tissue between the fascia lata and the semimembranosus tendon

Semimembranosus tendon

Fascia lata covering the ischiocrural muscles

FIGURE 8.16 Posterior view of the thigh. The fascia lata was cut and lifted medially to show the fascial insertions of the semimembranosus muscle. Over the tendon, the fascia lata is free to glide due to the presence of loose connective tissue.

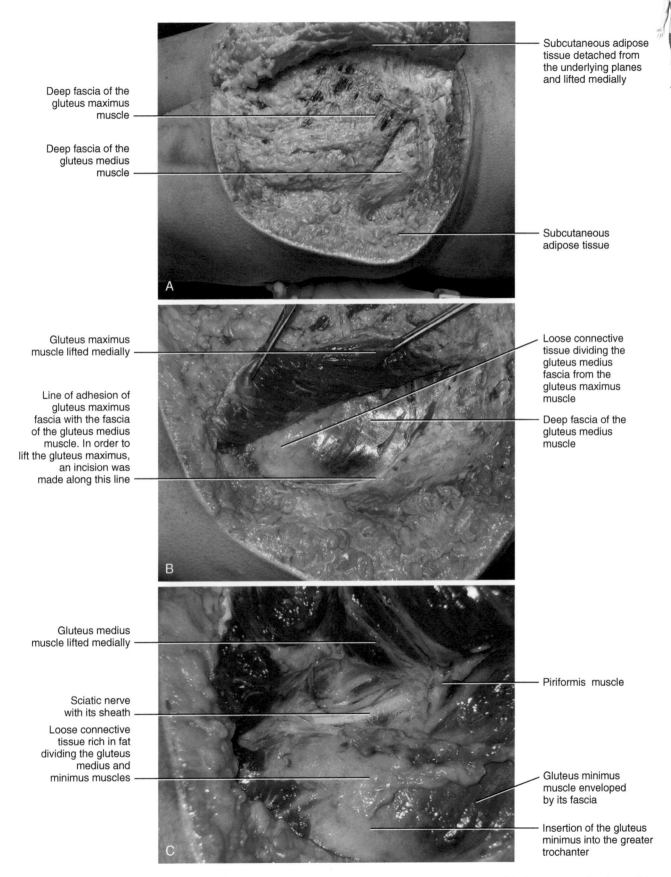

FIGURE 8.17 (A–C) Fasciomuscular planes of the gluteal region. The myofascial planes are partially separated by loose connective tissue. This permits the autonomous contraction of various muscles and stretching of their adjoining fascia, allowing correct proprioception of muscular tone.

Labels: Subcutaneous adipose tissue detached from the underlying planes and lifted medially; Deep fascia of the gluteus maximus muscle; Deep fascia of the gluteus medius muscle; Subcutaneous adipose tissue; Gluteus maximus muscle lifted medially; Line of adhesion of gluteus maximus fascia with the fascia of the gluteus medius muscle. In order to lift the gluteus maximus, an incision was made along this line; Loose connective tissue dividing the gluteus medius fascia from the gluteus maximus muscle; Deep fascia of the gluteus medius muscle; Gluteus medius muscle lifted medially; Sciatic nerve with its sheath; Loose connective tissue rich in fat dividing the gluteus medius and minimus muscles; Piriformis muscle; Gluteus minimus muscle enveloped by its fascia; Insertion of the gluteus minimus into the greater trochanter

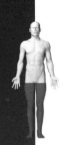

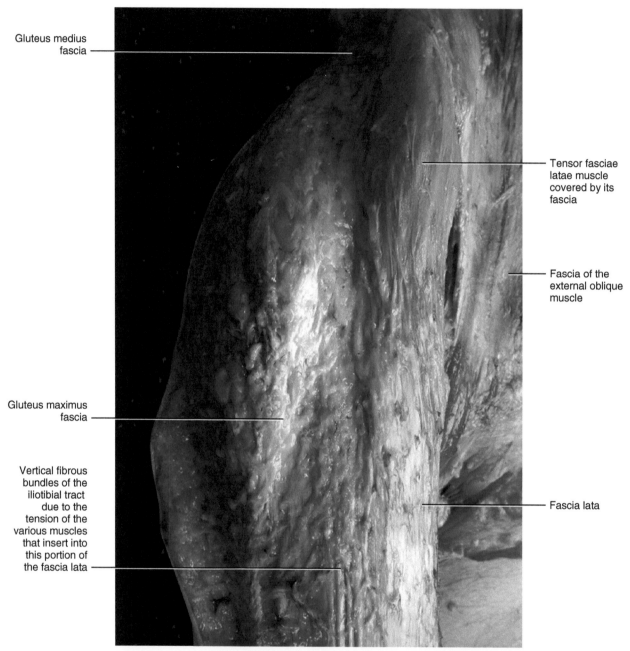

Gluteus medius fascia

Tensor fasciae latae muscle covered by its fascia

Fascia of the external oblique muscle

Gluteus maximus fascia

Fascia lata

Vertical fibrous bundles of the iliotibial tract due to the tension of the various muscles that insert into this portion of the fascia lata

FIGURE 8.18 Lateral view of the hip, with the lower limb adducted, to demonstrate the lines of forces inside the iliotibial tract (ITT). Note the continuity of the fasciae of gluteus maximus and medius and of the tensor fasciae latae muscle with the fascia lata. The ITT is a lateral reinforcement of the fascia lata created by the various muscular forces acting upon this portion of the fascia lata.

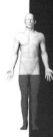

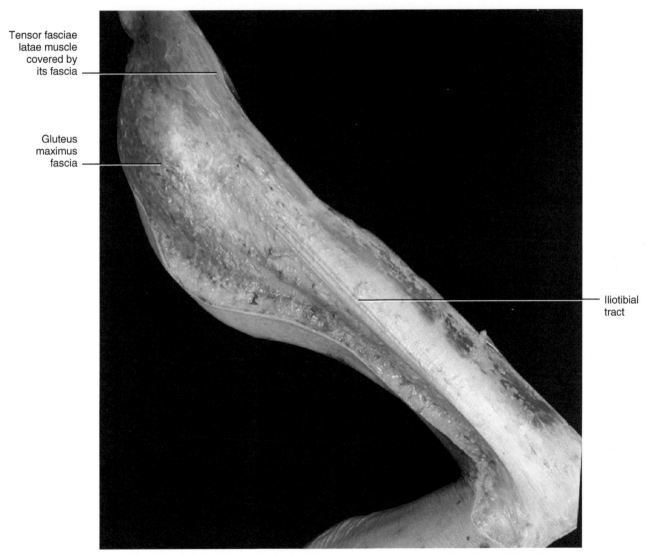

Tensor fasciae
latae muscle
covered by
its fascia

Gluteus
maximus
fascia

Iliotibial
tract

FIGURE 8.19 Lateral view of the thigh. The iliotibial tract is clearly visible along the lateral aspect of the thigh, but it is not possible to distinguish its medial and lateral border because it continues into the fascia lata, appearing just as its longitudinal reinforcement.

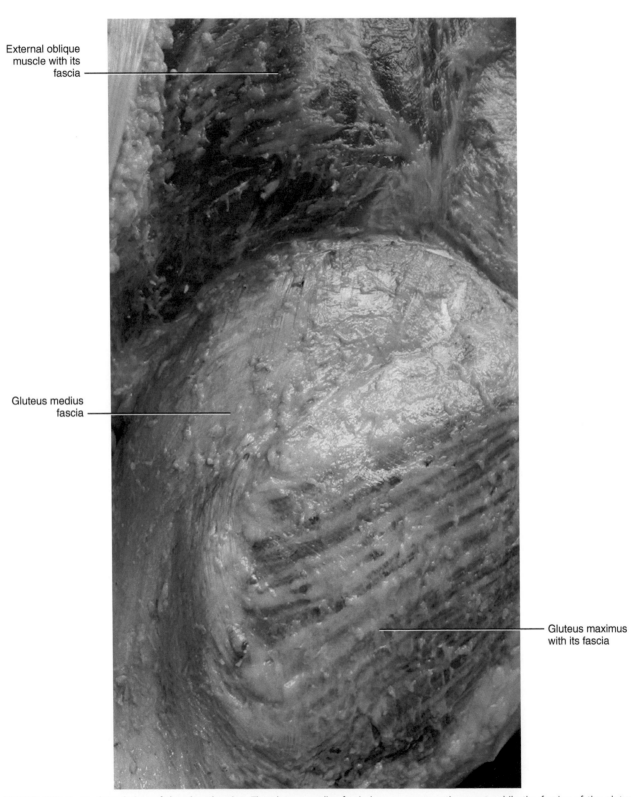

External oblique
muscle with its
fascia

Gluteus medius
fascia

Gluteus maximus
with its fascia

FIGURE 8.20 Posterolateral view of the gluteal region. The gluteus medius fascia has an aponeurotic aspect, while the fasciae of the gluteus maximus and external oblique muscles have epymisial features.

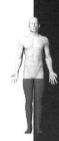

Insertions of the
gluteus maximus
muscle into the
fascia of the
gluteus medius

Superior gluteal
artery with
branches to the
gluteus maximus
muscle

Loose connective
tissue under the
gluteus maximus
muscle

Gluteus maximus
with its fascia

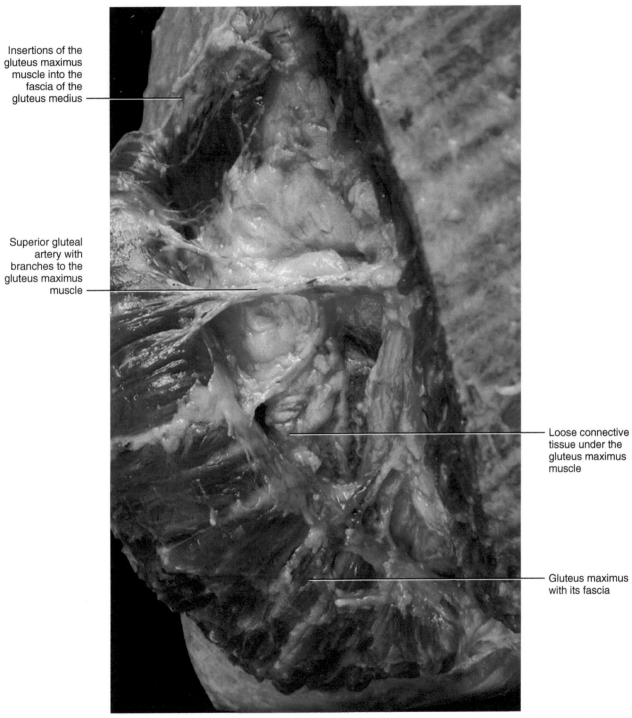

FIGURE 8.21 Posterior view of the gluteal region. The gluteus maximus was cut and lifted laterally to show the superior gluteal artery. Note the loose connective tissue rich in fat that creates a cushion around the artery, protecting it during muscular contraction.

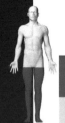

gluteus maximus this fascia is very thin and adheres to it by numerous intramuscular septa. There are also many muscular fibres originating from the inner side of this fascia. Such features are typical of an epimysial fascia and very different from those of the fascia lata (aponeurotic fascia). Between the gluteus medius and maximus, this fascia creates a perfect plane of gliding and permits the muscular fibres of these two muscles, in spite of their different orientations, to act autonomously. Laterally, the two layers of fascia enclosing the gluteus maximus muscle merge to pass over the gluteus medius muscle and then divide again to enclose the tensor fasciae latae muscle. Where the gluteus maximus does not cover the gluteus medius, this fascia becomes very thick and fibrous and has attachments from many muscular fibres of the gluteus medius. The tensor fasciae latae muscle is free to contract inside its compartment. Some loose connective tissue is present between this muscle and the deep fascia.

Proximally, the superficial layer of the gluteal fascia continues with the superficial layer of the posterior lamina of the thoracolumbar fascia, while its deep layer continues into the periosteum of the iliac crest. Distally, both layers continue with the fascia lata and the ITT, and become, together with the gluteus maximus muscle, one of the major proximal tensors of the fascia lata (Fig. 8.19). Medially, they adhere to the periostium of the sacrum and coccyx. Thus, the gluteal fascia and the gluteus maximus muscle connect the thoracolumbar fascia with the fascia lata. This arrangement is important for the coordination of the trunk and lower limb. The gluteal deep fascia is strongly connected to the overlying superficial fascia and then to the skin by many vertical septa. These septa become very strong at the level of the gluteal fold (Fig. 8.3).

Fascia of the Gluteus Medius Muscle

The fascia of the gluteus medius muscle is composed of a strongly adherent, thin connective tissue layer. This forms a perfect plane for gliding between the gluteus medius and maximus muscles. In addition, fat tissue is found between these two musculofascial planes. Distally, part of the gluteus medius fascia merges with the gluteus maximus fascia to form the iliotibial tract, and part continues to the periosteum of the femur. Proximally, it inserts into the iliac bone and, medially, it inserts into the sacrum. Where the gluteus maximus does not cover the gluteus medius, the gluteus medius fascia becomes thicker and more fibrous. On the inner aspect of the gluteus medius fascia many muscle fibres of the gluteus medius muscle have attachments.

Piriformis Fascia

The fascia of the piriformis consists of a very thin fibrous layer, which adheres firmly to the underlying muscle. It is attached medially to the front of the sacrum and the sides of the greater sciatic foramen. It extends laterally to cover the gluteus minimus muscle and finally merges with the periosteum of the iliac bone. The piriformis fascia is associated with, and ensheathes, the sacral nerves emerging from the sacral foramina. It is also associated with the sheath of the sciatic nerve.

Little is known of the structure and sonographic features of the sheath enveloping the sciatic nerve. Andersen et al (2012) studied this sheath by employing gross dissection, ultrasound and histological examinations. These authors identified a thin, transparent, fragile tissue layer surrounding the epineurium. Sonographically, this layer was identified as a hyperechoic layer separated from the surface of the sciatic nerve. Histologically, the sheath was seen as a multilayered circular fascia. Our dissections confirmed that the sciatic nerve is enveloped by a distinct fascial layer that is a continuation of the piriformis fascia (Fig. 8.22). This sheath usually follows the nerve up to the popliteal region but sometimes it ends in the proximal portion of the thigh.

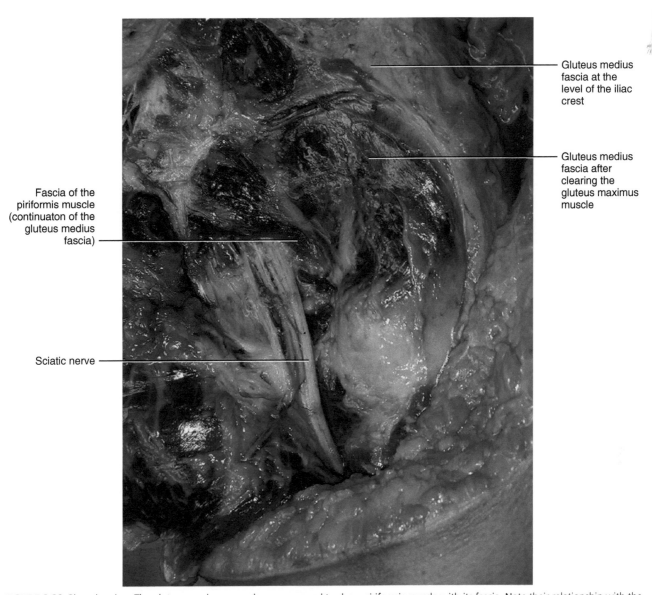

Gluteus medius fascia at the level of the iliac crest

Gluteus medius fascia after clearing the gluteus maximus muscle

Fascia of the piriformis muscle (continuaton of the gluteus medius fascia)

Sciatic nerve

FIGURE 8.22 Gluteal region. The gluteus maximus muscle was removed to show piriformis muscle with its fascia. Note their relationship with the sciatic nerve.

CLINICAL PEARL 8.4 PIRIFORMIS SYNDROME

This syndrome is still considered a controversial diagnosis and an uncommon cause of sciatic pain (Halpin 2009, Miller 2012). According to Miller, the proposed criteria for the classification of piriformis syndrome are:

- Buttock and leg pain made worse with sitting, stair climbing and/or leg crossing.
- Pain and tenderness to palpation of the sciatic notch area (piriformis muscle) and pain with increased piriformis muscle tension.
- No evidence of axonal loss to the sciatic nerve on electrophysiological testing.
- No evidence of abnormal imaging or other entity that could explain the presenting features of sciatica (e.g. radiculopathy, tumor, etc.).

- Reduction of >60% of buttock and leg pain with diagnostic injection into the piriformis muscle under radiographic imaging (fluoroscopic or ultrasound) and/or EMG guidance.

The sciatic nerve usually passes underneath the piriformis muscle, but many anatomical variations exist and the sciatic nerve could also travel through the piriformis muscle or pass over the piriformis muscle or split in two and pass directly around the piriformis muscle. Nobody has demonstrated an association of a topographic relationship between the sciatic nerve and piriformis muscle and the incidence of piriformis syndrome. Since the sciatic sheath is a continuation of the piriformis fascia, an increased tension in this fascia may alter the normal function of the sciatic sheath, causing symptoms similar to nerve compression.

Obturator Fascia

The obturator internus and gemelli are enveloped by the same thin fascia. This fascia has two intermuscular septa that separate each muscle. The obturator fascia originates in the pelvis as a continuation of the iliac fascia. Then, following the obturator internus muscle, it gradually separates from the iliac fascia and exits the pelvic cavity through the lesser sciatic foramen. It continues in the gluteal region, covering the superior and inferior gemelli muscles and attaches to the sacrotuberosus ligament. Distally, this fascia continues over the quadratus femoris muscle. Loose connective tissue, rich in fat cells, over this fascial layer allows a perfect plane of gliding between these muscles and overlying structures, such as the sciatic nerve.

In the pelvis, the obturator fascia forms the pudendal (Alcock's) canal. This canal contains the internal pudendal vessels and pudendal nerve. This fascial canal is located along the pelvic surface of the obturator internus muscle. Fibrosis of this fascia may cause a rare entrapment neuropathy of the pudendal nerve, called the Alcock's canal syndrome.

Iliopectineal Fascia

The iliacus, psoas and abdominal fasciae are described in Chapters 5 and 6. On the thigh, the iliacus and psoas fasciae form a single sheet termed the iliopectineal fascia (Fig. 8.23). This fascia covers the distal part of the iliopsoas muscle and connects it with the pectineus muscle. Where the external iliac vessels pass into the

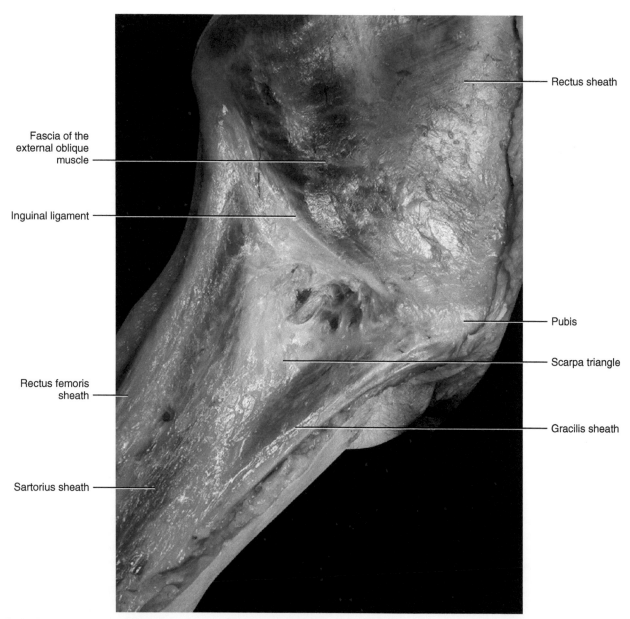

Fascia of the external oblique muscle

Inguinal ligament

Rectus femoris sheath

Sartorius sheath

Rectus sheath

Pubis

Scarpa triangle

Gracilis sheath

FIGURE 8.23 Anterior view of the inguinal region. The subcutaneous tissues were removed to show the continuity between the abdominal and limb deep fasciae. The rectus abdominis sheath inserts distally into the pubis, where the sheath of the gracilis muscle originate. The inguinal ligament gives insertion both to the fascia lata and the external oblique fascia. The sheath of the sartorius and gracilis are continuous with the fascia lata.

thigh, the iliopectineal fascia descends behind them, forming the posterior wall of the femoral sheath. The top portion of this sheath is formed by the cribiform fascia (see the paragraph about the fascia lata and the ITT below), which is a portion of the fascia lata. Distally, the iliopsoas muscle inserts into the lesser trochanter and its fascia continues with the portion of the fascia lata that covers the rectus femoris muscle (Figs 8.24 and 8.25). So, the iliopectineal fascia connects the flexor muscles of the hip (iliopsoas and pectineus), and then continues into the rectus femoralis muscle that participates in knee antepulsion[1]. The iliopsoas muscle is separated from the hip joint by the iliopectineal (or iliopsoas) bursa. This bursa, according to Van Dyke et al (1987), communicates with the hip joint in 15% of individuals.

Fascia Lata and the Iliotibial Tract

The fascia lata is the deep aponeurotic fascia of the thigh. Posteriorly, it is formed by the confluence of the myofascial expansions of the gluteus maximus and medius muscles. Laterally, it is formed by the tensor fasciae latae and, anteriorly, by the expansions of the iliopsoas fascia and the fasciae of the abdominal muscles.

The fascia lata forms a firm covering of the limb, strongest on the outer side where the iliotibial tract is present (Figs 8.26 and 8.27). On the medial surface of the thigh the fascia lata is thin. Over the iliopectineal fossa, the fascia lata is pierced by vessels and nerves, e.g., the great saphenous vein. This fascial area becomes very porous and is called the cribriform fascia. The fascia lata has a mean thickness of 1 mm and is generally easily separable from the underlying muscles due to the presence of loose connective tissue. Distally, part of the vastus medialis and lateralis insert directly into the inner aspect of the fascia lata (Figs 8.28 and 8.29).

In the thigh two main intermuscular septa, medial and lateral, are present (Fig. 8.27). They are attached to the whole length of the linea aspera with prolongations above and below. The lateral septum is the stronger one and, proximally, has attachments from many fibres of the gluteus maximus and short head of the biceps femoris. Distally, it attaches to the fibres of the vastus lateralis. The medial intermuscular septum is thinner and separates the vastus medialis from the adductor and pectineus muscles. In addition, there is a less evident septum between the adductor muscles and the hamstring muscles. Three muscular compartments of the thigh are thus formed: anterior, medial and posterior; each compartment is innerved by a specific nerve: the anterior compartment by the femoral

nerve, the posterior by the sciatic nerve and the medial by the obturator nerve.

The fascia lata creates almost two autonomous sheaths for the sartorius and gracilis muscles (Figs 8.30 and 8.31). The sartorius is completely free to glide inside its sheath (sartorius sheath) due to the presence of considerable loose connective tissue between the fascial sheath and the epimysium of the muscle. According to Burnet et al (2004), the fascia surrounding the sartorius fuses to both the fascia lata and the medial intermuscular septum. Distally, the sartorius muscle gives a myofascial expansion into the crural fascia. The sartorius sheath, therefore, allows this muscle partial autonomy and at the same time maintains a fascial continuity. Similarly, the gracilis muscle is enclosed in its own fascial sheath (gracilis sheath), which gives the muscle autonomy, but at the same time maintains continuities with the other fasciae.

The fascia lata also forms the adductor canal (Hunter's canal) that is an aponeurotic tunnel in the middle third of the thigh. It extends from the apex of the femoral triangle to the opening (adductor hiatus) in the adductor magnus. It runs between the anterior and the medial compartments of the thigh and is covered by the fascia lata that extends from the vastus medialis, across the femoral vessels to the adductor longus and magnus. This part of the fascia lata is usually called the, vastoadductor membrane, Tubbs et al (2007) suggest that, since compression of the femoral artery at the adductor hiatus is well recognized, the clinician may also try to explore potential compression of this vessel more proximally at the overlying vastoadductor membrane. The authors also hypothesize that the vastoadductor membrane creates a functional synergy between the adductor magnus and vastus medialis.

The fascia lata is an aponeurotic fascia formed by two or three fibrous layers. Its spatial orientation of the collagen fibres differs from layer to layer. Usually, the longitudinal and oblique directions are prevalent, while the transverse orientation is uncommon (Figs 8.32–8.35). This permits the fascia to adapt to the volume variations of the muscle, while connecting the hip, knee and ankle like a belt. The more important longitudinal fibres are on the lateral side and are so thick and resistant that they merit their own name: the iliotibial tract (ITT). This is not actually an autonomous structure, in spite of being so described in many anatomical textbooks. Rather, it is part of a whole fascial stocking completely encircling the thigh and is extensively connected to the lateral intermuscular septum and anchored to the lower part of the femur (Figs 8.13, 8.19 and 8.26). The action of the ITT and its associated muscles is to flex and abduct the hip. In addition, the ITT contributes to lateral knee stabilization. The ITT also serves as a distal tendon insertion for the tensor fasciae latae and gluteus maximus muscles. Distally, the ITT is attached to the lateral condyle of the tibia and gives an oblique myofascial expansion that passes under the patella, contributing to the formation of the anterior knee retinaculum. This attachment allows stretching of

---

[1]We prefer the term 'antepulsion' because the anterior direction of movement of the lower extremity corresponds to hip flexion and knee extension. These two movements appear antagonistic, but both correspond to a forward motion and are coordinated by the longitudinal fibrous bundles of the deep fascia of the anterior region of the thigh.

Text continued on p. 328

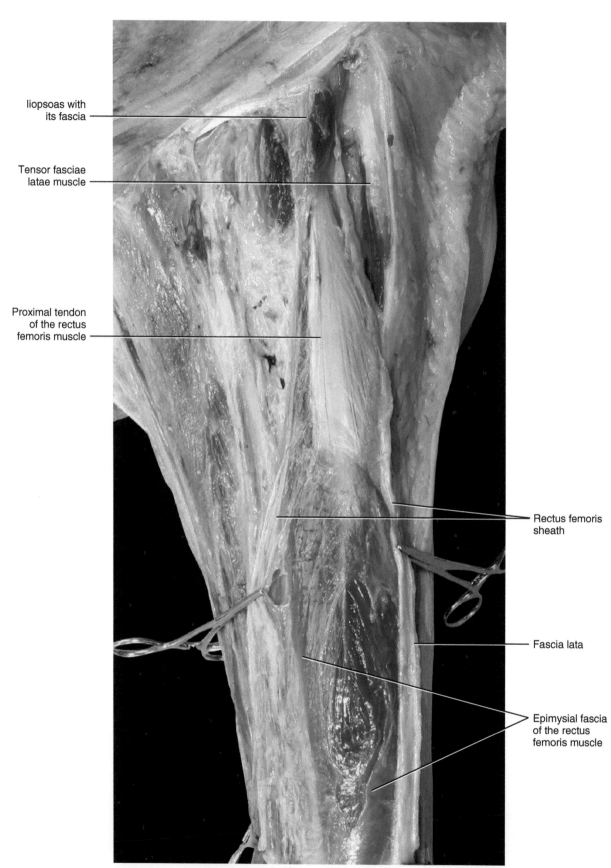

Iliopsoas with its fascia

Tensor fasciae latae muscle

Proximal tendon of the rectus femoris muscle

Rectus femoris sheath

Fascia lata

Epimysial fascia of the rectus femoris muscle

FIGURE 8.24 Anterior view of the thigh. The fascia lata is cut to show the rectus femoris. Note the continuity between the rectus femoris sheath and the fascia of the iliopsoas. The fascia lata connects the rectus femoris muscle with the tensor fasciae latae muscle. The muscles involved in antepulsion of the hip are all joined together by the fascia.

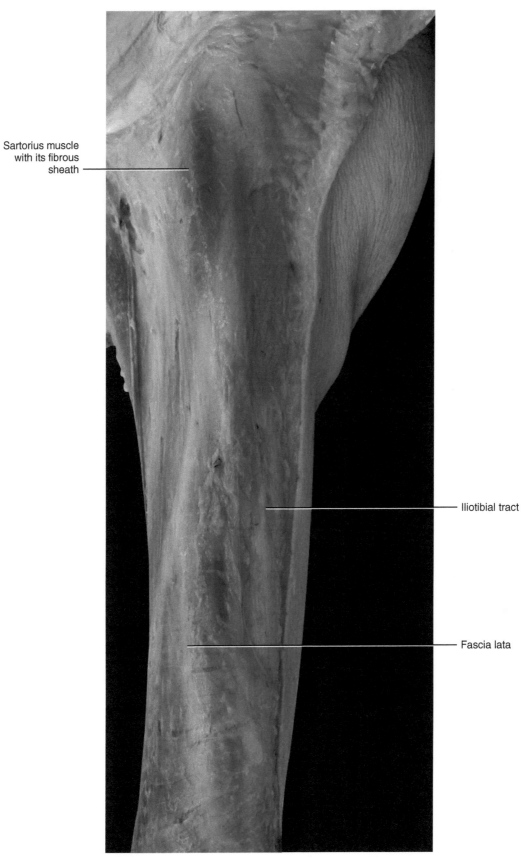

Sartorius muscle
with its fibrous
sheath

Iliotibial tract

Fascia lata

FIGURE 8.25 Anterior view of the thigh. The subcutaneous tissue was removed to show the fascia lata. Note that the sartorius sheath and the iliotibial tract are in continuity with the fascia lata.

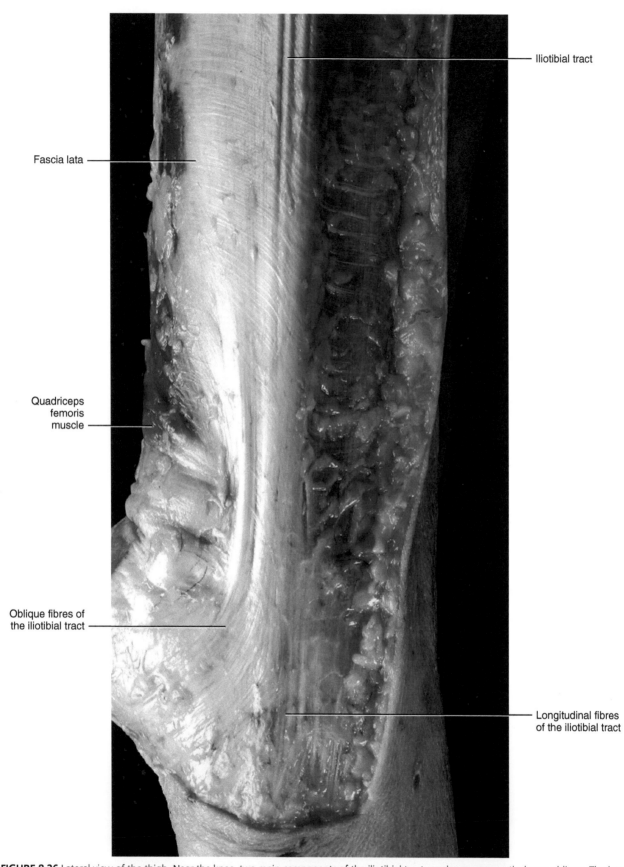

Iliotibial tract

Fascia lata

Quadriceps
femoris
muscle

Oblique fibres of
the iliotibial tract

Longitudinal fibres
of the iliotibial tract

FIGURE 8.26 Lateral view of the thigh. Near the knee, two main components of the iliotibial tract are shown: one vertical, one oblique. The latter collaborates in the formation of the anterior knee retinaculum, joining with the myofascial expansions of the pes anserinus muscles.

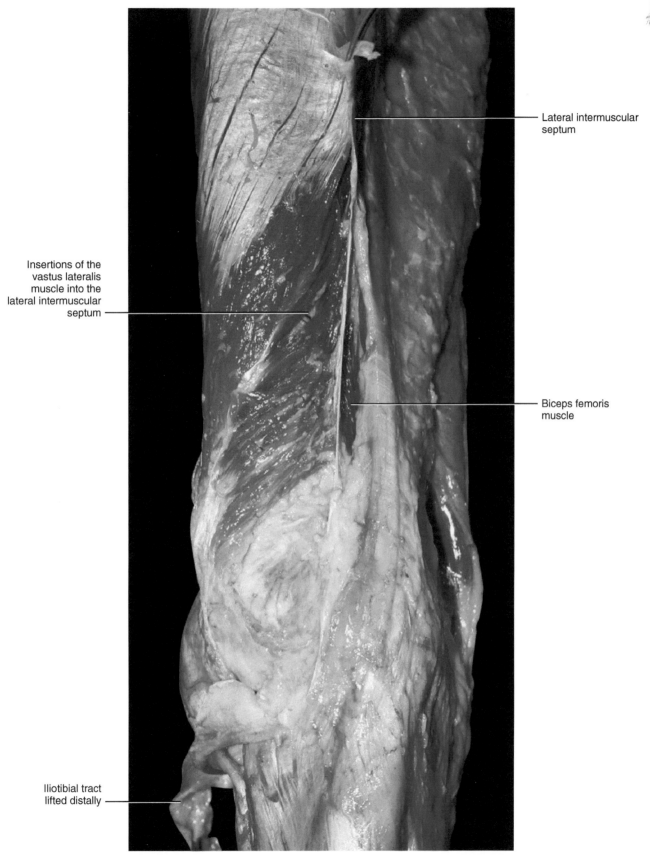

Lateral intermuscular septum

Insertions of the vastus lateralis muscle into the lateral intermuscular septum

Biceps femoris muscle

Iliotibial tract lifted distally

FIGURE 8.27 Lateral view of the thigh. The fascia lata was removed to show the vastus lateralis muscle and its insertion into the lateral intermuscular septum. The biceps femoris muscle also has many fibres that originate from this septum. The lateral intermuscular septum originates from the inner side of the fascia lata, just under the iliotibial tract.

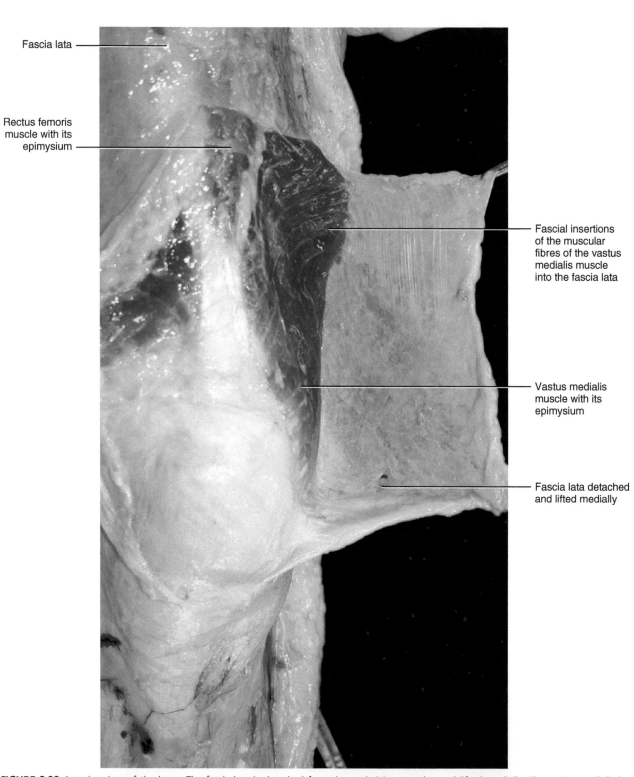

Fascia lata

Rectus femoris muscle with its epimysium

Fascial insertions of the muscular fibres of the vastus medialis muscle into the fascia lata

Vastus medialis muscle with its epimysium

Fascia lata detached and lifted medially

FIGURE 8.28 Anterior view of the knee. The fascia lata is detached from the underlying muscles and lifted medially. The vastus medialis has some fibres inserted into the fascia lata, while distally it is autonomous and free to glide with respect to the fascia lata (due to the presence of its epimysial fascia).

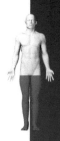
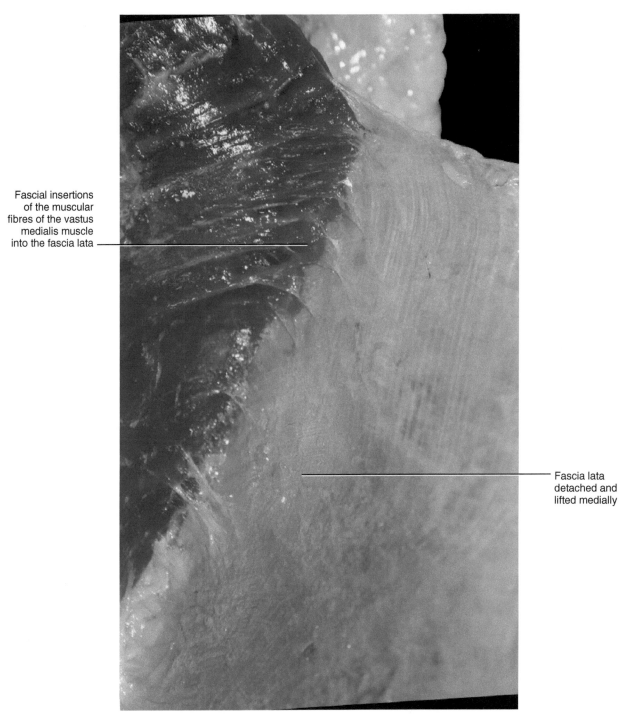

Fascial insertions of the muscular fibres of the vastus medialis muscle into the fascia lata

Fascia lata detached and lifted medially

FIGURE 8.29 Enlargement of the fascial insertions of the vastus medialis into the inner aspect of the fascia lata.

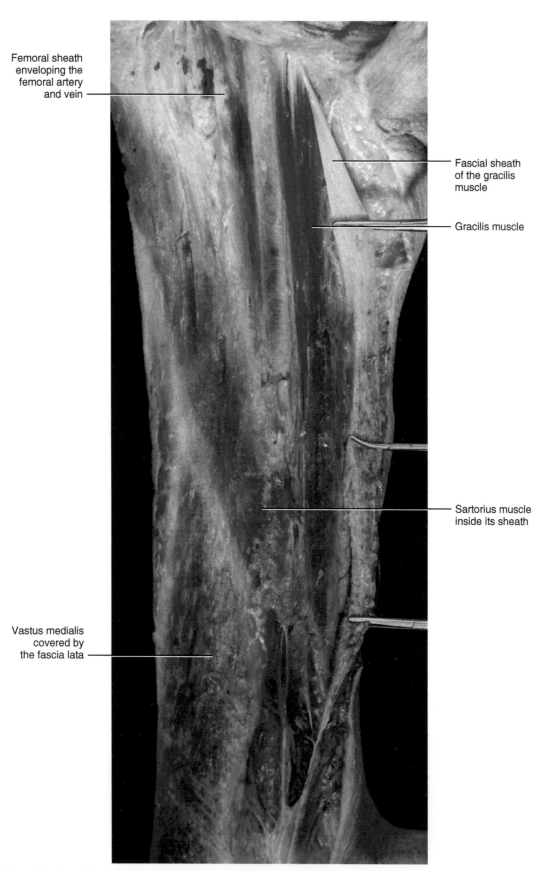

Femoral sheath
enveloping the
femoral artery
and vein

Fascial sheath
of the gracilis
muscle

Gracilis muscle

Sartorius muscle
inside its sheath

Vastus medialis
covered by
the fascia lata

FIGURE 8.30 Medial view of the right thigh. The sheath of the gracilis muscle is opened to show the muscle. Note the continuity of the gracilis, sartorius and femoral sheath with the fascia lata.

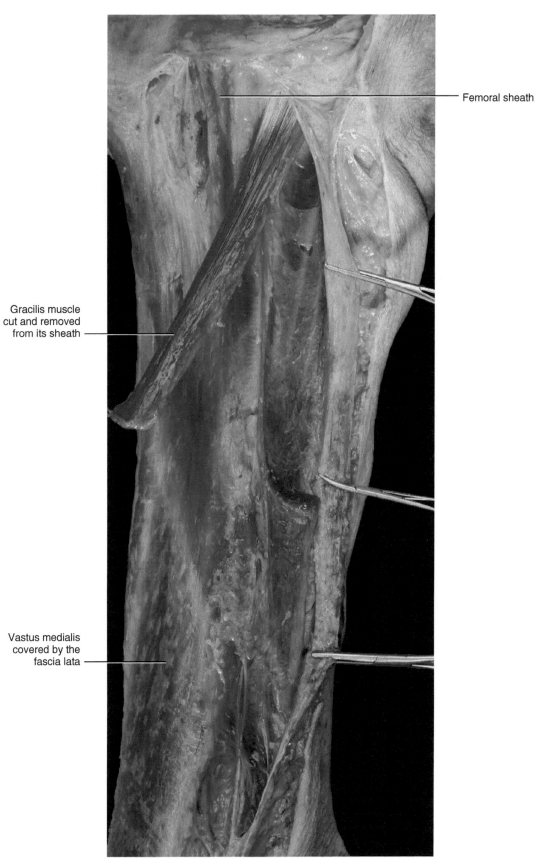

Femoral sheath

Gracilis muscle
cut and removed
from its sheath

Vastus medialis
covered by the
fascia lata

FIGURE 8.31 Medial view of the right thigh. The gracilis muscle is partially removed to show its sheath. The gracilis muscle is a biarticular muscle and is separated from the deeper monoarticular muscles by its sheath.

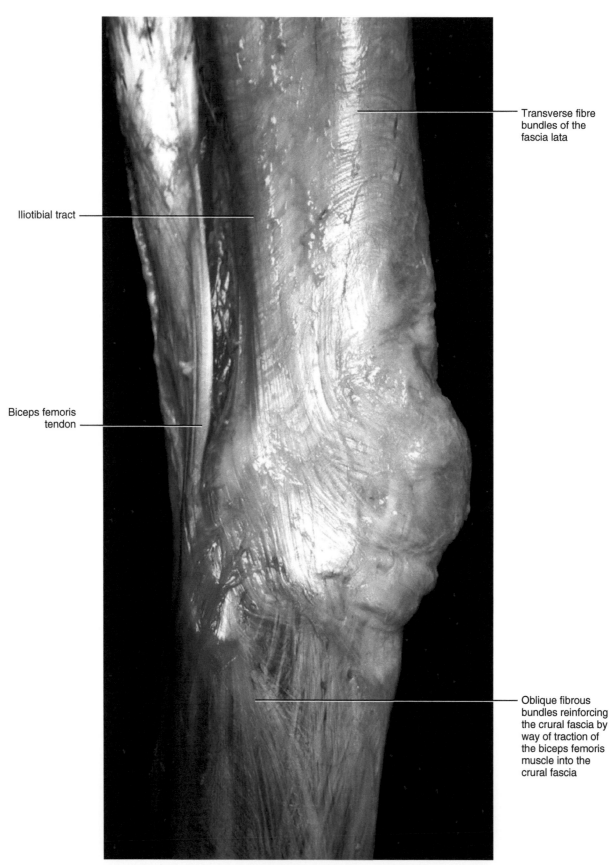

Transverse fibre
bundles of the
fascia lata

Iliotibial tract

Biceps femoris
tendon

Oblique fibrous
bundles reinforcing
the crural fascia by
way of traction of
the biceps femoris
muscle into the
crural fascia

FIGURE 8.32 Lateral region of the knee. The various reinforcements of the deep fascia are clearly visible.

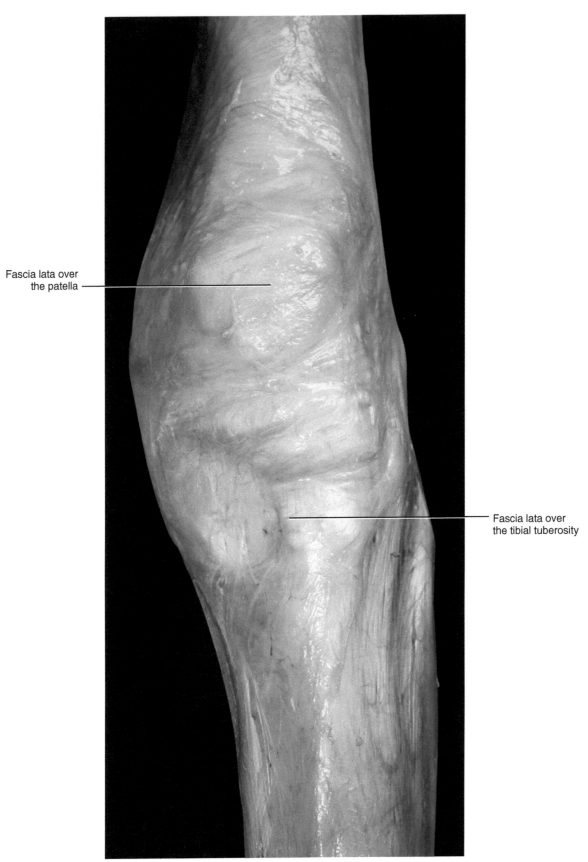

Fascia lata over
the patella

Fascia lata over
the tibial tuberosity

FIGURE 8.33 Anterior view of the knee. The fascia lata and crural fascia form a unique structure that crosses the knee, covering the patella and quadriceps tendon.

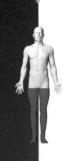

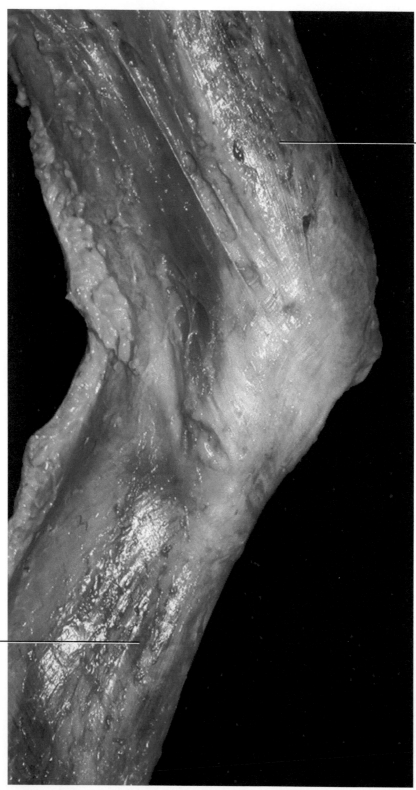

Fascia lata covering the vastus medialis muscle

Crural fascia

FIGURE 8.34 Medial view of the knee.

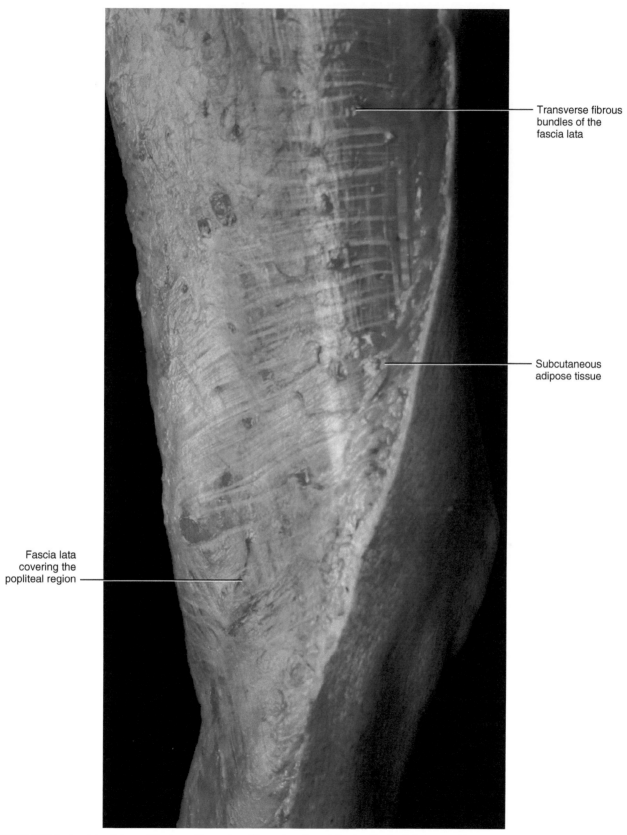

Transverse fibrous bundles of the fascia lata

Subcutaneous adipose tissue

Fascia lata covering the popliteal region

FIGURE 8.35 Posterolateral view of the knee. The various fibrous bundles reinforcing the fascia lata are evident.

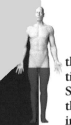
the crural fascia in a mediolateral direction. In addition, this connection can explain the results of Wu and Shih (2004) who reported significant improvement in the congruence angle and lateral patellofemoral angle in patients with patellar malalignment after surgical release of an ITT contracture in the trochanteric area. These authors conclude (confirming our idea) that the ITT affects patellar tracking and dominates lateral patellar supporting structures. Finally, Vieira et al (2007) emphasize the importance of the ITT as a lateral stabilizer or brace for the knee. The ITT also has extensive attachments to the lateral intermuscular septum in the thigh and terminates at Gerdy's tubercle at the upper end of the tibia (Fairclough et al 2007).

Specific oblique reinforcements of the fascia lata (knee retinacula) could be recognized both in the anterior and posterior parts (Figs 8.36–8.41). The anterior knee retinaculum is formed by two or three fibrous layers, each separated by thin layers of loose connective tissue. The most superficial is formed by the fascia lata that pass in front of the patella and continue into the crural fascia. Under it there are the expansions of the vasti (medialis and lateralis) that present an oblique direction. The deep layer is formed by the longitudinal expansion of the rectus femoris and the vastus intermedius muscles. This layer partially adheres to the periosteum of the patella and partially continues into the crural fascia. Wangwinyuvirat et al (2009) found that at the proximal pole of the patella the entire quadriceps tendon had an average thickness of 8.54 mm, but only a percentage of these fibres (7.87 mm) insert into the proximal patellar pole, while some fibres (0.68 mm) pass over the anterior patellar surface. Histological analysis showed that the fibres that continue over the patella were the distal extensions of the longitudinal fibres of the rectus femoris tendon. This study confirmed that some fibres of the rectus femoris tendon pass over the patella, connecting the quadriceps and patellar tendons.

The medial part of the anterior knee retinaculum was the specific focus of Thawait et al (2012). Their study confirmed that it is composed of the following three layers:

- Layer I (superficial) in continuity with the deep crural fascia.

- Layer II (middle) receives expansions from the superficial portion of the medial collateral ligament.

- Layer III (deep) in continuity with the joint capsule.

Layers I and II fuse together along the anterior aspect of the medial side of the knee, whereas layers II and III fuse along the posterior aspect of the joint. The lateral part of the anterior patellar retinaculum is also formed by several fascial layers: the expansion of the ITT, the myofascial expansions of the lateral vasti, and the capsular ligaments.

Based on MR imaging the knee retinacula appear as low-signal intensity bands with a mean thickness of 0.8–1 mm. In patients affected by anterior knee pain

CLINICAL PEARL 8.5 ILIOTIBIAL BAND SYNDROME

The iliotibial tract (ITT) connects the muscles of the pelvis with the knee. It stabilizes the knee both in extension and in partial flexion and is used constantly during walking and running. In leaning forward with a slightly flexed knee, the tract is the main support of the knee against gravity. Many fibres of the gluteus maximus are inserted into the ITT and into the posterior aspect of the lateral intermuscular septum (which is continuous with the ITT). Other gluteus maximus fibres have an oblique direction and so pass over the ITT to continue into the fascia over the vastus lateralis. Many fibres of the vastus lateralis also insert into the anterior aspect of the lateral intermuscular septum and, finally, merge at the knee with the anterior knee retinaculum. Thus, the ITT together with the lateral intermuscular septum coordinates the action of both the gluteus maximus and vastus lateralis.

Iliotibial band syndrome (ITBS) is a common thigh injury generally associated with running, but can also result from cycling or hiking. Other risk factors for ITBS include gait abnormalities, such as hyperpronation, leg length discrepancies, or bow-leggedness. It is considered an overuse syndrome of the distal ITT near the lateral femoral condyle at Gerdy's tubercle, and is believed to be associated with excessive friction between the ITT and the lateral femoral epicondyle, i.e. friction that 'inflames' the ITT or the underlying bursa. But Fairclough et al (2007) suggest that the ITT cannot create frictional forces by moving forwards and backwards over the epicondyle during flexion and extension of the knee. The perception of movement of the ITB across the epicondyle is an illusion due to changing tension in its anterior and posterior fibres. They propose that ITBS is caused by increased compression of the highly vascularized and innervated layer of fat and loose connective tissue that separates the ITT from the epicondyle. Therefore, the aetiology of ITT can be related to a chronic increased tension of the ITT caused by increased tension of the tensor fasciae latae or gluteus maximus muscles. To check ITT tension, the Ober test could be useful, but we suggest also checking the gluteus maximus and the tensor fasciae latae muscles as they are the main tensors of the ITT. Chen et al (2006) have demonstrated with MRI that gluteal contracture causes a posteromedial displacement of the ITT. The resolution of the ITBS can only be properly achieved when the biomechanics of hip muscle function are properly addressed.

or patellofemoral malalignment it is often possible to highlight a difference in thickness between the medial and lateral portions of the anterior knee retinaculum. Tight lateral patellar retinaculum may cause abnormal lateral patellar tilt and exaggerated pressure in the lateral aspect of the patellofemoral joint (known as the

Text continued on p. 334

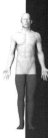

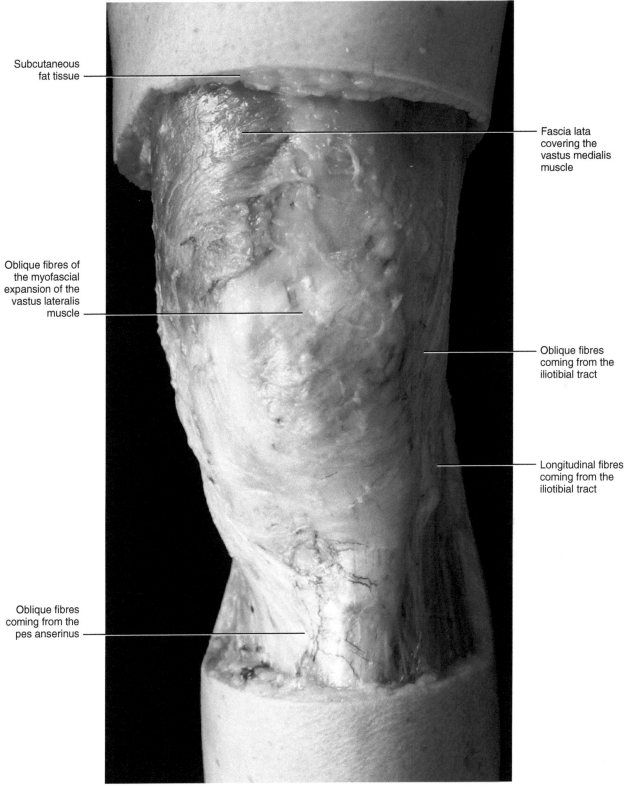

Subcutaneous fat tissue

Fascia lata covering the vastus medialis muscle

Oblique fibres of the myofascial expansion of the vastus lateralis muscle

Oblique fibres coming from the iliotibial tract

Longitudinal fibres coming from the iliotibial tract

Oblique fibres coming from the pes anserinus

FIGURE 8.36 Anterior view of the knee. The collagen fibre bundles of the deep fascia present many orientations, forming the anterior knee retinaculum.

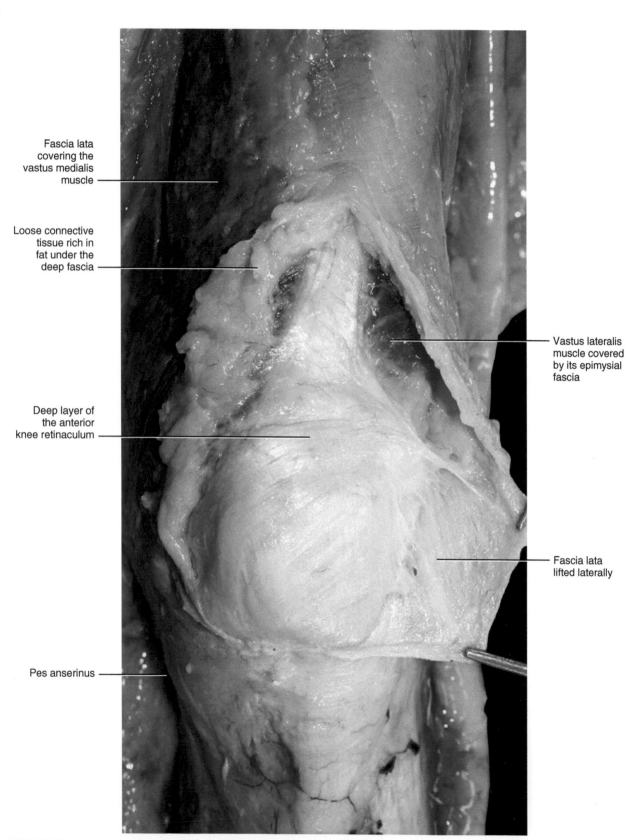

Fascia lata covering the vastus medialis muscle

Loose connective tissue rich in fat under the deep fascia

Deep layer of the anterior knee retinaculum

Pes anserinus

Vastus lateralis muscle covered by its epimysial fascia

Fascia lata lifted laterally

FIGURE 8.37 Anterior view of the knee. The anterior knee retinaculum consists of two fibrous layers: a deep layer formed by the oblique tendinous expansions of the two vasti, and a superficial one, formed by the fascia lata. The joint capsule also may collaborate in the formation of the retinaculum, forming a third fibrous layer.

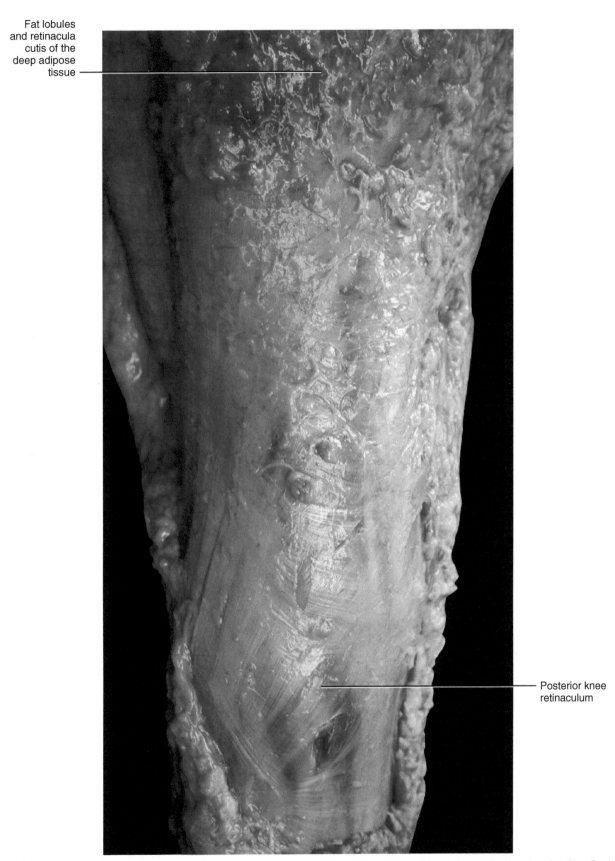

Fat lobules
and retinacula
cutis of the
deep adipose
tissue

Posterior knee
retinaculum

FIGURE 8.38 Posterior view of the knee. The honeycombed structure of the DAT is clearly visible. In the popliteal region the deep fascia is reinforced by oblique fibrous bundles that form the posterior knee retinacula.

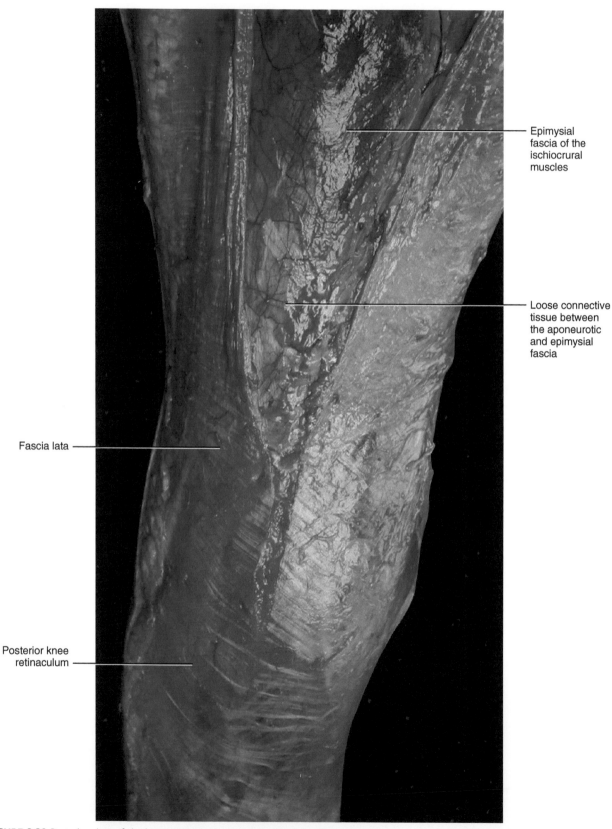

Epimysial fascia of the ischiocrural muscles

Loose connective tissue between the aponeurotic and epimysial fascia

Fascia lata

Posterior knee retinaculum

FIGURE 8.39 Posterior view of the knee. Note the loose connective tissue between the aponeurotic fascia (fascia lata) and the epimysial fascia (epimysium). In this way the fascia lata can work like a bridge between the hip and knee.

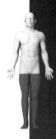

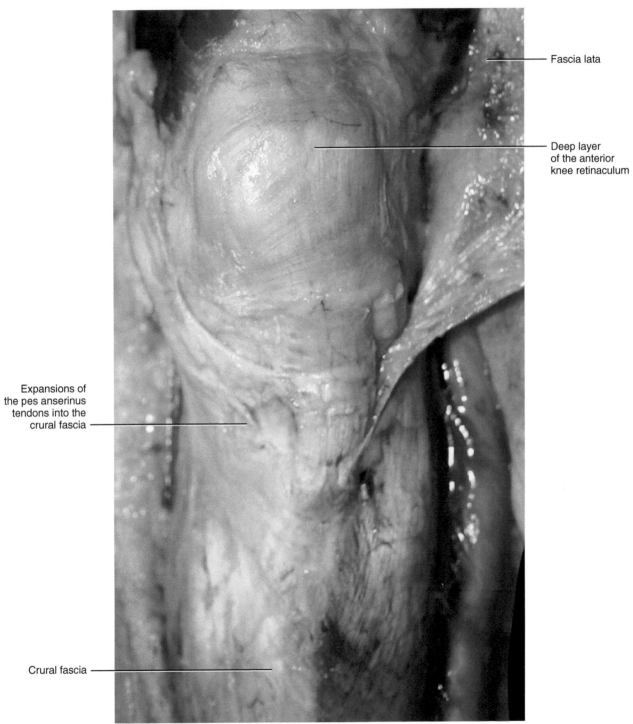

Fascia lata

Deep layer
of the anterior
knee retinaculum

Expansions of
the pes anserinus
tendons into the
crural fascia

Crural fascia

FIGURE 8.40 Anterior knee retinaculum.

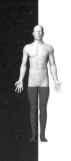

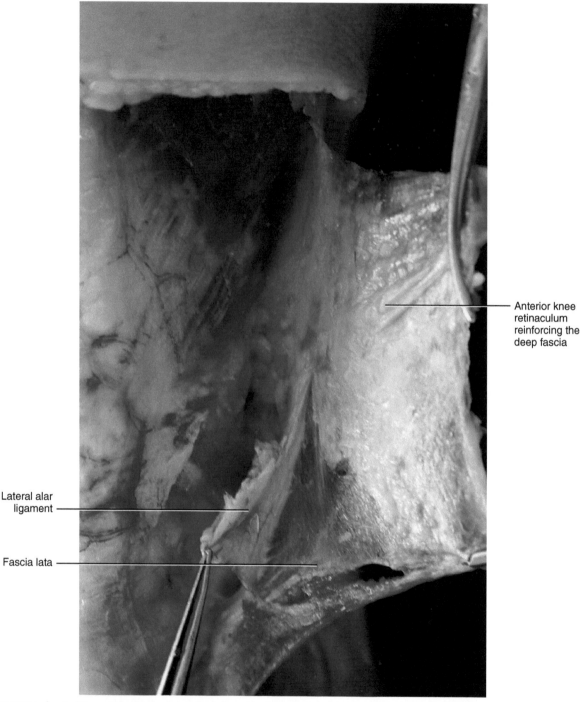

Anterior knee retinaculum reinforcing the deep fascia

Lateral alar ligament

Fascia lata

FIGURE 8.41 In front of the patella, the fascia lata is reinforced by the anterior knee retinaculum. The alar ligaments are strongly adherent to the deep fascia.

excessive lateral pressure syndrome), friction-related superolateral Hoffa's fat pad oedema, and early patellofemoral osteoarthrosis. Other possible alterations of the retinaculum are fibrosis, thickening, attenuated retinaculum, bony productive changes at a retinacular attachment and ossification of the retinacular layers. Thawait et al (2012) showed some chronic cases where altered stresses led to thickening of the retinaculum on one side with attenuation of the contralateral retinaculum.

Specific fascial reinforcements are also present in the posterior aspect of the knee. Other authors do not describe a posterior knee retinaculum and only a few (Terry & La Prade 1996) speak about the arcuate ligamentous complex of the knee. This complex could be considered the deeper part of the posterior knee retinaculum which is formed by the myofascial expansions of the sartorius, popliteus, semimembranous and biceps muscles. Tubbs et al (2006) found that the tendon of the biceps femoris muscle has both medial and lateral slips, each with an anterior and posterior component, attaching not only into the lateral condyle of the femur, but also into the popliteus tendon and arcuate popliteal ligament. These authors hypothesize that these myofascial expansions could function as a synergistic link between the biceps femoris and the popliteus muscles. In the rabbit, the function of fascial tensor of the biceps femoris is extremely important. Crum et al (2003) analysed the distal insertion of the biceps femoris in the rabbit and found that this muscle has no attachment to the fibula at all and is attached only to the anterior compartment fascia of the leg. This probably improves its springing and jumping ability.

Medially, the myofascial expansions of the sartorius, gracilis and semitendinosus form the pes anserinus superficialis. The myofascial expansions of the semimembranosus form the pes anserinus profundis (Figs 8.42–8.47). According to Mochizuki et al (2004), the distal parts of the tendons of the gracilis and semitendinosus always have longitudinal fascial expansions that fuse with the crural fascia. The semimembranosus has a small oblique myofascial expansion that fuses with the crural fascia covering the medial head of the gastrocnemius. These authors suggest that due to the considerable tension from the sartorius, gracilis, semitendinosus, semimembranosus, and gastrocnemius muscles, these myofascial expansions may act as complex fascial tensors and play a significant role as stabilizers of the medial side of the knee joint in the upright posture.

Finally, the posterior portion of the fascia lata is stretched caudally by the fascial insertions of the gastrocnemius muscles, and the anterior portion is stretched caudally by the insertion of the tibialis anterior into the crural fascia. In this case the insertion is not directly into the fascia lata, but into the crural fascia, that is continuous with the fascia lata. We should always be aware that the division between the two structures is only didactic.

Crural Fascia

The muscles of the leg are ensheathed by the crural fascia (Figs 8.48–8.51). It is continuous with the fascia lata and the deep fasciae of the foot. It fuses with the periosteum of the tibial crest, the tibial condyles, the head of the fibula, and the medial and lateral malleoli. The crural fascia has a mean thickness of 900 µm and is thicker and denser in the upper and anterior part of the leg. It is reinforced laterally by the myofascial expansions of the biceps femoris and ITT, anteriorly by the myofascial expansions of the quadriceps muscle and medially by the tendons of the sartorius, gracilis, semitendinosus and semimembranosus muscles. Proximally, the crural fascia provides attachment from its deep surface to the tibialis anterior and extensor digitorum longus muscles (Figs 8.52 and 8.53).

De Maeseneer et al (2000) found that the crural fascia at the medial aspect of the knee adheres to the superficial layer of the medial collateral ligament and it adheres posteriorly to the knee capsule. In the distal ⅓ of the leg, it is completely separated from the surrounding muscles and their tendons due to loose connective tissue. Around the ankle, the crural fascia is strengthened by transverse and oblique fibres of the retinacula. Posteriorly, the crural fascia is thinner and easily separated from the underlying muscles. In the popliteal region, the fascia is perforated by the small saphenous vein.

The crural fascia forms two strong intermuscular septa: the anterior and posterior peroneal septa. These septa bound the lateral compartment of the leg and separate the fibularis longus and brevis from the muscles of the anterior and posterior crural compartments. In addition, the crural fascia forms the transverse intermuscular septum, also called the deep transverse fascia of the leg, that *separates* the superficial and deep posterior crural muscles. The deep transverse fascia gives insertion to many muscular fibres of the soleus. In the leg, each compartment formed by these septa is innervated by a specific nerve: the anterior compartment by the deep fibular nerve, the lateral compartment by the superficial fibular nerve, the posterior compartment by the tibial nerve.

Near the ankle, the retinacula are clearly distinguishable but not separable from the crural fascia or the deep fasciae of the foot (Stecco et al 2010). Thus, describing their exact limits is difficult, although it is possible to identify the main bundles, with their bone and muscular insertions and relation to tendons. Four main retinacula may be identified, even though other fascial reinforcements with retinacular features may be recognized in different subjects.

The superior extensor retinaculum appears as a transverse, fibrous thickening of the crural fascia, about 3 cm proximal to the tibiotarsal joint (Figs 8.54 and 8.55). It is attached medially to the anterior surface of the tibia, continuing with its periosteum, and to the lateral fibula. Its anatomical landmarks are more clearly defined distally. Proximally, however, the retinaculum tapers gradually into the crural fascia and it is not possible to identify the proximal border of the retinacula in all subjects. Where such identification is possible, the proximal border was about 9 cm from the tibiotarsal joint. The superior extensor retinaculum shows great variability in thickness and orientation of fibres among subjects. In most, the fibres are orientated transversely, but in some the fibres are oblique and ascend medially. The tendons of the tibialis anterior, extensor digitorum longus and extensor hallucis longus muscles slide under the superior extensor retinaculum.

The inferior extensor retinaculum is the most easily identifiable retinaculum of the ankle (Figs 8.54–8.56). It is commonly described as having a Y-shaped form, with the two branches of the Y medially directed. The stem of the Y is set about 1.5 cm distal to the distal tibiofibular joint and is attached to the volar surface of the talus and to the capsule of the ankle joint. The lateral branch of the retinaculum has two distinct parts: one superficial, continuing with the inferior

Text continued on p. 350

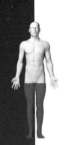

Fat tissue
between the
iliotibial tract and
the epimysial
fascia (*epimysium*)
of the vastus
lateralis muscle —

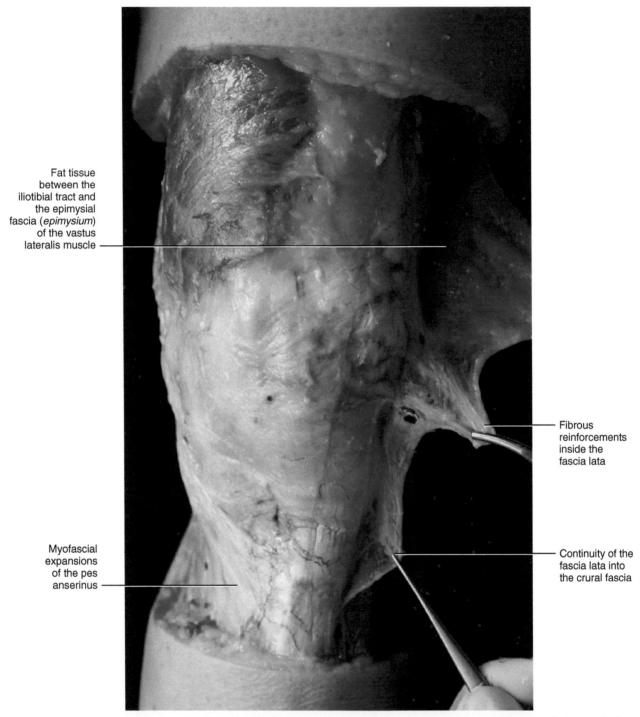

— Fibrous
reinforcements
inside the
fascia lata

Myofascial
expansions
of the pes
anserinus —

— Continuity of the
fascia lata into
the crural fascia

FIGURE 8.42 Anterior view of the knee. The fascia lata continues into the crural fascia. When the vasti contract they stretch the anterior knee retinaculum and thus the crural fascia.

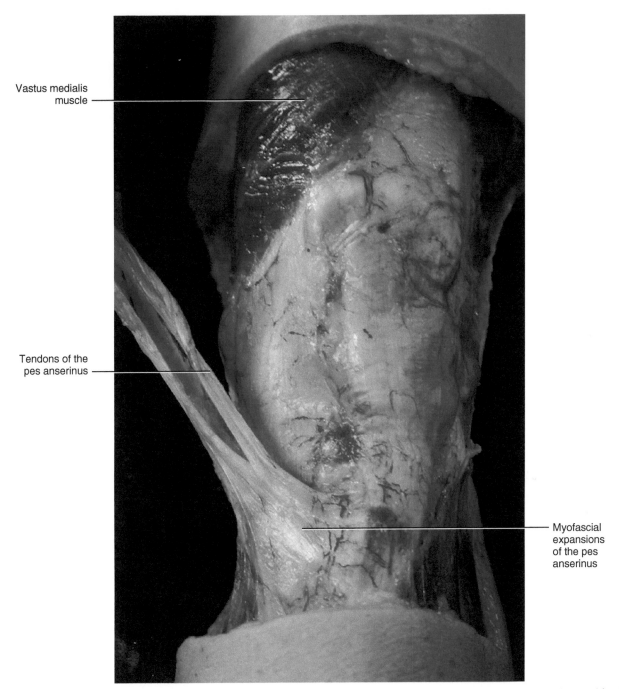

Vastus medialis
muscle

Tendons of the
pes anserinus

Myofascial
expansions
of the pes
anserinus

FIGURE 8.43 Pes anserinus muscles detached from their proximal insertions and stretched. They have myofascial expansions into the crural fascia. The pes anserinus and the ITT stabilize the knee in the frontal plane, even through the knee does not have movement in this plane.

Sartorius muscle

Oblique myofascial expansion of the sartorius muscle into the crural fascia

Longitudinal myofascial expansion of the sartorius muscle into the crural fascia

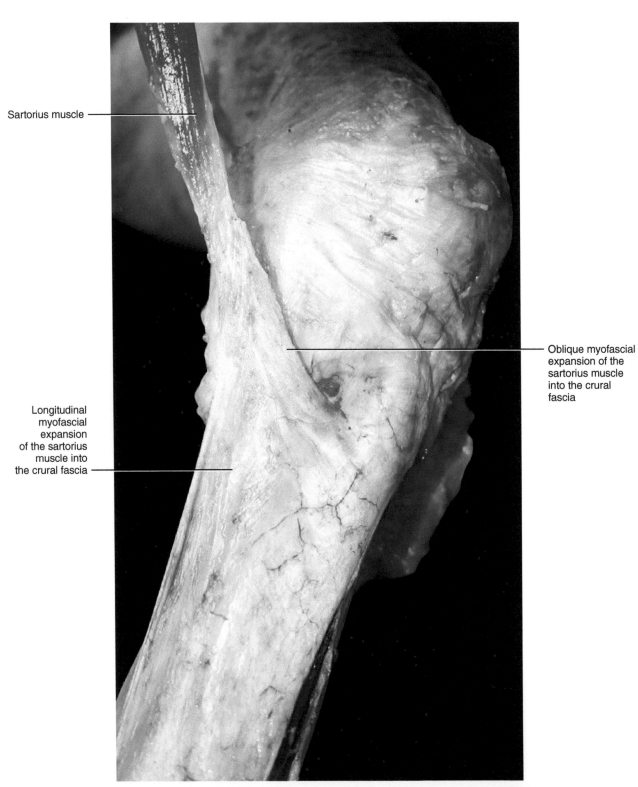

FIGURE 8.44 Anteromedial view of the knee. The sartorius muscle forms the superficial layer of the pes anserinus. Upon stretching the sartorius muscle which simulates its contraction, two lines of force into the crural fascia appear: one longitudinal and one oblique. This occurs due to the myofascial expansions of this muscle. The sartorius tendon takes an oblique course and has an expansion that crosses the midline to join with the oblique expansion of the ITT. Thus, the tensor fasciae latae and sartorius muscles strongly connect the hip and the knee during movements.

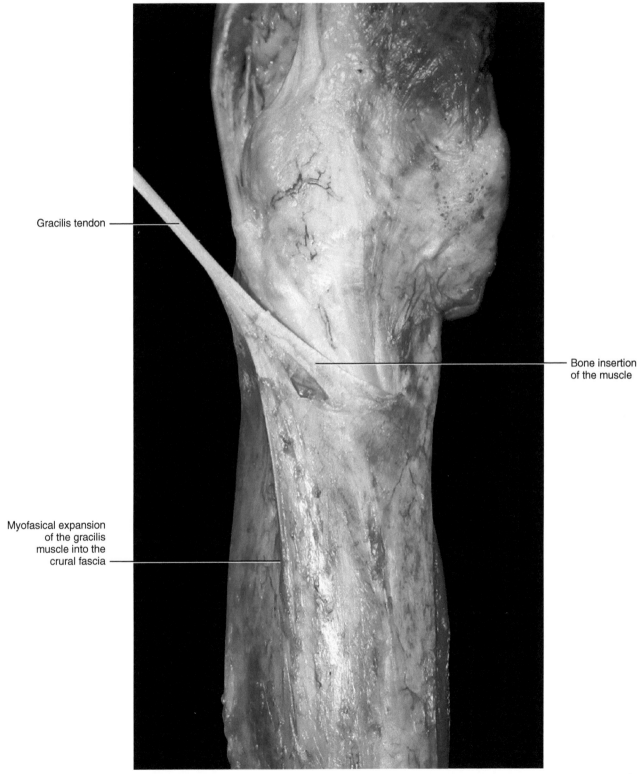

Gracilis tendon

Bone insertion
of the muscle

Myofasical expansion
of the gracilis
muscle into the
crural fascia

FIGURE 8.45 Anteromedial view of the knee. The gracilis muscle is deeper with respect to the sartorius muscle. It gives an expansion into the medial portion of the crural fascia.

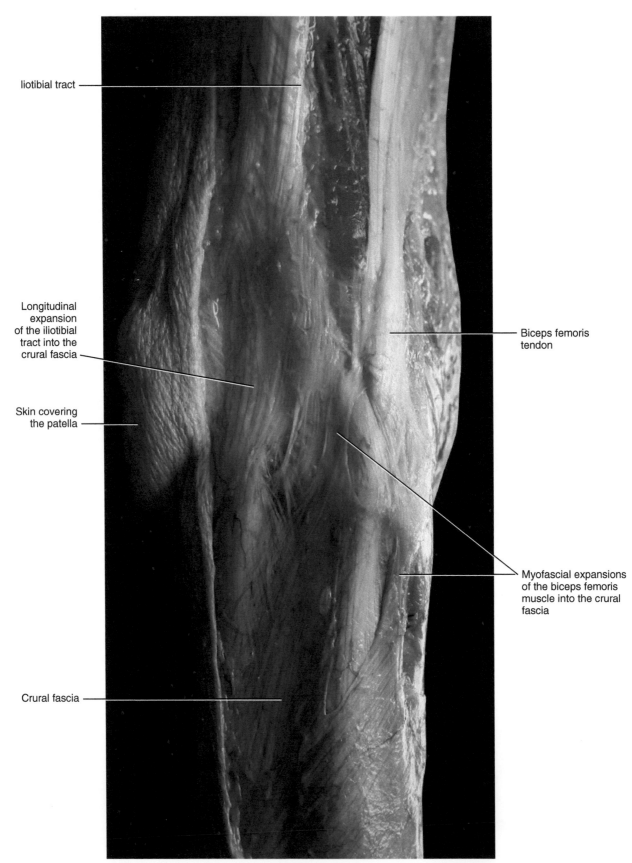

liotibial tract

Longitudinal
expansion
of the iliotibial
tract into the
crural fascia

Skin covering
the patella

Crural fascia

Biceps femoris
tendon

Myofascial expansions
of the biceps femoris
muscle into the crural
fascia

FIGURE 8.46 Lateral view of the knee. Note the longitudinal expansions of the iliotibial tract and the biceps femoris muscle into the crural fascia.

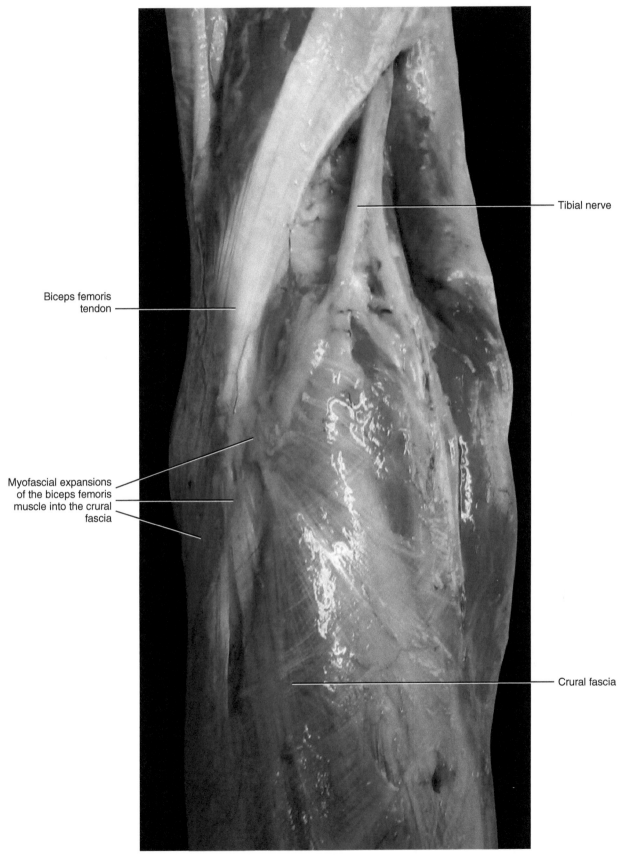

Tibial nerve

Biceps femoris
tendon

Myofascial expansions
of the biceps femoris
muscle into the crural
fascia

Crural fascia

FIGURE 8.47 Posterior region of the knee. The biceps femoris muscle has several myofascial expansions into the crural fascia: one longitudinal and two oblique. The first stretches the lateral portion of the crural fascia, the other stretches the posterior region of the crural fascia. In this way, the contracting biceps femoris stretches the entire fibular sheath.

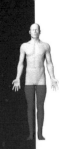

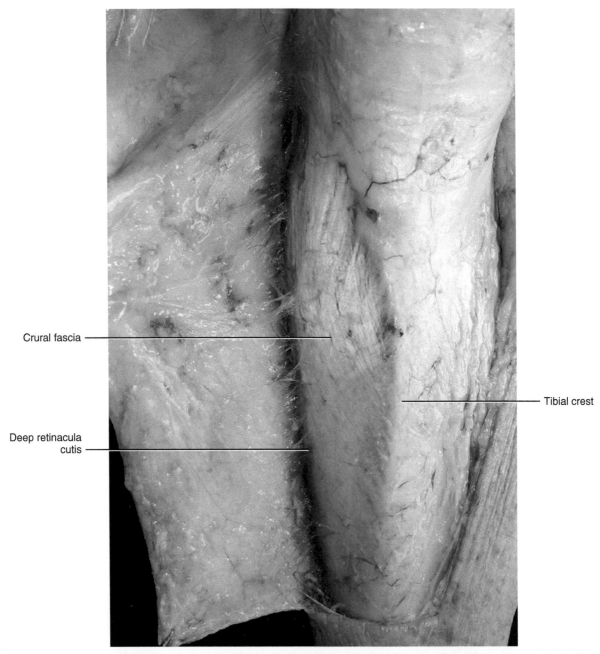

Crural fascia

Deep retinacula cutis

Tibial crest

FIGURE 8.48 Anterolateral view of the leg. The superficial fascia was detached from the deep fascia together with the skin and the SAT. The crural fascia appears as a very fibrous layer, covering all the muscles and bones. Over the tibial crest, it adheres to the periosteum.

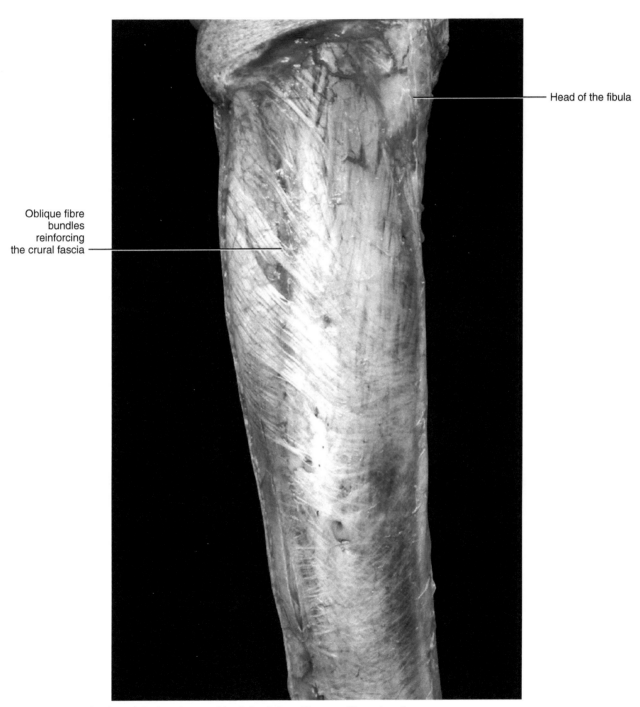

Head of the fibula

Oblique fibre
bundles
reinforcing
the crural fascia

FIGURE 8.49 Posterior view of the leg. The crural fascia is reinforced by many fibrous bundles.

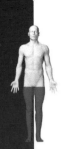

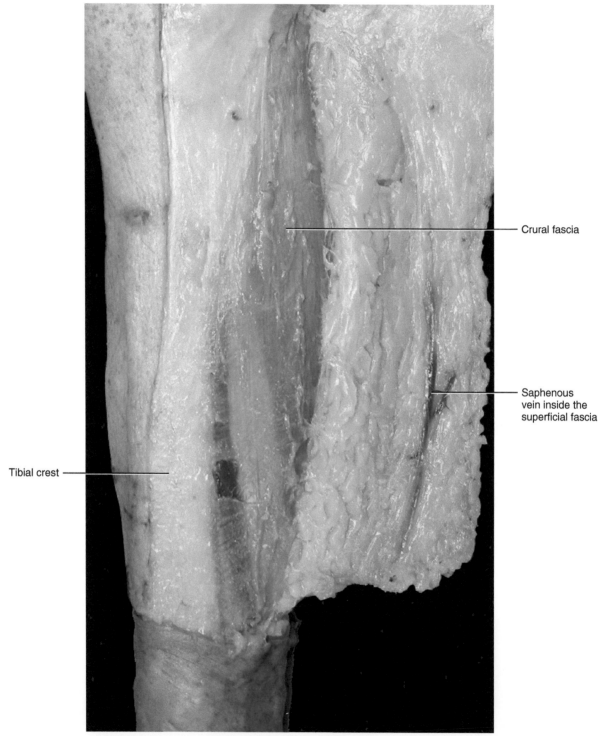

Crural fascia

Saphenous vein inside the superficial fascia

Tibial crest

FIGURE 8.50 Deep fascia (crural) of the anteromedial region of the leg.

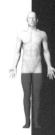

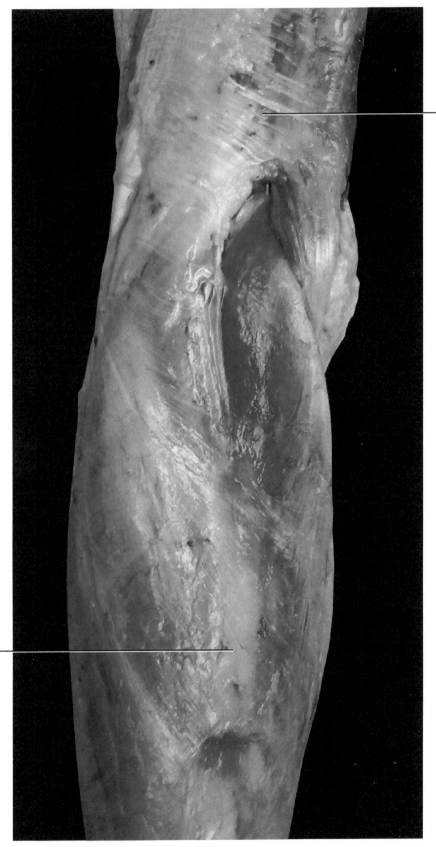

Fibrous bundles
reinforcing the
fascia lata

Crural fascia
covering the
triceps muscle

FIGURE 8.51 Deep *(aponeurotic)* fascia of the posterior region of the leg.

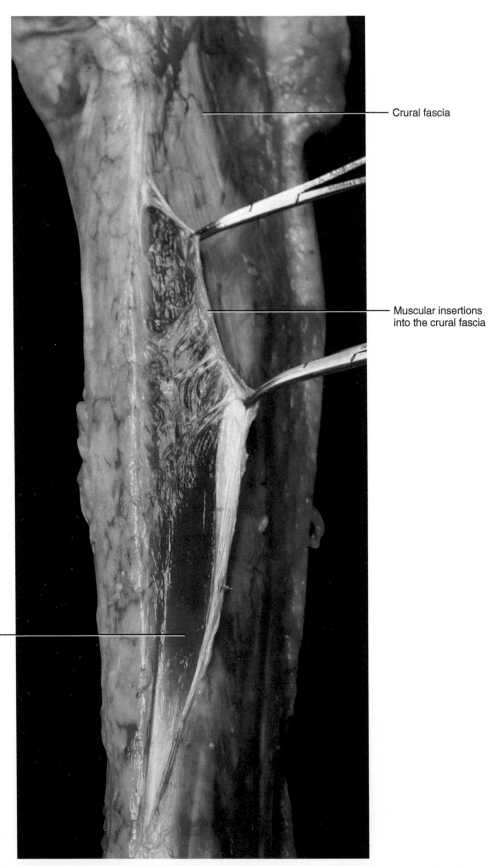

Crural fascia

Muscular insertions
into the crural fascia

Tibialis
tibialis anterior
muscle enveloped
by its epimysial
fascia (epimysium)

FIGURE 8.52 Anterolateral view of the leg. The crural fascia is detached from the underlying planes and lifted laterally. The tibialis anterior muscle has many muscular fibres inserted into the inner aspect of the crural fascia, while its distal portion is enveloped by epimysial fascia and is completely free to glide under the crural fascia.

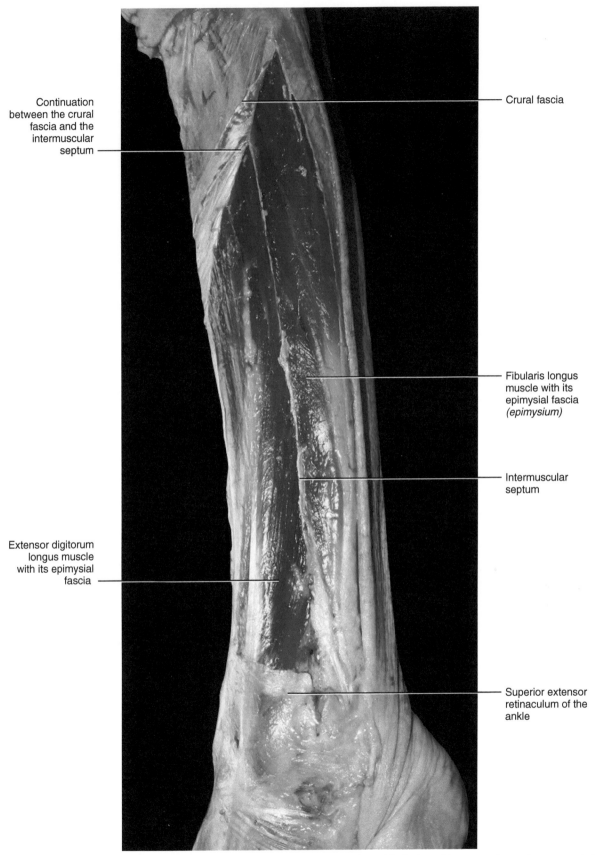

Continuation between the crural fascia and the intermuscular septum

Crural fascia

Fibularis longus muscle with its epimysial fascia *(epimysium)*

Intermuscular septum

Extensor digitorum longus muscle with its epimysial fascia

Superior extensor retinaculum of the ankle

FIGURE 8.53 Anterolateral view of the leg. To remove the crural fascia, its connection with the lateral intermuscular septum was cut. Many muscular fibres of the fibularis muscles and the extensor digitorum longus muscle are inserted into this septum.

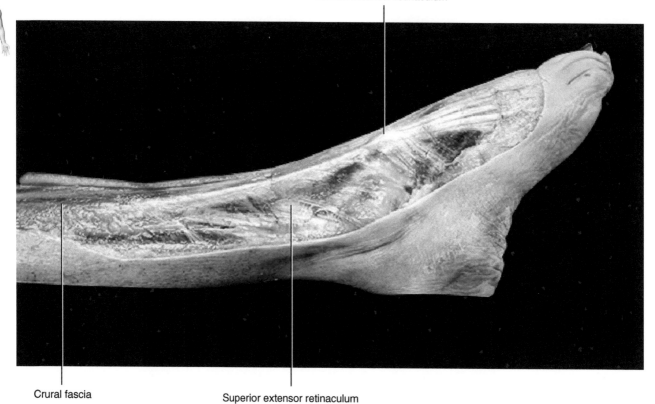

Inferior extensor retinaculum

Crural fascia

Superior extensor retinaculum

FIGURE 8.54 Anterolateral view of the leg and foot. The subcutaneous tissue is removed to show the deep fascia. The crural fascia continues in the dorsal fascia of the foot. Some fibrous reinforcements (ankle retinacula) are present around the ankle. These reinforcements follow the direction of the mechanical forces acting upon the deep fascia.

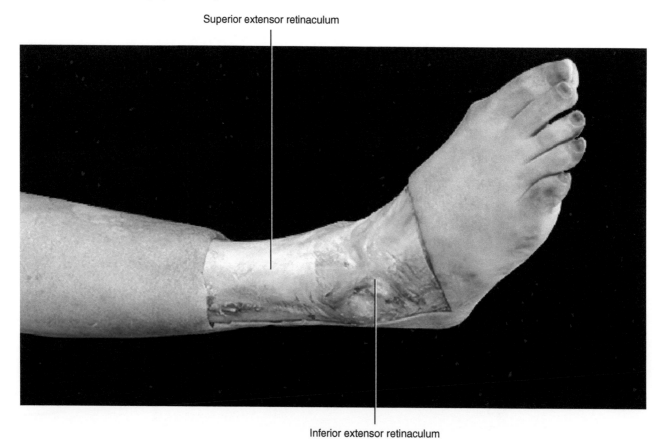

Superior extensor retinaculum

Inferior extensor retinaculum

FIGURE 8.55 Anterolateral view of the right ankle. Note the different aspect of the superior extensor retinaculum in comparison with the Figure 8.54. Here the retinaculum is thicker and shows a transverse disposition of the collagen fibre bundles. The other figure shows a superior extensor retinaculum that is thin and has fibres orientated obliquely.

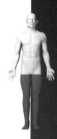

Inferior extensor retinaculum

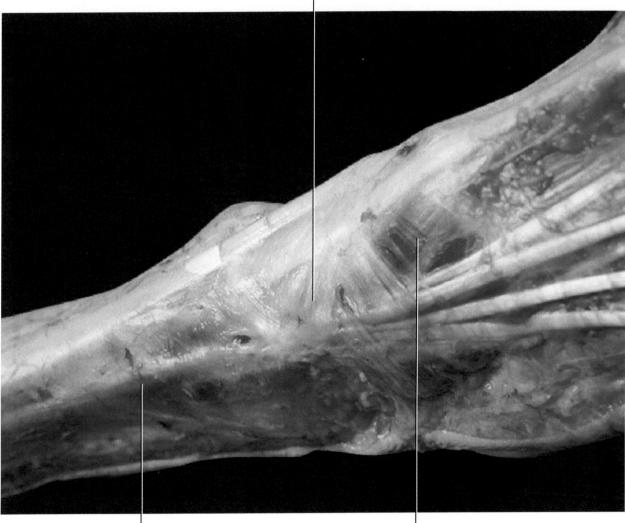

Superior extensor retinaculum   Deep fascia of the foot

FIGURE 8.56 Anterior view of the ankle. This inferior extensor retinaculum has the collagen fibre bundles arranged in various directions. It is evident that the retinacula are shaped by the forces acting on the deep fasciae.

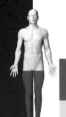

CLINICAL PEARL 8.6 COMPARTMENT SYNDROME

Compartment syndrome is a clinical condition in which increased pressure within a closed anatomical space compromises the circulation and function of the tissues within that space. This compromise in circulation may result in temporary or permanent damage to muscles and nerves. Compartment syndrome may be acute or chronic.

Acute compartment syndrome is usually caused by trauma, i.e. closed leg fracture or contusion, although the trauma may be relatively minor. The acute type is a medical emergency requiring prompt diagnosis and treatment (fasciotomy). The aponeurotic fascia, which is not very elastic, resists the excessive increase of volume in the compartment and the internal pressure increases rapidly and excessively. This alters the venous return and then the arterial flow.

Chronic compartment syndrome is an exercise-induced condition characterized by recurrent pain and disability, due to the temporary ischaemia of the muscles of that compartment. Symptoms subside when the offending activity is stopped but return when the activity is resumed. Anyone can develop chronic exertional compartment syndrome, but it is more common in athletes who participate in sports that involve repetitive movements. The most involved fascial compartment is the anterior compartment of the leg and it is most common in runners. However, any compartment formed by aponeurotic fasciae could be affected. Orava et al (1998), for example, describe this syndrome in the anterior thigh compartment in nine subjects (four power lifters, three body builders, one endurance walker and one cyclist; the use of anabolic steroids was admitted by four of the nine patients). Leppilahti et al (2002) describe acute bilateral exercise-induced medial compartment syndrome of the thigh. In chronic compartment syndrome, a building pressure within the compartment sheath is described. This may be due to excessive development of the muscular mass (e.g. this syndrome is typical for sports men, especially if they use anabolic steroids). It may also result from increased stiffness of the aponeurotic fascia that then becomes unable to adapt to muscular volume variations during activities. Increased pressure may, therefore, be due to a combination of surface alteration (stiffened aponeurosis) or content (increased muscular mass).

fibular retinaculum to attach to the anterolateral part of the calcaneus, and one deeper, inserted in the tarsal sinus. Medially, the two branches of the Y diverge: one is directed upwards, to attach to the tibial malleolus (superomedial branch), and the other extends downwards, to continue with the superficial part of the flexor retinaculum and then attaches to the border of the plantar aponeurosis (inferomedial branch). The superomedial branch passes over the extensor hallucis longus muscle, vessels and nerves; its fibres then split to enclose the tibialis anterior. The inferomedial branch is also inserted by a group of fibres of the abductor hallucis muscle, and it becomes thicker nearer this muscle. Many muscular fibres of the extensor digitorum brevis and extensor hallucis brevis muscles originate from the inner side of the inferior extensor retinaculum.

The flexor retinaculum extends from the medial malleolus to the medial calcaneal surface to form the tarsal tunnel. In the tarsal tunnel the tendons of the flexor digitorum longus, flexor hallucis longus and tibialis posterior muscles, the posterior tibial vessels and tibial nerve pass. The anterior margin of the flexor retinaculum is thicker, forming a fibrous ring where the abductor hallucis muscle inserts (Fig. 8.57). Posteriorly, the flexor retinaculum envelops the Achilles tendon and then continues with the superior fibular retinaculum. The deep layer of the flexor retinaculum provides attachment for the quadratus plantae muscle.

The superior fibular retinaculum and inferior fibular retinaculum are fibrous bands in the lateral side of the ankle, binding the tendons of the fibularis longus and brevis muscles. The superior fibular retinaculum appears as a quadrilateral lamina extending, distally and posteriorly, from the lateral malleolus to the lateral calcaneal surface (Fig. 8.58). Posteriorly, it splits into two layers: superficial and deep. The superficial layer envelops the Achilles tendon and then continues into the flexor retinaculum. Its anatomical boundaries are not sharply defined, particularly towards the superior, where it tapers gradually into the crural fascia. The deep layer of the superior fibular retinaculum passes between the achilles tendon and the flexor hallucis longus muscle. It represents a reinforcement of the deep lamina of the crural fascia. The inferior fibular retinaculum is continuous with the superficial layer of the lateral branch of the inferior extensor retinaculum. It appears as a vertical fibrous band passing over the tendons of the fibularis longus and brevis muscles (Fig. 8.59). Some of its fibres are attached to the calcaneus and form a septum between the two tendons.

Many muscle fibres of the intrinsic muscles of the foot are inserted into the ankle retinacula. They stretch the crural fascia in a distal direction due to the continuity between the ankle retinacula and the crural fascia. The anterior portion of the crural fascia is stretched caudally by the extensor digiti brevis muscle, which is inserted into the dorsal fascia of the foot and into the inferior extensor retinaculum (Fig. 8.60). The medial portion of the crural fascia is stretched by the abductor hallucis muscle, which has a substantial insertion into the flexor ankle retinaculum (Fig. 8.57). Laterally, the abductor digiti minimi creates stretching as it has many muscular fibres that insert into the deep fascia that envelops this muscle. This fascia is also continuous with the crural fascia. Consequently, every time the abductor digiti minimi contracts, it stretches its deep fascia tensioning the lateral portion of the crural fascia in a longitudinal direction. The posterior portion of the

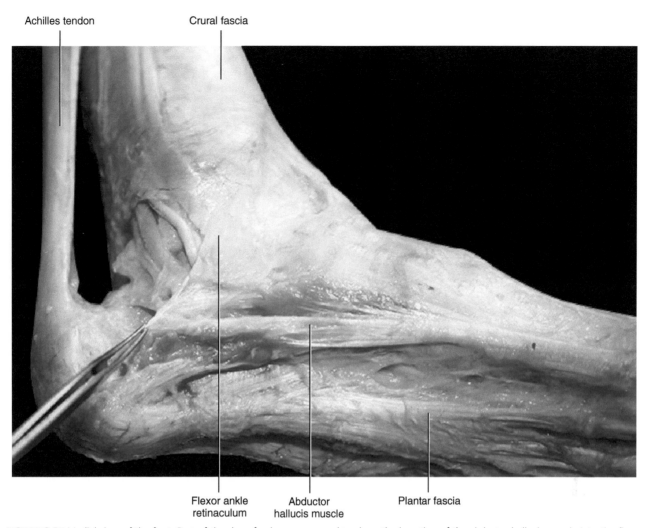

Achilles tendon   Crural fascia

Flexor ankle
retinaculum   Abductor
hallucis muscle   Plantar fascia

FIGURE 8.57 Medial view of the foot. Part of the deep fascia was removed to show the insertion of the abductor hallucis muscle into the flexor retinaculum.

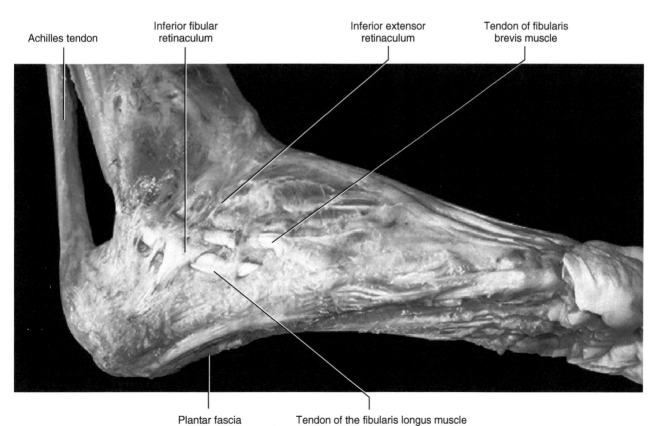

Inferior fibular
retinaculum   Inferior extensor
retinaculum   Tendon of fibularis
brevis muscle

Achilles tendon

Plantar fascia   Tendon of the fibularis longus muscle

FIGURE 8.58 Lateral view of the ankle and foot. The inferior fibular retinaculum covers the fibularis (*longus or brevis*) tendons and, in the dorsum of the foot, continues with the inferior extensor retinaculum. Note the continuity of the plantar fascia and the Achilles tendon.

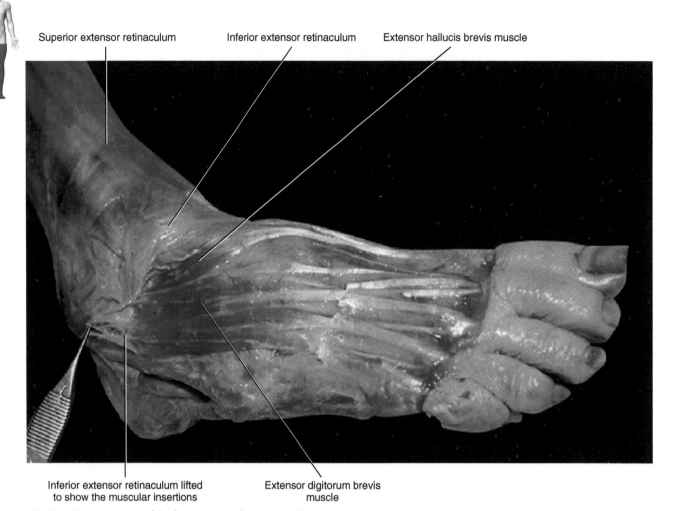

Superior extensor retinaculum   Inferior extensor retinaculum   Extensor hallucis brevis muscle

Inferior extensor retinaculum lifted
to show the muscular insertions

Extensor digitorum brevis
muscle

FIGURE 8.59 Dorsal region of the foot. The deep fascia is partially removed to show the intrinsic muscles of the foot. This figure shows the fascial insertions of the extensor digitorum brevis muscle. Many muscular fibres of this muscle originate from the inner side of the inferior extensor retinaculum. The fibre disposition and thickness of the retinaculum may be the result of traction into the fascia of this muscle.

crural fascia is stretched distally due to the continuity between it and the plantar fascia. The plantar fascia gives insertions to many intrinsic muscles and traction occurs between the heel and the posterior region of the crural fascia.

Finally, a paragraph must be dedicated to the plantaris muscle because it might be considered more of a fascial tensor than a muscle of force (Fig. 8.61). The plantaris muscle originates from the lateral supracondylar line of the femur and from the capsule of knee joint. In some cases the origin is only from the knee capsule and crural fascia, without any bone insertions. Distally, Nayak et al (2010) found that the plantaris tendon inserted into the flexor retinaculum of the foot in 29% of cases, into the os calcaneum in 29% of cases and into the crural fascia around the Achilles tendon in 27% of cases. This means that both the origin and insertion of this muscle could be into fascial structures. In 8% of cases the plantaris muscle could be completely absent. When this muscle contracts it stretches the posterior portion of the capsule of the knee and the popliteal fascia in a caudal direction, and it stretches the flexor retinaculum, or the posteromedial portion of the crural fascia, in a proximal direction. It thus coordinates the movement of the knee and foot.

Fasciae of the Foot

The foot contains many myofascial connections the dorsal fascia (which continues laterally with the abductor digiti minimi fascia and medially with the abductor hallucis fascia), the plantar fascia in the sole and the fascia of the interossei muscles. Another thin fascial layer is located under the flexor digitorum brevi that separates it from the quadratus plantae muscle. This fascial layer provides a fascial plane where the tendon of the flexor digitorum longus, the lateral plantar vessels and nerve flow. Under the quadratus plantae muscle are the flexor hallucis brevis of the hallux, *abductor digiti minimi* and adductor hallucis muscles, that are all enveloped by a very thin fascial layer.

Currently there is still no agreement on the number and location of the myofascial compartments. Ling and Krumar (2008) identified three tough, vertical fascial septa that extended from the hindfoot to the midfoot on the plantar surface. These septa separate the

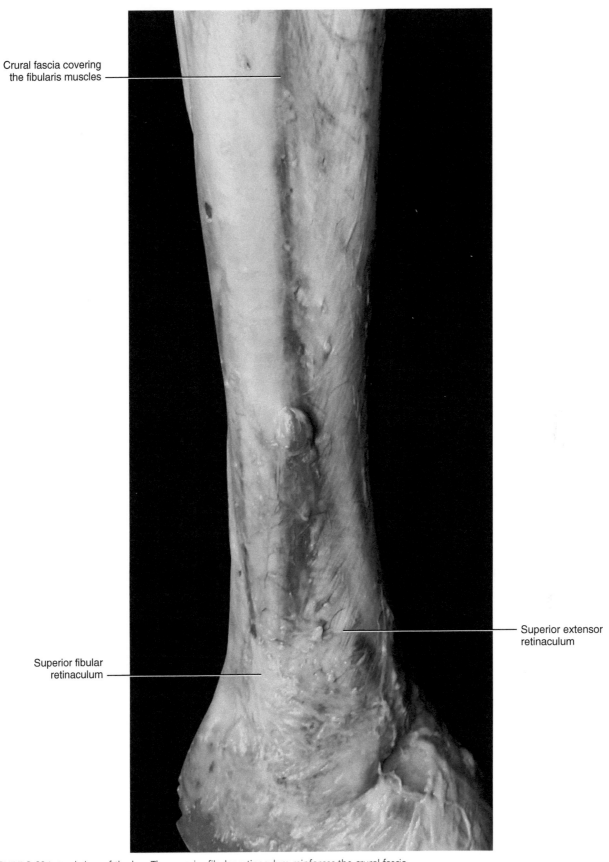

Crural fascia covering
the fibularis muscles

Superior extensor
retinaculum

Superior fibular
retinaculum

FIGURE 8.60 Lateral view of the leg. The superior fibular retinaculum reinforces the crural fascia.

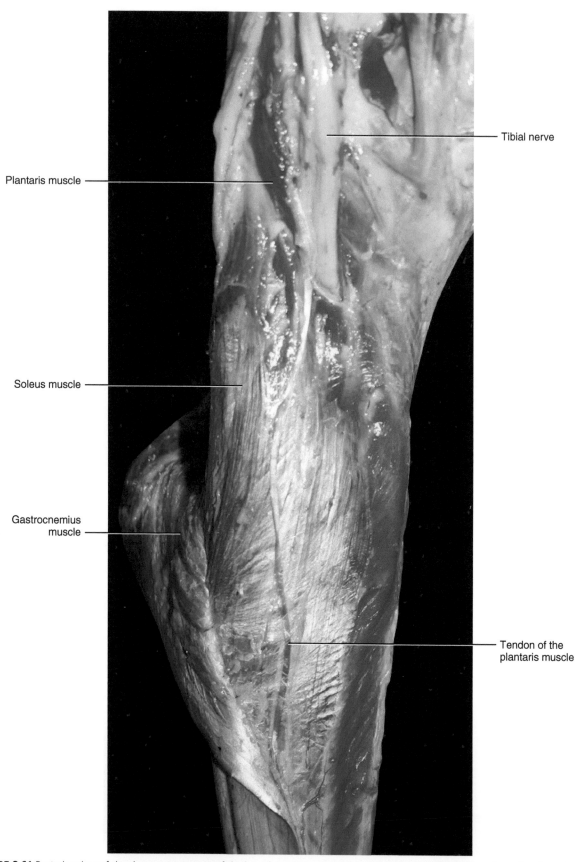

Tibial nerve

Plantaris muscle

Soleus muscle

Gastrocnemius
muscle

Tendon of the
plantaris muscle

FIGURE 8.61 Posterior view of the deep compartment of the leg. The gastrocnemius muscle is detached and lifted to show the plantaris muscle and soleus.

CLINICAL PEARL 8.7 TARSAL TUNNEL SYNDROME

Tarsal tunnel syndrome is a compression syndrome of the distal branches of the posterior tibial nerve as it runs beneath the flexor retinaculum (Fig. 8.62). Pain and/or paraesthesia along the medial plantar surface of the foot reaching the first three toes are common. A positive Tinel's sign posterior to the medial malleolus and impaired two-point discrimination may be present. Passive maximal eversion and dorsiflexion of the ankle, while all of the metatarsophalangeal joints are maximally dorsiflexed, and holding this position for 5–10 s might elicit the symptoms.

This syndrome can be due to trauma, autoimmune disease, pronation, tendonitis and ganglionic cysts, among others. An increased tension of the deep fascia and flexor retinaculum could also cause this syndrome, and may be due to trauma or overuse, or to excessive tension of the abductor hallucis muscle that inserts many fibres into the retinaculum. Hudes K (2010) treated this syndrome using cross-friction massage and instrument assisted fascial stripping techniques applied to the lateral heel over the tarsal tunnel, and over the plantar and dorsal surfaces of the forefoot.

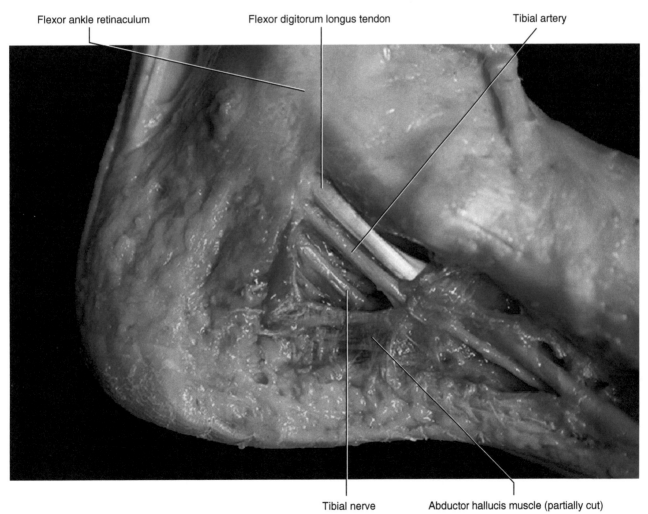

Flexor ankle retinaculum   Flexor digitorum longus tendon   Tibial artery

Tibial nerve   Abductor hallucis muscle (partially cut)

FIGURE 8.62 Medial view of the ankle. The deep fascia and abductor hallucis muscle are partially removed to show the structures inside the tarsal tunnel.

posterior half of the foot into three compartments: the medial compartment (containing the abductor hallucis and flexor hallucis brevis muscles), the intermediate compartment (central or calcaneal compartment) containing the flexor digitorum brevis, quadratus plantae and adductor hallucis muscles (located more deeply), and the lateral compartment (containing the abductor digiti minimi and flexor digiti minimi brevis muscles). Finally, there is an intrinsic compartment formed by the four intrinsic muscles between the first and fifth metatarsals.

DORSAL FASCIA OF THE FOOT

The fascia on the dorsum of the foot consists of a thin fibrous layer, continuous above with the inferior extensor ankle retinaculum (Fig. 8.63). It forms a sheath for the tendons on the dorsum of the foot (extensor digitorum longus and extensor hallucis longus) (Fig. 8.64). Inserted at its inner side are some muscle fibres of the extensor digitorum brevis and extensor hallucis brevis muscles. When these muscles contract they stretch this fascia and the inferior extensor retinaculum in a caudal direction. The dorsal fascia of the foot is also stretched in a cranial direction by the myofascial

expansions of the tibialis anterior and fibularis tertius muscles (Figs 8.65–8.68)

In the medial region of the foot the fascia continues with the abductor hallucis fascia that envelops the abductor hallucis muscle. This muscle has many fascial insertions. Some of its fibres arise from the flexor retinaculum of the ankle, others from the plantar fascia and from the intermuscular septum between it and the flexor digitorum brevis. Thus, the abductor hallucis muscle could be considered a key muscle for the fascial tension of the foot, as it connects the fascia of the dorsum with the plantar fascia, and these fasciae with the crural fascia in the leg.

Laterally, the dorsal fascia of the foot forms the fascial compartment of the abductor digiti minimi. The abductor digiti minimi has some fibres that originate from the plantar fascia and others from the intermuscular septum between it and the flexor digitorum brevis.

FASCIA OF THE INTEROSSEI

Kalin and Hirsch (1987) found that the dorsal and plantar interosseous muscles arise not only from the metatarsal bones, but also from ligamentous tissue

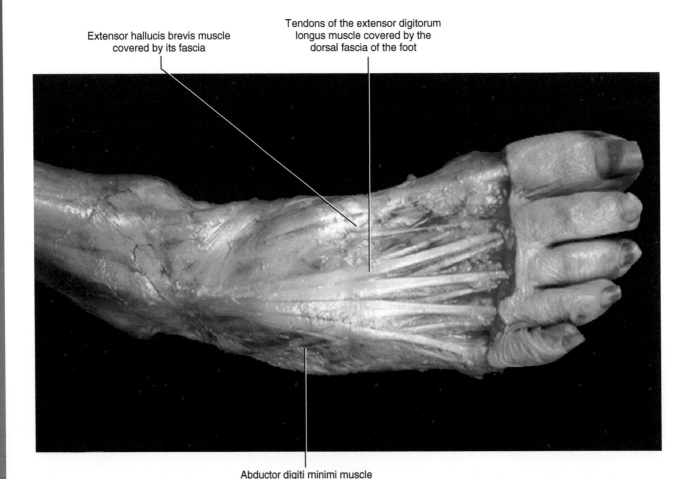

Extensor hallucis brevis muscle covered by its fascia

Tendons of the extensor digitorum longus muscle covered by the dorsal fascia of the foot

Abductor digiti minimi muscle covered by its fascia

FIGURE 8.63 Dorsal region of the foot. The deep fascia covers all the tendons and muscles and continues laterally with the fascia of the abductor digiti minimi muscle. Proximally, the dorsal fascia of the foot continues with the crural fascia.

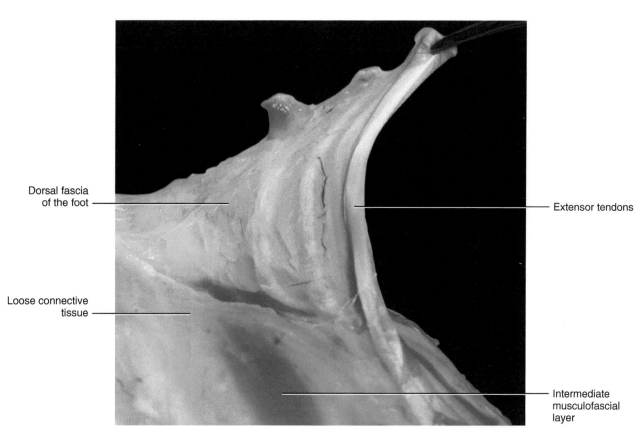

Dorsal fascia
of the foot

Extensor tendons

Loose connective
tissue

Intermediate
musculofascial
layer

FIGURE 8.64 Dorsal region of the foot. All the tendons of the extensor digitorum longus muscle and the extensor hallucis longus muscle are embedded in the dorsal fascia of the foot. This deep fascia splits around each tendon, creating individual sheaths. Underneath this fascial layer is another myofascial layer. This layer is formed by the extensor digitorum brevis and extensor hallucis brevis muscles. Between these two myofascial layers loose connective tissue is present.

CLINICAL PEARL 8.8 MORTON'S DISEASE (NEUROMA AND METATARSALGIA)

A fibrosis and thickening of the connective tissue around the intermetatarsal plantar nerve occurs, and most often affects the second and third intermetatarsal spaces (between 2nd–3rd and 3rd–4th metatarsal heads). Microscopically, the affected nerve appears markedly distorted with extensive concentric perineural fibrosis. The main symptoms are pain on weight bearing and/or numbness, sometimes relieved by removing footwear. Direct pressure between the metatarsal heads will replicate the symptoms, as will compression of the forefoot between the finger and thumb so as to compress

the transverse arch of the foot (Mulder's sign). One of the major contributors in neuroma formation is the deep transverse metatarsal ligament, but the mechanism is unclear. Mariano De Prado (2003) proposes a deep transverse metatarsal ligament release, associated with metatarsal shortening by osteotomy, to treat Morton's neuroma without cutting the nerve. This decompression relieves pain by reducing the tension acting on the nerve. Similar results may be possible with some manual techniques as suggested by Davis (2012).

---

proximal to the tarsometatarsal joints and from the fascia of adjacent muscles. Oukouchi et al (1992) revealed that the plantar and dorsal interosseous muscles often contain some accessory smaller tendons that continue into the dorsal fascia. Due to these fascial connections, it is possible that the tension created by the contraction of one muscle triggers the contraction

of others, so that they function as a unit in a coordinated manner. It is necessary that the foot be flexible and adaptable in order to adjust to uneven terrain. At other times it serves best as a rigid structure, and the extensive connections among the interossei indicate that they could also be important stabilizers of the foot when rigidity is required.

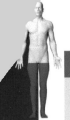

Fasciae of the Lower Limb

CLINICAL PEARL 8.9 HEEL PAIN

Heel pain is a common condition in adults that may cause significant discomfort and disability. A variety of soft tissue, osseous, and systemic disorders can cause heel pain. Narrowing the differential diagnosis begins with a history and physical examination of the lower extremity to pinpoint the anatomical origin of the heel pain. The most common cause of heel pain in adults is plantar fasciitis. Patients with plantar fasciitis report increased heel pain with their first steps in the morning or when they stand up after prolonged sitting. Tenderness at the calcaneal tuberosity is usually apparent on examination and is increased with passive dorsiflexion of the toes. Achilles tendonitis or tendinosis may be associated with posterior heel pain. In addition, bursae adjacent to the Achilles tendon insertion may become inflamed and cause pain. Calcaneal stress fractures are

more likely to occur in athletes who participate in sports that require running and jumping. Patients with plantar heel pain accompanied by tingling, burning, or numbness may have tarsal tunnel syndrome. Heel pad atrophy may present with diffuse plantar heel pain, especially in patients who are older and obese. Since there is a definite fascial continuity between the paratenon of the calcaneal tendon and the plantar fascia, it is evident that heel pain could also be due to increased tension from either or both the plantar fascia or triceps surae muscle. Carlson et al (2000) demonstrated that excessive stretching and/or tightness of the Achilles tendon are risk factors for plantar fasciitis. Every physical examination of a patient with heel pain should include evaluation of the plantar fascia and triceps surae for tissue tightness and fascial restrictions (Stecco et al 2013).

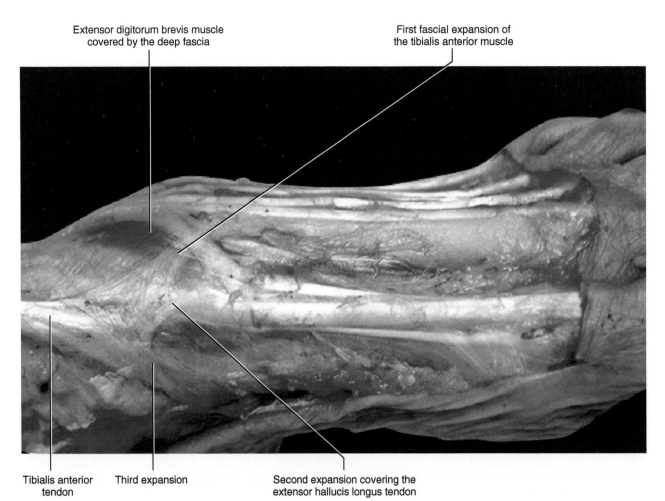

Extensor digitorum brevis muscle covered by the deep fascia

First fascial expansion of the tibialis anterior muscle

Tibialis anterior tendon

Third expansion

Second expansion covering the extensor hallucis longus tendon

FIGURE 8.65 Medial view of the dorsal region of the foot. The tibialis anterior muscle has three myofascial expansions for the dorsal fascia of the foot. Every time this muscle contracts, it stretches the dorsal fascia of the foot. The first expansion inserts exactly where the dorsal fascia of the foot gives insertions, on the inner side, to the extensor digitorum brevis muscle. The second expansion covers the extensor hallucis longus muscle; the third expansion runs medially to join with the abductor hallucis muscle.

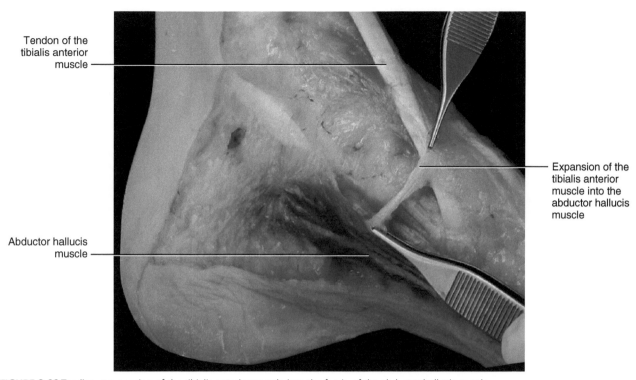

Tendon of the tibialis anterior muscle

Abductor hallucis muscle

Expansion of the tibialis anterior muscle into the abductor hallucis muscle

FIGURE 8.66 Tendinous expansion of the tibialis anterior muscle into the fascia of the abductor hallucis muscle.

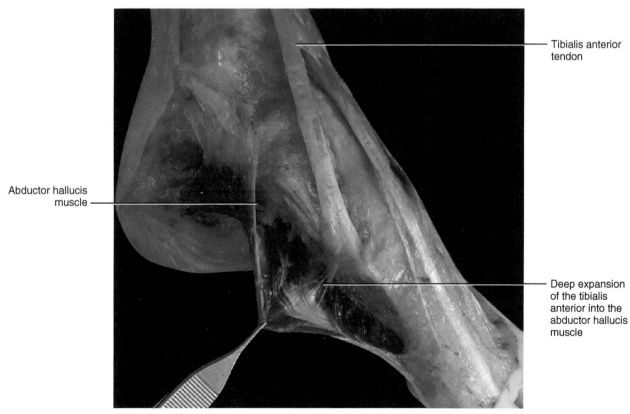

Abductor hallucis muscle

Tibialis anterior tendon

Deep expansion of the tibialis anterior into the abductor hallucis muscle

FIGURE 8.67 Deep tendinous expansion of the tibialis anterior muscle into the fascia of the abductor hallucis muscle.

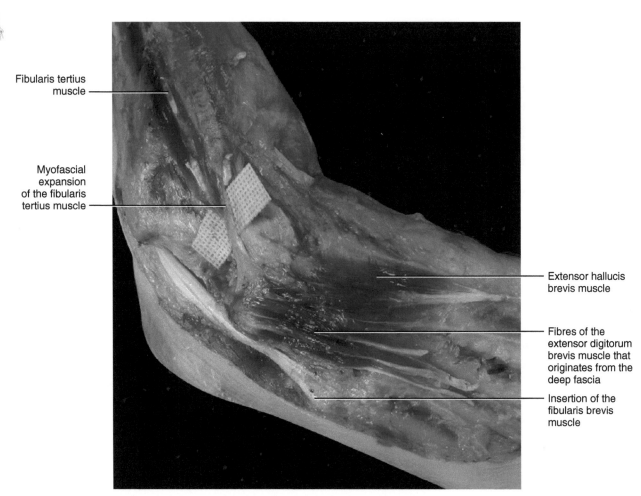

Fibularis tertius muscle

Myofascial expansion of the fibularis tertius muscle

Extensor hallucis brevis muscle

Fibres of the extensor digitorum brevis muscle that originates from the deep fascia

Insertion of the fibularis brevis muscle

FIGURE 8.68 Lateral view of the dorsal region of the foot. The deep fascia was removed, together with the tendons of the extensor digitorum longus muscle, to show the deeper planes. The extensor digitorum brevis and extensor hallucis brevis muscles are enveloped by their fascia. This fascia is stretched by the myofascial expansion of the fibularis tertius muscle. Deeper to these muscles, the deep dorsal fascia covers the interosseous muscles.

PLANTAR FASCIA[2]

The plantar fascia has probably been investigated more frequently than most of the fasciae of the human body, thanks to its key role in foot biomechanics and to its involvement in several pathologies. The plantar fascia is composed of densely compacted collagen fibres mostly orientated longitudinally (Fig. 8.69). It has two fibrous layers: superficial and deep. The superficial layer is formed by longitudinal fibres, which originate from the medial process of the calcaneal tuberosity, and diverge distally to form five bands that continue into the fascial sheets of the five toes. The deep layer is thinner and is not present throughout all the plantar fascia. It is formed by bundles of collagen fibres with a transverse disposition. The deep layer is easier to identify over the heads of the metatarsal bones. From this point some vertical septa anchor the deep aspect of the plantar fascia to the metatarsal bones. This organization corresponds to the palmar aponeurosis[3], so we can affirm that the superficial layer of the plantar fascia corresponds to the superficial fascia and the deep layer to the deep fascia. In the foot these two layers fuse to form the plantar fascia. From the superficial aspect of the plantar fascia, many vertical fibrous septa

---

[2]Investigators debate whether this structure is deep fascia or aponeurosis. *Dorland's Medical Dictionary* defines an aponeurosis as a white, flattened tendinous expansion, connecting a muscle with the parts that it moves, while fascia is defined as a sheet or band of fibrous tissue investing muscles and various body organs. Because the plantar fascia covers and protects the intrinsic muscles of the foot it can be considered as a fascia. In addition, the aponeurosis has all the collagen fibres parallel to each other, while the plantar fascia is formed by longitudinal and transverse collagen bundles (which happens to be the typical structure of aponeurotic fascia).

---

[3]For the reason given in the first footnote the palmar aponeurosis should be called 'palmar fascia', but in the common terminology it is known as the 'palmar aponeurosis'. We adopt this nomenclature, but consider this structure as aponeurotic fascia.

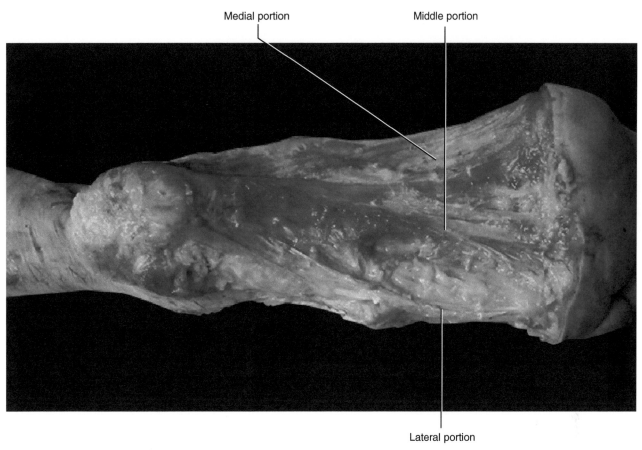

Medial portion   Middle portion

Lateral portion

FIGURE 8.69 Sole of the foot. The subcutaneous tissues are removed to show the plantar fascia. The plantar fascia has a middle portion and two thinner parts: a medial one that continues with the fascia of the abductor hallucis muscle, and a lateral one that continues with the fascia of the abductor digiti minimi muscle. Note that all the collagen fibre bundles of the plantar fascia converge into the calcaneous.

(retinaculum cutis superficialis) originate, strongly connecting the plantar fascia with the skin. Between these septa, fat lobules are present which act as shock absorbers.

The mean thickness of the plantar fascia varies from 2.2 to 3.9 mm depending on the study. According to Pascual Huerta et al (2008), the mean plantar fascia thickness evaluated with ultrasonography was 1.99±0.65 mm, 3.33±0.69 mm at the insertion, 2.70±0.69 mm at 1 cm distal from the insertion and 2.64±0.69 mm at 2 cm distal from the insertion. According to Moraes do Carmo et al (2008), the plantar fascia, evaluated by dissection, presented a mean thickness of 4.4 mm in its central part, of 2.7 mm in its lateral part, while its medial portion was thin. The thickness of the plantar fascia could vary with the patient's sex, weight and different pathologies (plantar fasciitis, diabetes, etc.), but it seems to remain constant with age. In plantar fasciitis different studies have found an increased thickness of the plantar fascia, varying from 2.9 to 6.2 mm, depending on the study and the points evaluated (Fig. 8.70).

The plantar fascia can be divided into three parts: the middle part is the strongest and thickest, while the medial and lateral portions continue with the deep fasciae enveloping the intrinsic muscles of the hallux and

fifth toe respectively. Two intermuscular septa, medial and lateral, extend in oblique vertical planes between the medial, intermediate and lateral groups of plantar muscles to reach bone. The central part of the plantar aponeurosis covers the long and short flexors of the digits, the lateral part covers the abductor digiti minimi, while the medial part covers the abductor hallucis muscle. Medially, the plantar aponeurosis is continuous with the flexor retinaculum and, laterally, with the inferior peroneal retinaculum.

Several authors (Benjamin 2009, Benninghoff & Goerttler 1978, Erdemir et al 2004, Shaw et al 2008, Wood Jones 1944) have found that the plantar fascia is continuous with the Achilles tendon. Thus, the plantar fascia contributes to a more homogeneous distribution of Achilles stress and permits transmission of force from the hind to the forefoot and vice versa. Snow et al (1995) have demonstrated that aging produces a continued diminution of the number of fibres connecting the Achilles tendon and the plantar fascia. The neonate has a thick continuation of fibres, the middle aged foot has only superficial periosteal fibres that continue from tendon to fascia, while in elderly feet no connections could be found at all. Our recent study (Stecco et al 2013) has demonstrated that a connection between plantar fascia and the paratenon of

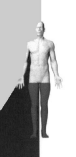

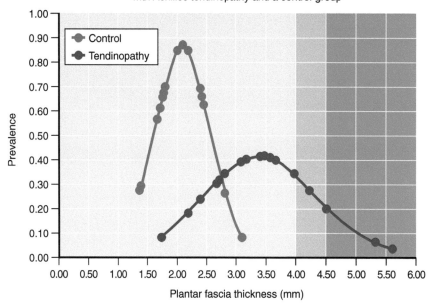

FIGURE 8.70 Comparison of the thickness of the plantar fascia in healthy subjects (blue) and in patients with Achilles tendinopathy (red). It is evident that the patients with Achilles tendinopathy had thicker plantar fascia. This data suggests that the plantar fascia should always be examined in patients with Achilles tendinopathy as the plantar fascia is continuous with the Achilles paratenon.

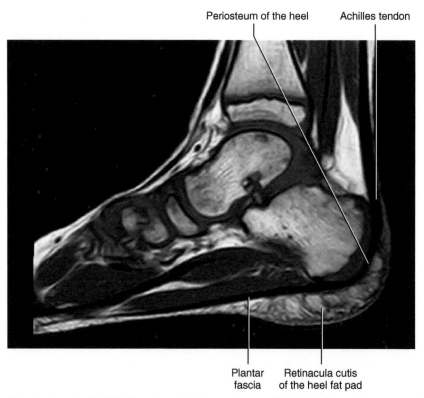

FIGURE 8.71 MRI of the foot of a six-year-old child. The plantar fascia appears as a visible black line and is connected clearly with the Achilles tendon via the periosteum of the calcaneous. MRI allows us to visualize the retinacula cutis of the heel fat pad.

the Achilles tendon, via a fascial sheet over the calcaneous bone, is present at all ages (Figs 8.71 and 8.72).

The plantar fascia helps to maintain the medial longitudinal arch and transmit forces from the hind to the forefoot (Erdemir et al 2004). It can act both as a beam and a truss (Hicks 1954, Salathe et al 1986): a beam during propulsion when the metatarsals are subject to significant bending force and a truss when the foot absorbs impact force during landing and during the stance phase of gait. Its function as a tie beam for the

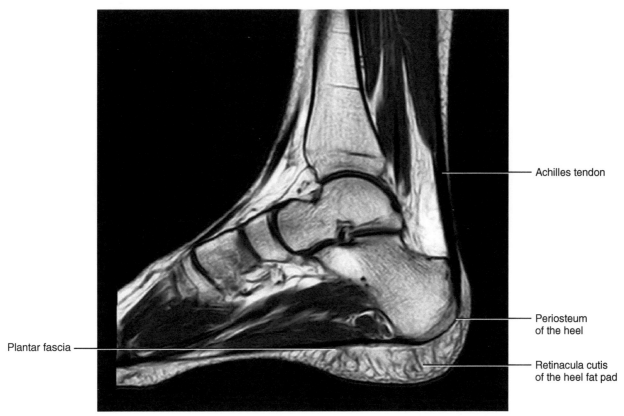

Achilles tendon

Periosteum
of the heel

Plantar fascia

Retinacula cutis
of the heel fat pad

FIGURE 8.72 MRI of an adult foot. The connection between the plantar fascia and the Achilles tendon via the periosteum of the calcaneous is always present, but thinner.

foot is clearly explained by Sarrafian (1987) who likens the foot to a twisted plate in which the hindfoot lies in the sagittal plane and the forefoot lies horizontally. It is the twist that occurs between hind and forefoot that creates the characteristic arch. When the foot is loaded by body weight acting through the ankle joint, the dorsum of the foot experiences compressive loading and the plantar side is subject to tensile loading. The plantar fascia thus acts as a tie beam in the sole to relieve the tensile loading to which this area is subject. The plantar fascia carries 14% of the total load of the foot. In cadavers, plantar fascia fails at average loads of 1189±244 N. Surgical release is often performed to reduce plantar tension. Creating release in cadaver models results in an average decrease in arch height of 7.4±4.1 mm and an average increase in horizontal elongation of the foot of 15%. In addition, the plantar fascia plays a role in the dissipation of impact and muscular force, thereby protecting the plantar vessels and nerves.

The presence of Pacini's and Ruffini's corpuscles, usually considered responsible for mechanoreception, suggests that plantar fascia innervations have a role in proprioception, stability and control of foot movements. Thanks to the many muscle insertions, the plantar fascia is capable of perceiving both the foot's position and the state of contraction of the various intrinsic muscles. If these muscles contract excessively,

CLINICAL PEARL 8.10 PATHOLOGIES OF THE PLANTAR FASCIA

Plantar fasciitis is an inflammation of the plantar fascia especially at its calcaneal insertion. It is particularly common in runners (Warren 1990) and in workers that require a lot of walking on hard surfaces. It is also commonly associated with weight bearing, shoes with little or no arch support, and alteration of the plantar support. It is usually considered an overuse syndrome caused by excessive stretching, repetitive and abnormal stress, excessive pronation of the foot, flat or high-arched foot structures and tight Achilles tendon. Stretching exercises and dorsiflexion night splints are often prescribed to relieve the plantar fascia tension. Less frequently a traumatic rupture could be the cause. The plantar fascia may be altered in different systemic pathologies. For example, in type I diabetes the plantar fascia is susceptible to glycation, oxidation and thickening. For some authors this thickening is used as an alternative index of tissue glycation and as a marker of microvascular disease. The plantar fascia may also be involved in psoriasis, ankylosing spondylitis and fibromatosis (morbus Ledderhose). It may also appear in degenerative alterations such as calcification and cartilaginous metaplasia.

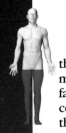

the plantar fascia (and the nerve endings it contains) might be overstretched. These properties of the plantar fascia shed new light on this complex tissue. The fascia could be seen as a coachman guiding the muscles in the sole of the foot and helping to coordinate all these structures during movement.

References

Andersen, H.L., Andersen, S.L., Tranum-Jensen, J., 2012. Injection inside the paraneural sheath of the sciatic nerve: Direct comparison among ultrasound imaging, macroscopic anatomy, and histologic analysis. Reg. Anesth. Pain Med. 37 (4), 410–414.

Benjamin, M., 2009. The fascia of the limbs and back: A review. J. Anat. 214 (1), 1–18.

Benninghoff, A., Goerttler, K., 1978. Lehrbuch der Anatomie des Menschen, vol. 1, second ed. Urban & Schwarzenberg, München, pp. 430–450.

Burnet, N.G., Bennett-Britton, T., Hoole, A.C., Jefferies, S.J., Parkin, I.G., 2004. The anatomy of sartorius muscle and its implications for sarcoma radiotherapy. Sarcoma 8 (1), 7–12.

Caggiati, A., 2000. Fascial relations and structure of the tributaries of the saphenous veins. Surg. Radiol. Anat. 22 (3–4), 191–196.

Canoso, J.J., Stack, M.T., Brandt, K.D., 1983. Hyaluronic acid content of deep and subcutaneous bursae of man. Ann. Rheum. Dis. 42 (2), 171–175.

Carlson, R.E., Fleming, L.L., Hutton, W.C., 2000. The biomechanical relationship between the tendoachilles, plantar fascia and metatarsophalangeal joint dorsiflexion angle. Foot Ankle Int. 21 (1), 18–25.

Chen, C.K., Yeh, L., Chang, W.N., Pan, H.B., Yang, C.F., 2006. MRI diagnosis of contracture of the gluteus maximus muscle. AJR Am. J. Roentgenol. 187 (2), W169–W174.

Cichowitz, A., Pan, W.R., Ashton, M., 2009. The heel: anatomy, blood supply, and the pathophysiology of pressure ulcers. Ann. Plast. Surg. 62 (40), 423–429.

Crum, J.A., La Prade, R.F., Wentorf, F.A., 2003. The anatomy of the posterolateral aspect of the rabbit knee. J. Orthop. Res. 21 (4), 723–729.

Davis, F., 2012. Therapeutic massage provides pain relief to a client with morton's neuroma: A case report. Int. J. Ther. Massage. Bodywork. 5 (2), 12–19.

De Maeseneer, M., Van Roy, F., Lenchik, L., Barbaix, E., De Ridder, F., Osteaux, M., 2000. Three layers of the medial capsular and supporting structures of the knee: MR imaging – anatomic correlation. Radiographics 20, Spec No, S83–S89.

De Prado, M., 2003. Cirugía percutánea del pie. Masson, Barcellona, pp. 213–220.

Dunn, T., Heller, C.A., McCarthy, S.W., Dos Remedios, C., 2003. Anatomical study of the "trochanteric bursa". Clin. Anat. 16 (3), 233–240.

Dye, S.F., Campagna-Pinto, D., Dye, C.C., Shifflett, S., Eiman, T., 2003. Soft-tissue anatomy anterior to the human patella. J. Bone Joint Surg. Am. 85-A (6), 1012–1017.

Erdemir, A., Hamel, A.J., Fauth, A.R., Piazza, S.J., Sharkey, N.A., 2004. Dynamic loading of the plantar aponeurosis in walking. J. Bone Joint Surg. Am. 86-A (3), 546–552.

Fairclough, J., Hayashi, K., Toumi, H., et al., 2007. Is iliotibial band syndrome really a friction syndrome? J. Sci. Med. Sport 10 (2), 74–76.

Halpin, R.J., Ganju, A., 2009. Piriformis syndrome: a real pain in the buttock? Neurosurgery 65 (4 Suppl.), A197–A202.

Hicks, J.H., 1954. The mechanics of the foot. II. The plantar aponeurosis and the arch. J. Anat. 88 (1), 25–30.

Hudes, K., 2010. Conservative management of a case of tarsal tunnel syndrome. J. Can. Chiropr. Assoc. 54 (2), 100–106.

Kalin, P.J., Hirsch, B.E., 1987. The origins and function of the interosseous muscles of the foot. J. Anat. 152 (June), 83–91.

Kimani, J.K., 1984. The structural and functional organization of the connective tissue in the human foot with reference to the histomorphology of the elastic fibre system. Acta Morphol. Neerl. Scand. 22 (4), 313–323.

Leppilahti, J., Tervonen, O., Herva, R., Karinen, J., Puranen, J., 2002. Acute bilateral exercise-induced medial compartment syndrome of the thigh. Correlation of repeated MRI with clinicopathological findings. Int. J. Sports Med. 23 (8), 610–615.

Ling, Z.X., Kumar, V.P., 2008. The myofascial compartments of the foot: A cadaver study. J. Bone Joint Surg. Br. 90 (8), 1114–1118.

Miller, T.A., White, K.P., Ross, D.C., 2012. The diagnosis and management of piriformis syndrome: Myths and facts. Can. J. Neurol. Sci. 39 (5), 577–583.

Mochizuki, T., Akita, K., Muneta, T., Sato, T., 2004. Pes anserinus: layered supportive structure on the medial side of the knee. Clin. Anat. 17 (1), 50–54.

Moraes do Carmo, C.C., Fonseca de Almeida Melão, L.I., Valle de Lemos Weber, M.F., Trudell, D., Resnick, D., 2008. Anatomical features of plantar aponeurosis: cadaveric study using ultrasonography and magnetic resonance imaging. Skeletal Radiol. 37 (10), 929–935.

Nayak, S.R., Krishnamurthy, A., Ramanathan, L., et al., 2010. Anatomy of plantaris muscle: a study in adult Indians. Clin. Ter. 161 (3), 249–252.

Orava, S., Laakko, E., Mattila, K., Mäkinen, L., Rantanen, J., Kujala, U.M., 1998. Chronic compartment syndrome of the quadriceps femoris muscle in athletes. Diagnosis, imaging and treatment with fasciotomy. Ann. Chir. Gynaecol. 87 (1), 53–58.

Oukouchi, H., Murakami, T., Kikuta, A., 1992. Insertions of the lumbrical and interosseous muscles in the human foot. Okajimas Folia Anat. Jpn 69 (2–3), 77–83.

Pascual Huerta, J., García, J.M., Matamoros, E.C., Matamoros, J.C., Martínez, T.D., 2008. Relationship of body mass index, ankle dorsiflexion, and foot pronation on plantar fascia thickness in healthy, asymptomatic subjects. J. Am. Podiatr. Med. Assoc. 98 (5), 379–385.

Salathe, E.P., Jr., Arangio, G.A., Salathe, E.P., 1986. A biomechanical model of the foot. J. Biomech. 19 (12), 989–1001.

Sarrafian, S.K., 1987. Functional characteristics of the foot and plantar aponeurosis under tibiotalar loading. Foot Ankle 8 (1), 4–18.

Schweighofer, G., Mühlberger, D., Brenner, E., 2010. The anatomy of the small saphenous vein: fascial and neural relations, saphenofemoral junction, and valves. J. Vasc. Surg. 51 (4), 982–989.

Shaw, H.M., Vázquez, O.T., McGonagle, D., Bydder, G., Santer, R.M., Benjamin, M., 2008. Development of the human Achilles tendon enthesis organ. J. Anat. 213 (6), 718–724.

Silva, F., Adams, T., Feinstein, J., Arroyo, R.A., 2008. Trochanteric bursitis: refuting the myth of inflammation. J. Clin. Rheumatol. 14 (2), 82–86.

Snow, S.W., Bohne, W.H., 2006. Observations on the fibrous retinacula of the heel pad. Foot Ankle Int. 27 (8), 632–635.

Snow, S.W., Bohne, W.H., Di Carlo, E., Chang, V.K., 1995. Anatomy of the Achilles tendon and plantar fascia in relation to the calcaneus in various age groups. Foot Ankle Int. 16 (7), 418–421.

Stecco, C., Corradin, M., Macchi, V., et al., 2013. Plantar fascia anatomy and its relationship with Achilles tendon and paratenon. J. Anat. 223 (6), 665–676.

Stecco, C., Macchi, V., Porzionato, A., et al., 2010. The ankle retinacula: morphological evidence of the proprioceptive role of the fascial system. Cells Tissues Organs 192 (3), 200–210.

Terry, G.C., LaPrade, R.F., 1996. The posterolateral aspect of the knee. Anatomy and surgical approach. Am. J. Sports Med. 24 (6), 732–739.

Thawait, S.K., Soldatos, T., Thawait, G.K., Cosgarea, A.J., Carrino, J.A., Chhabra, A., 2012. High resolution magnetic resonance imaging of the patellar retinaculum: normal anatomy, common injury patterns, and pathologies. Skeletal Radiol. 41 (2), 137–148.

Tubbs, R.S., Caycedo, F.J., Oakes, W.J., Salter, E.G., 2006. Descriptive anatomy of the insertion of the biceps femoris muscle. Clin. Anat. 19 (6), 517–521.

Tubbs, R.S., Loukas, M., Shoja, M.M., Apaydin, N., Oakes, W.J., Salter, E.G., 2007. Anatomy and potential clinical significance of the vastoadductor membrane. Surg. Radiol. Anat. 29 (7), 569–573.

Van Dyke, J.A., Holley, H.C., Anderson, S.D., 1987. Review of iliopsoas anatomy and pathology. Radiographics 7 (1), 53–84.

Vieira, E.L., Vieira, E.A., da Silva, R.T., Berlfein, P.A., Abdalla, R.J., Cohen, M., 2007. An anatomic study of the iliotibial tract. Arthroscopy 23 (3), 269–274.

Vleeming, A., Pool-Goudzwaard, A.L., Stoeckart, R., van Wingerden, J.P., Snijders, C.J., 1995. The posterior layer of the thoracolumbar fascia. Its function in load transfer from spine to legs. Spine 20 (7), 753–758.

Wangwinyuvirat, M., Dirim, B., Pastore, D., et al., 2009. Prepatellar quadriceps continuation: MRI of cadavers with gross anatomic and histologic correlation. Am. J. Roentgenol. 192 (3), W111–W116.

Warren, B.L., 1990. Plantar fasciitis in runners: Treatment and prevention. Sports Med. 10 (5), 338–345.

Wood Jones, F., 1944. Structure and Function as Seen in the Foot. Baillière, Tindall and Cox, London, pp. 1–324.

Woodley, S.J., Mercer, S.R., Nicholson, H.D., 2008. Morphology of the bursae associated with the greater trochanter of the femur. J. Bone Joint Surg. Am. 90 (2), 284–294.

Wu, C.C., Shih, C.H., 2004. The influence of iliotibial tract on patellar tracking. Orthopedics 27 (2), 199–203.

Bibliography

Aguiar, R.O., Viegas, F.C., Fernandez, R.Y., Trudell, D., Haghighi, P., Resnick, D., 2007. The prepatellar bursa: cadaveric investigation of regional anatomy with MRI after sonographically guided bursography. Am. J. Roentgenol. 188 (4), W355–W358.

Campanelli, V., Fantini, M., Faccioli, N., Cangemi, A., Pozzo, A., Sbarbati, A., 2011. Three-dimensional morphology of heel fat pad: an in vivo computed tomography study. J. Anat. 219 (5), 622–631.

Cardinal, E., Chhem, R.K., Beauregard, C.G., Aubin, B., Pelletier, M., 1996. Plantar fasciitis: sonographic evaluation. Radiology 201 (1), 257–259.

Cheng, H.Y., Lin, C.L., Wang, H.W., Chou, S.W., 2008. Finite element analysis of the plantar fascia under stretch: The relative contribution of windlass mechanism and Achilles tendon force. J. Biomech. 41 (9), 1937–1944.

Cheung, J.T., Zhang, M., An, K.N., 2006. Effect of Achilles tendon loading on plantar fascia tension in the standing foot. Clin. Biomech. 21 (2), 194–203.

Cheung, J.T.M., Zhang, M., An, K.N., 2004. Effects of plantar fascia stiffness on the biomechanical responses of the ankle–foot complex. Clin. Biomech. 19 (8), 839–846.

Evans, P., 1979. The postural function of the iliotibial tract. Ann. R. Coll. Surg. Engl. 61 (4), 271–280.

Gerlach, U.J., Lierse, W., 1990. Functional construction of the superficial and deep fascia system of the lower limb in man. Acta. Anat. 139 (1), 11–25.

Gibbon, W.W., Long, G., 1999. Ultrasound of the plantar aponeurosis (fascia). Skeletal Radiol. 28 (1), 21–26.

Jahss, M.H., Michelson, J.D., Desai, P., et al., 1992. Investigations into the fat pads of the sole of the foot: Anatomy and histology. Foot Ankle 13 (5), 233–242.

Kitaoka, H.B., Luo, Z.P., An, K.N., 1997. Effect of plantar fasciotomy on stability of arch of foot. Clin. Orthop. Relat. Res. (344), 307–312.

Kitaoka, H.B., Luo, Z.P., An, K.N., 1997. Mechanical behavior of the foot and ankle after plantar fascia release in the unstable foot. Foot Ankle Int. 18 (1), 8–15.

Marotel, M., Cluzan, R.V., Pascot, M., Alliot, F., Lasry, J.L., 2002. Lymphedema of the lower limbs: CT staging. Rev. Med. Interne 23 (Suppl. 3), 398s–402s.

Murphy, G.A., Pneumaticos, S.G., Kamaric, E., Noble, P.C., Trevino, S.G., Baxter, D.E., 1998. Biomechanical consequences of sequential plantar fascia release. Foot Ankle Int. 19 (3), 149–152.

Natali, A.N., Fontanella, C.G., Carniel, E.L., 2012. A numerical model for investigating the mechanics of calcaneal fat pad region. J. Mech. Behav. Biomed. Mater. 5 (1), 216–223.

Ozdemir, H., Yilmaz, E., Murat, A., Karakurt, L., Poyraz, A.K., Ogur, E., 2005. Sonographic evaluation of plantar fasciitis and relation to body mass index. Eur. J. Radiol. 54 (3), 443–447.

Reina, N., Abbo, O., Gomez-Brouchet, A., Chiron, P., Moscovici, J., Laffosse, J.M., 2013. Anatomy of the bands of the hamstring tendon: How can we improve harvest quality? Knee 20 (2), 90–95.

Sayegh, F., Potoupnis, M., Kapetanos, G., 2004. Greater trochanter bursitis pain syndrome in females with chronic low back pain and sciatica. Acta Orthop. Belg. 70 (5), 423–428.

Starok, M., Lenchik, L., Trudell, D., Resnick, D., 1997. Normal patellar retinaculum: MR and sonographic imaging with cadaveric correlation. AJR Am. J. Roentgenol. 168 (6), 1493–1499.

Stecco, A., Stecco, C., Macchi, V., et al., 2011. RMI study and clinical correlations of ankle retinacula damage and outcomes of ankle sprain. Surg. Radiol. Anat. 33 (10), 881–890.

Stecco, C., Pavan, P.G., Macchi, V., et al., 2009. Mechanics of crural fascia: from anatomy to constitutive modeling. Surg. Radiol. Anat. 31 (7), 523–529.

Tsai, W.C., Chiu, M.F., Wang, C.L., Tang, F.T., Wong, M.K., 2000. Ultrasound evaluation of plantar fasciitis. Scand. J. Rheumatol. 29 (4), 255–259.

Williams, B.S., Cohen, S.P., 2009. Greater trochanteric pain syndrome: A review of anatomy, diagnosis and treatment. Anesth. Analg. 108 (5), 1662–1670.

Wright, D.G., Rennels, D.C., 1964. A study of elastic properties of plantar fascia. J. Bone Joint Surg. Am. 46, 482–492.

Index

Page numbers followed by 'f' indicate figures and 'b' indicate boxes.

369